D0072329

LONG-TERM CARE AND THE LAW

A Legal Guide for Health Care Professionals

George D. Pozgar, MBA

Instructor, Graduate Program in Health Care Administration
New School for Social Research
New York, New York
Instructor, Undergraduate Program in Health Care Administration
St. Joseph's College
Patchogue, New York

President
G.P. Management Consulting Intl.
East Northport, New York

Legal Review:
Nina Santucci Pozgar, Esq.
Deputy Bureau Chief, White Collar Crime
Suffolk County District Attorney's Office
Hauppauge, New York

Editorial Review:
Richard B. Wallace, MSW, NHA
Administrator, Arden House Nursing Home
Hamden, Connecticut

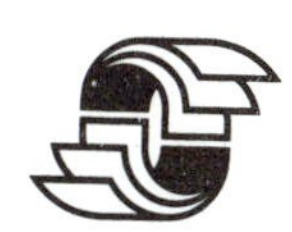

AN ASPEN PUBLICATION®
Aspen Publishers, Inc.
Gaithersburg, Maryland
1992

Library of Congress Cataloging-in-Publication Data

Pozgar, George D.
Long-term care and the law: a legal guide for health care professionals / George D. Pozgar.
p. cm.
"Adapted from the author's text on the Legal aspects of health care administration"—Pref.
Kept up to date with periodically issued newsletters.
Includes bibliographical references and index.
ISBN: 0-8342-0289-1
1. Aged—Long-term care—Law and legislation—United States.
2. Long-term care facilities—Law and legislation—United States
I. Pozgar, George D. Legal aspects of health care administration. II. Title.
[DNLM: 1. Long Term Care—in old age—United States—legislation.
2. Nursing Homes—United States—legislation. WT 33 AA1 P8L]
KF3608.A4P69 1992
344.73'03216—dc20
[347.3043216]
DNLM/DLC
for Library of Congress
91-41445
CIP

Editorial Services: Ruth Bloom

Library of Congress Catalog Card Number: 91-41445
ISBN: 0-8342-0289-1

Printed in the United States of America

1 2 3 4 5

Table of Contents

Preface ix

Acknowledgments xi

Chapter 1—Introduction to Law 1
Sources of Law 2
Common Law 2
Statutory Law 7
Administrative Law 8
Government Organization 13
Administrative Departments and Agencies 20

Chapter 2—Tort Law 29
Negligence 30
Corporate Negligence 45
Intentional Torts 47
Products Liability 58

Chapter 3—Criminal Aspects of Long-Term Care 60
Arrest 61
Arraignment 61
Conference 61
The Prosecutor 62
The Defense Attorney 62
The Criminal Trial 62
Drugs 63
Criminal Negligence 63
Falsification of Records 64
Fraud 64

Murder 69
Operating without an Operating Certificate 70
Resident Abuse 70
Petty Theft 78
Sexual Improprieties 79
Conclusion 79

Chapter 4—Civil Procedure and Trial Practice 81
Pleadings 81
Discovery/Examination before Trial 85
Motions 87
Notice of Trial 89
Memorandum of Law 89
The Court 89
The Jury 90
Subpoenas 90
Opening Statements 91
Burden of Proof 91
Evidence 95
Defenses against Recovery 100
Closing Statements 107
Judge's Charge to the Jury 108
Damages 109
Appeals 112
Execution of Judgments 112

Chapter 5—Introduction to Long-Term Care 114
The Aging Population 114
Long-Term Care Services 116
Health Planning 126
House Select Committee on Aging 128
Omnibus Budget Reconciliation Acts 130
Longevity and Quality Living 137
Conclusion 139

Chapter 6—Liability of Long-Term Care Facilities 143
Authority of Long-Term Care Corporations 144
Doctrine of Respondeat Superior 145
Duties of Long-Term Care Corporations 147
Medical Staff 160
CEO/Administrator's Role and Responsibility 161
Conclusion 165

Chapter 7—The Medical Staff 166
Physician Services 166
Medical Director 173
Medical Staff Privileges 176
The OBRA Survey 180
Physician Liability 182
Conclusion 189

Chapter 8—Nursing and the Law 190
Historical Perspective 191
The Practice of Nursing 192
Nurse Licensure 195
American Nurses Association 197
National League for Nursing 199
Director of Nurses and Nursing Supervisors 199
Nurse Practitioner 200
Clinical Nurse Specialist 202
Special Duty Nurse 202
Nursing Assistants 203
Student Nurses 205
Adequate Nursing Services 205
Administration of Drugs 208
Duties of the Nursing Staff 211
Duty To Take Safety Precautions 215
Conclusion 216

Chapter 9—Nursing Facility Services 218
Dental Services 219
Dietary Services 219
Laboratory Services 221
Occupational Therapy 221
Pharmaceutical Services 221
Physical Therapy 227
Physician's Assistant 228
Recreation Services 229
Radiology Services 229
Rehabilitative Services 229
Respiratory Therapy 230
Certification of Health Care Professionals 232
Licensing of Health Care Professionals 232
Conclusion 233

Chapter 10—Consent 235
Informed Consent 236

Proof of Consent ... 237
Nursing Facility Liability ... 240
Who May Consent ... 240
Implied Consent ... 242
Refusal of Treatment ... 244

Chapter 11—Resident Rights and Responsibilities ... 245
Resident Rights ... 245
Resident Responsibilities ... 262
Resident Ombudsman ... 263

Chapter 12—Long-Term Care Records and Legal Reporting Obligations ... 266
Contents of the Medical Record ... 267
Legal Requirements ... 268
Legal Proceedings and the Medical Record ... 269
Confidential Communications ... 270
Ownership and Release of Medical Records ... 271
Privacy Act of 1974 ... 272
Computerized Medical Records ... 273
Medical Record Battleground ... 273
Falsification of Records ... 274
Charting—Some Helpful Advice ... 274
Retention of Records ... 275
Legal Reporting Obligations ... 275

Chapter 13—Euthanasia, Death, and Dying ... 282
Defining Euthanasia ... 282
Classifying Euthanasia ... 283
Constitutional Considerations ... 286
Defining Death ... 289
The Legislative Response ... 294
Feeding Tubes ... 298
Do Not Resuscitate Orders ... 302
Health Care Ethics ... 302
Conclusion ... 305

Chapter 14—Autopsy and Donation ... 310
Right of Suit for Improper Action ... 311
Autopsy ... 311
Organ Donations ... 314
Unclaimed Dead Bodies ... 316

Chapter 15—Financing Long-Term Care **318**
Federal Program for the Elderly 322
Medicare 322
Medicaid 324
Private Insurance 331
Life Care Contracts 333
Financial Obligations of the Spouse 336
Avoiding Legal Pitfalls 337
DRGs and Nursing Facilities 337
RUGs—The Case Mix Reimbursement System 338

Chapter 16—Malpractice Insurance **342**
The Insurance Policy 343
Liability of the Professional 344
Liability Insurance 345
Medical Liability Insurance 349
Medical Malpractice Insurance Associations 350
Self-Insurance 350
Other Insurance Coverages 351
Trustee Coverage 351
Mandated Medical Staff Insurance Coverage 352
Investigation and Settlement of Claims 352
Risk Management 353

Chapter 17—Labor Relations **355**
Unions and Nursing Facilities 355
Federal Labor Acts 356
State Laws 364
Labor's Rights 368
Management Rights 368
Equal Employment Opportunity or Affirmative Action Plan 371
Resident Rights during Labor Disputes 372
Injunction 372
Administering a Collective Bargaining Agreement 372
Occupational Safety and Health Act 373

Chapter 18—Employment, Discipline, and Discharge **377**
Employment-at-Will 377
Termination 392
Employment Practices 400

Chapter 19—Medical Malpractice—The Crisis—The Solution? **402**
Mediation and Arbitration 404

Pretrial Screening Panel 405
Collateral Source Rule 406
Contingency Fee Limitations 407
Precalendar Conference 408
Discovery Proceedings 408
Expert Witnesses 408
Statutes of Limitations 408
Frivolous Claims 408
Joint and Several Liability 409
Malpractice Caps 410
No-Fault System 411
Peer Review Organizations 411
Professional Misconduct 413
Regulation of Insurance Practices 414
Structured Awards 414
Conclusion 415

Chapter 20—Miscellaneous Topics 417
Quality Assurance 417
Risk Management 421
Utilization Review 423
Acquired Immunodeficiency Syndrome 424
Certificate of Need 430

Appendix A—Glossary 435

Appendix B—Consent to Use of Restraints 448

Appendix C—Residents' Bill of Rights 450

Appendix D—National Practitioner Data Bank Forms 457

Appendix E—Living Will Forms 462

Appendix F—Durable Power of Attorney Forms 466

Appendix G—Health Care Proxy 473

Index of Cases 477

Index 483

Preface

The motivation for preparation of this textbook has been the observed need to provide health care professionals and students with a description of the legal aspects of long-term care. The text has been written to provide sufficient information to ensure a basic understanding of the legal system and its increasing interface with and impact on the long-term care industry.

The trend in health care for older persons is unmistakable—an aging population, inadequate funding, fewer caregivers, and sicker patients. Without a doubt, the health care needs of the elderly, the nation's greatest resource and often the most forgotten, is the fastest growing segment of the health care delivery system.

According to a report by the Office of Technology Assessment on *Life-Sustaining Technology and the Elderly*, more than 70 percent of all deaths occurred in hospitals or other institutions by the 1970s. While the percentage of persons who die in hospitals decreases with age, the percentage of persons who die in nursing facilities increases with age. The percentage of all elderly people living in nursing facilities grew from less than 2 percent in 1950 to about 5 percent in 1980. Approximately 25 percent of those over 85 are in nursing facilities and many die there. For example, in 1978, 38 percent of those decedents over 85 died in nursing facilities.

Despite numerous technological advances and the growing interest in the quality of health care for the elderly in the United States, a significant gap exists in our knowledge about how to define and enhance such care. Acute care has been the primary focus of such efforts to date, while long-term care, as well as ambulatory care, have received less attention, even though most health care occurs in these sectors.

The failure to diagnose disease is most likely more prevalent with those over age 65 than statistics would have us believe. The physical and psychological complaints of the elderly are often ignored and diseases undiagnosed simply because of their age and because of those who believe it is their time to die. The aged are like everyone else—they die of disease, not old age. Early detection and prevention is as important with the aged as with any other age group.

Increases in the complexity of treating long-term patients and unawareness of their needs will most likely increase the probability of lawsuits. The early discharge of the elderly from acute care facilities because of irrational reimbursement schemes, such as DRGs, has only served to exacerbate the problem by effecting the admission of sicker patients to nursing facilities. Although the plethora of negligence law affecting acute care institutions has not plagued the long-term care industry, the fallout of skyrocketing malpractice claims, exorbitant awards, and astronomical insurance premiums has and continues to play havoc on the nation's health care system.

Growing public concern regarding the welfare of the elderly and disabled has resulted in the enactment of comprehensive statutory and administrative schemes for the licensing and regulation of nursing facilities on both the federal and state levels. Nursing facilities face ever-increasing demands from regulatory and accreditation bodies, as well as from the public, to account for the quality of care they provide. The programs that are in place do not adequately respond to these demands.

Many of the statutes and regulations quoted in this text are representative of areas of concern expressed by regulatory bodies. Future additions or revisions in existing regulations will most likely lead to a refining and tightening of regulations. It should be noted that the law affecting the long-term care industry continues to evolve and will most likely do so into the foreseeable future. As with most legal texts, no in-depth study of any particular state is addressed in this volume. Health professionals should familiarize themselves with those regulations specific to their own state.

This text has been adapted from the author's text on the *Legal Aspects of Health Care Administration*, 4th edition, an Aspen publication. It has been prepared primarily to assist health care professionals, students, and non-specialists in understanding many of the legal aspects of long-term care. It is hoped that through this understanding, the quality of care in the nation's long-term care facilities will continue in the direction of excellence. There are more than 150 cases specifically involving long-term care facilities included in this text. Although a variety of other cases discussed in this text involve an acute care setting, the principles upon which the courts reached their decisions are applicable to long-term care facilities and are, therefore, included here. As with any review of case law, it must be remembered that one state court's decision is not binding in another state.

Although nursing home administrators may be somewhat familiar with the contents of certain topics discussed in this text, the book is intended to provide some background to students and other health care professionals who may have limited knowledge of long-term care.

Because of the rapidly changing legal environment in long-term care, this text will be periodically supplemented with new materials in the form of a newsletter. The newsletter will review the continuing changes in the law and legal aspects of long-term care. It will be available from Aspen Publishers, Inc.

Acknowledgments

The author wishes to especially acknowledge Aspen Publishers, Inc., whose guidance and assistance was so important in making this publication a reality. Many thanks to Aspen for permitting use of special adaptions from its publications, the *Legal Aspects of Health Care Administration*, 4th Edition, and the *Nursing Home Law Manual.*

Special thanks to Touro College, Jacob D. Fuchsberg Law Center, and Daniel P. Jordan, Jr., Head Law Librarian and Assistant Professor of Law, for use of the college's library facilities.

There are numerous government and professional organizations I am grateful to for providing me with pertinent research materials (e.g., the Administration on Aging, American Association of Homes for the Aging, National Council on Aging, American Medical Directors Association, Society for the Right to Die, National Practitioner Data Bank).

Many thanks to those whom I have instructed in the legal aspects of health care at C. W. Post College, St. Joseph's College, St. Francis College, Molloy College, and the New School for Social Research, as well as those whom I have instructed through the years at various seminars and workshops, for their continuing inspiration.

Many thanks to Jay Bolnick, M.B.A., M.P.H., Columbia University Lecturer, Graduate School of Public Health, for his review of the New York RUGs reimbursement system; my graduate students Rita Agulla, Cathy Mulroney, and Theresa A. Murray for their review of Chapter 8, Nursing and the Law; and Eileen Houlihan for her review of Chapter 16, Malpractice Insurance.

Chapter 1

Introduction to Law

> Laws are the very bulwarks of liberty; they define every man's rights, and defend the individual liberties of all men.
>
> J.G. Holland (1819-81)

This chapter provides health care professionals with some elementary information regarding the law, the functioning of the legal system, and the roles of the various branches of government in creating, administering, and enforcing the law in the United States.

Supreme Court Justice Oliver Wendell Holmes said that the law is a magic mirror in which we see reflected not only our own lives but also the lives of those who went before us. Thus a history of American law is a history of the United States and the internal stresses of its society.[1] "The government of the United States has been emphatically termed a government of laws, and not of men. It will certainly cease to deserve this high appellation, if the laws furnish no remedy for the violation of a vested right." *Marbury v. Madison*, 5 U.S. (1 Cranch) 137, 163 (1803).

Most definitions of law describe it as a system of principles and processes by which people in a society deal with their disputes and problems, seeking to solve or settle them without resort to force. Simply stated, laws are general rules of conduct that are enforced by government, which imposes penalties when prescribed laws are violated.

Laws govern the relationships between private individuals and organizations and between both of these parties and government. Law that governs the relationships between private parties may be termed private law. Public law deals with the relationships between private parties and government. Laws regulate the activities of individuals in international situations as well as in federal, state, local, and municipal settings.

One important segment of public law is criminal law, which prohibits conduct deemed injurious to public order and provides for punishment of those found to have engaged in such conduct. Public law also consists of countless regulations designed to advance societal objectives by requiring private individuals and organizations to adopt specified courses of action in their activities and undertakings. The thrust of most public law is to attain what society deems valid public goals.

Private law is concerned with the recognition and enforcement of the rights and duties of private individuals and organizations. Tort and contract actions are two basic types of private law. In a tort action, one party asserts that the wrongful conduct of another has caused harm, and the injured party seeks compensation for the harm suffered. Generally, a contract action involves a claim by one party that another party has breached an agreement by failing to fulfill an obligation. Either remuneration or specific performance of the obligation may be sought as a remedy.

SOURCES OF LAW

The basic sources of law are constitutional law; statutory law, which emanates from the federal and state legislatures; administrative law, prescribed by administrative agencies; and common law, which is derived from judicial decisions. In those instances where the written laws are either silent, vague, or contradictory to other laws, the judicial system is often called upon to resolve those disputes until such time as appropriate legislative action can be taken to clear up a particular legal issue.

COMMON LAW

The term common law is applied to the body of principles that has evolved and continues to evolve and expand from judicial decisions that arise during the trial of actual court cases. Many of the legal principles and rules applied today by courts in the United States had their origins in English common law.

It is impossible to have a law that covers every potential human event that might occur in society. The judicial system is thus doubly necessary: it not only serves as a mechanism for reviewing legal disputes that arise in the written law, but it is also an effective review mechanism for those issues on which the written law is silent or in instances where there is a mixture of issues involving both written law and common law decisions. For example, in the Cruzan case, discussed in Chapter 13, "Euthanasia, Death and Dying," the issue decided by the U.S. Supreme Court revolved around the consideration of existing statutory law and prior judicial decisions.

Common Law in England

> Law reflects to a large degree the civilization of those that live under it. Its progress and development are mirrors not merely of material prosperity but of the method of thought and of the outlook of the age.[2]

The common law of England is much like its language. It is as various as the nations that have peopled its land in different parts and different periods. Some of it is derived from the Britons, the Romans, the Saxons, the Danes, and the Normans.

> To recount what innovations were made by the succession of these different nations, or estimate what proportion of the customs of each go to the composing of our body of common law, would be impossible at this distance of time. As to a great part of this period, we have no monuments of antiquity to guide us in our inquiry; and the lights which gleam upon the other part afford but a dim prospect. Our conjectures can only be assisted by the history of the revolutions effected by these several nations.[3]

It appears certain that the Romans had governed the island, as a province, since the time of Claudius, 43 A.D., and that they did not leave until the year A.D. 448. It was a time of peace and cultivation of the arts. Roman laws were administered as laws of the country. When the Romans left Britain to attend to their own domestic safety, the Picts and Scots broke in upon the inhabitants of the south. Unable to oppose the attack, they appealed to the Saxons for assistance. The Saxons came from German lands and drove the northern invaders back inside their own borders.[4] They contended with the Danish raiders from the 8th to the 11th centuries.

The law, prior to the Norman Conquest in A.D. 1066, was dispensed primarily on the basis of tradition and local customs and dealt, for the most part, with violent crimes. The kings during this period were concerned more with enforcing customary law than with amending it. The courts basically consisted of open-air meetings where no records were maintained. "For the Anglo-Saxons justice was a local matter, administered chiefly in the shire courts, and was largely dependent upon local customs, preserved in the memory of those persons who declared the law in the court."[5] The Saxons turned against the Britons and forced great numbers of them into the mountains of Wales, subjecting the rest of the dominion into seven independent kingdoms.[6]

> The circumstances of this revolution are related to be of a kind differing from most others. The Saxons are described as a rude and bloody race; who beyond any other tribe of northern people, set themselves to exterminate the original inhabitants, and destroy every monument and remains of their establishment. In so general a ruin, it cannot be imagined that the customs of the native Britons, or the laws ingrafted upon them by the Romans, could meet with any favour.[7]

The kingdoms were for a time independent of one another and a variety of laws grew among the Saxons themselves. During the reign of Alfred, the Danes, who had long harassed the kingdom, were by treaty settled in Northumberland. The Danes were considered in some measure to be part of the nation. They enjoyed their own laws within their district. When their own kings sat upon the English throne, their laws pervaded, in some degree, all parts of the country. Toward the latter part of the Saxon times, the kingdom was governed by several different laws and local customs.[8]

> The most general of these were the three following: the Mercian Law, the West-Saxon Law, and the Danish Law. If any of the British or Roman customs still subsisted, they were sunk into, and lost in one of these laws; which governed the whole kingdom and have since received the general appellation of The Common Law.[9]

The Normans, following their conquest in A.D. 1066, had little regard for Anglo-Saxon laws. They considered themselves apart from such laws.

> It is obviously impossible to attempt an adequate picture of Anglo-Saxon life. It was a wild time. Men lived in terror of the vast forests, where it was easy to be lost and succumb to starvation, of their fellow man who would plunder and slay, and above all of the Unknown, whose inscrutable ways seemed constantly to be bringing famine and disaster. The uncertainties of modern life pale into insignificance when regarded from the standpoint of these men. It is natural, therefore, that their law should reflect their reaction against the environment. It was conservative and harsh. Violence, robbery and death formed its background.[10]

Land disputes involved the Saxons who held the land before the conquest and the Normans who dispossessed them. Evidence in such disputes was often the result of oral testimony from neighboring landowners.

> The principal change introduced by the Norman Conquest, so far as the central jurisdiction was concerned, was that the King's court now became, for the first time, the court in which disputes relating to land-tenure among the King's tenants-in-chief were regularly decided . . . there is no hint of any professional judiciary at this period. The trials were held locally in the presence of the county court or several county courts by the king's representatives, sent out from Curia Regis (the King's Court) and the tenants-in-chief. The presiding officer was often a cleric.[11]

Following the Norman Conquest, in A.D. 1066 a system of national law began to develop, based on custom, foreign literature, and the rule of strong kings. The first royal court was established in A.D. 1178. This court, enlisting the aid of a jury, heard the complaints of the kingdom's subjects. Since there were few written laws, a body of principles evolved from these court decisions, which became known as "common law." These decisions were used by judges in deciding subsequent cases. As Parliament's power to legislate grew, the initiative for developing new laws passed from the king to Parliament.

Medical malpractice litigation is not a new problem, only its current magnitude is. "The first recorded case of medical malpractice in English common law was noted in 1329. By 1518 when the College of Physicians of London was incorporated, malpractice litigation was common enough for the charter to include disciplinary provisions for malpractice."[12]

Common Law in the United States

During the colonial period, English common law began to be applied in the colonies. According to John Dickinson in his Letters from a Farmer in Pennsylvania in 1768,

> The common law of England is generally received . . .; but our courts EXERCISE A SOVEREIGN AUTHORITY, in determining what parts of the common and statute law ought to be extended: For it must be admitted, that the difference of circumstances necessarily require us, in some cases to REJECT the determination of both . . . . Some of the English rules are adopted, others rejected.[13]

Joseph Story in an 1829 Supreme Court decision wrote, "The common law of England is not to be taken in all respects to be that of America. Our ancestors brought with them its general principles, and claimed it as their birthright but they brought with them and adopted only that portion which was applicable to their situation."[14]

> The size of the country and the abundance of its natural resources made impossible the importation of the common law exactly as it had been developed in England. Measured by English standards, America had superabundant land, timber, and mineral wealth. American law had to serve the primary need of the new society—to master the vast land areas of the American continent. The decisive facts upon which the law had to be based were the seemingly limitless expanses of land and the wealth and variety of natural resources.[15]

After the Revolution each state, with the exception of Louisiana, adopted all or part of the existing English common law and added to it as needed. Louisiana civil law is based to a great extent on the French and Spanish laws and, especially, on the Code of Napoleon. As a result, there is no national system of common law in the United States, and common law on specific subjects may differ from state to state.

> Case law—court decisions—did not easily pass from colony to colony. There were no printed reports to make transfer easy, though in the 18th century some manuscript materials did circulate among lawyers. These

> could have hardly been very influential. No doubt custom and case law slowly seeped from colony to colony. Travelers and word of mouth spread knowledge of living law. It is hard to say how much; thus it is hard to tell to what degree there was a common legal structure.[16] Judicial review started to become part of the living law during the decade before the adoption of the federal Constitution. During that time American courts first began to assert the power to rule on the constitutionality of legislative acts and to hold unconstitutional statutes void.[17]

Cases are tried on common law principles unless a statute governs. Even though statutory law has affirmed many of the legal rules and principles initially established by the courts, new issues continue to arise, especially in private law disputes, which require decision making according to common law principles. Common law actions are basically initiated to recover money damages and/or possession of real or personal property.

The first common law case in the United States where physicians were held legally responsible for a negligence-related action occurred as early as 1794. Since that time, physicians have experienced recurring periods of substantial increases in the number of malpractice cases. The first such increase occurred in the fifteen years prior to the Civil War.[18]

> Distinct periods of increases in malpractice cases and concern about them occurred at the beginning of this century and again in the years prior to World War II. In 1941, *The Journal of the American Medical Association* published studies showing that 1,296 malpractices had occurred between 1900 and 1940, with more than 500 between 1930 and 1940. The explanations for these increases in malpractice cases are similar to opinions expressed about the current malpractice situation: increased patient expectations, improvements in diagnostic procedures, and erosion of the patient–physician relationship, particularly in large urban centers.[19]

The Harvard Medical Practice study commissioned by New York State, which cost $3.1 million and ran 1,200 pages, revealed that 3.7 percent of patients entering New York Hospitals in 1984 were injured by the care provided, ". . . but only a tenth of those who were treated negligently filed malpractice suits."[20]

When a common law principle has been enunciated by a higher state court, that principle must be followed by the lower courts within the state where the decision was rendered. A decision in a case that sets forth a new legal principle establishes a precedent. Trial courts or those on equal footing are not bound by the decisions of other trial courts. Also, a principle established in one state does not set precedent for another state. Rather, the rulings in one jurisdiction may be used by the courts of other jurisdictions as guides to the legal analysis of a particular legal problem. Decisions found to be reasonable will be followed.

The position of a court or agency, relative to other courts and agencies, determines the place assigned to its decision in the hierarchy of decisional law. The decisions of the U.S. Supreme Court are highest in the hierarchy of decisional law with respect to federal legal questions. Because of the parties or the legal question involved, most legal controversies do not fall within the scope of the Supreme Court's decision-making responsibilities. On questions of purely state concern—such as the interpretation of a state statute that raises no issues under the U.S. Constitution or federal law—the highest court in the state has the final word on proper interpretation.

The legal principle stare decisis ("let the decision stand") provides that when a decision is rendered in a lawsuit involving a particular set of facts, another lawsuit involving an identical or substantially similar situation is to be resolved in the same manner as the first lawsuit. The resolution of later lawsuits will be arrived at by applying the rules and principles of preceding cases. In this manner, courts arrive at comparable rulings. Sometimes slight factual differences may provide a basis for recognizing distinctions between the precedent and the current case. In some cases, even when such differences are absent, a court may conclude that a particular common law rule is no longer in accord with the needs of society and may depart from precedent. It should be understood that principles of law are subject to change, whether they originate in statutory or in common law. Common law principles may be modified, overturned, abrogated, or created by new court decisions in a continuing process of growth and development to reflect changes in social attitudes, public needs, judicial prejudices, or contemporary political thinking.

STATUTORY LAW

A statute is a written law emanating from a legislative body. Although a statute can abolish any rule of common law, it can do so only by express words. The principles and rules of statutory law are set in hierarchical order. The Constitution of the United States adopted at the Constitutional Convention in Philadelphia in 1787 at Independence Hall and ratified by the states, with its duly ratified amendments, is highest in the hierarchy of enacted law. Article VI of the Constitution declares:

> This Constitution, and the Laws of the United States which shall be made in Pursuance thereof; and all Treaties made, or which shall be made, under the Authority of the United States, shall be the supreme Law of the Land; and the Judges in every State shall be bound thereby, any Thing in the Constitution or Laws of any State to the Contrary notwithstanding.

The clear import of these words is that the U.S. Constitution, federal law, and federal treaties take precedence over the constitutions and laws of states and local jurisdictions.

Statutory law may be amended, repealed, or expanded by action of the legislature. States and local jurisdictions may enact and enforce laws that do not conflict with federal law. Statutory laws may be declared void by a court for a variety of reasons. For example, a statute may be found unconstitutional because it does not comply with a state or federal constitution, because it is vague or ambiguous, or, in the case of a state law, because it is in conflict with a federal law.

In many cases involving statutory law, the court is called on to interpret how a statute applies to a given set of facts. For example, a statute may merely state that no person may discriminate against another person because of race, creed, color, or sex. A court may then be called on to decide whether certain actions by a person are discriminatory and therefore violate the law.

ADMINISTRATIVE LAW

Administrative law is the extensive body of public law issued by administrative agencies to administer the enacted laws of the federal and state governments. It is the branch of law that controls the administrative operations of government. Congress and state legislative bodies cannot realistically oversee their many laws; therefore, they delegate implementation and administration of the law to an appropriate administrative agency.

The Administrative Procedures Act[21] describes the various procedures under which federal administrative agencies must operate.[22] The Act prescribes the procedural responsibilities and authority of administrative agencies and provides for legal remedies for those wronged by agency actions. The regulatory power exercised by administrative agencies includes the power to license, the power of rate–setting (e.g., Health Care Finance Administration), and power over business practices (e.g., National Labor Relations Board).

Administrative agencies have both legislative and judicial functions. They have the authority to formulate rules and regulations considered necessary to carry out the intent of legislative enactments.

> [A] "rule" means the whole or a part of an agency statement of general or particular applicability and future effect designed to implement, interpret, or prescribe law or policy or describing the organization, procedure, or practice requirements of an agency and includes the approval or prescription for the future of rates, wages, corporate or financial structures or reorganizations thereof, prices, facilities, appliances, services or allowances therefor or of valuations, costs, or accounting, or practices bearing on any of the foregoing[.][23]

Agencies have the authority to prescribe generally what shall or shall not be done in a given situation, as well as the power to administer and enforce their rules and regulations.

Rules and regulations that are established by an administrative agency must be administered within the scope of authority delegated to it by Congress. An agency must comply with its own regulations. *Lipp v. United States*, 181 Ct.Cl. 355 (1967). An executive regulation which defines some general statutory term in too restrictive or unrealistic manner is invalid. *Tasker v. United States*, 178 Ct.Cl. 56 (1976). Agency regulations and administrative decisions are subject to review by the courts when questions arise as to whether or not an agency has overstepped its bounds in its interpretation of the law.

§702. Right To Review

> A person suffering legal wrong because of agency action, or adversely affected or aggrieved by agency action within the meaning of a relevant statute, is entitled to judicial review thereof. An action in a court of the United States seeking relief other than money damages and stating a claim that an agency or an officer or employee thereof acted or failed to act in an official capacity or under color of legal authority shall not be dismissed nor relief therein be denied on the grounds that it is against the United States or that the United States is an indispensable party. The United States may be named as a defendant in any action, and a judgment or decree may be entered against the United States: Provided, That any mandatory or injunctive decree shall specify the Federal officer or officers (by name or by title), and their successors in office, personally responsible for compliance. Nothing herein (1) affects other limitations on judicial review or the power or the duty of the court to dismiss any action or deny relief on any other appropriate legal or equitable ground; or (2) confers authority to grant relief if any other statute that grants consent to suit expressly or impliedly forbids the relief which is sought.[24]

§703. Form and Venue of Proceeding

> The form of proceeding for judicial review is the special statutory review proceeding relevant to the subject matter in a court specified by statute or, in the absence or inadequacy therof, any applicable form of legal action . . . . If no special statutory review proceeding is applicable, the action for judicial review, may be brought against the United States, the agency by its official title, or the appropriate officer.[25]

§704. Actions Reviewable

> Agency action made reviewable by statute and final agency action for which there is no other adequate remedy in a court are subject to judicial review. A preliminary, procedural, or intermediate agency action or ruling not directly reviewable is subject to review on the review of the final

agency action. Except as otherwise expressly required by statute, agency action otherwise final is final for the purposes of this section . . . .[26]

§705. Relief Pending Review

When an agency finds that justice so requires, it may postpone the effective date of action taken by it, pending judicial review. On such conditions as may be required and to the extent necessary to prevent irreparable injury, the reviewing court, including the court to which a case may be taken on appeal from or on application for certiorari or other writ to a reviewing court, may issue all necessary and appropriate process to postpone the effective date of an agency action or to preserve status or rights pending conclusion of the review proceedings.[27]

§706. Scope of Review

To the extent necessary . . . the reviewing court shall decide all relevant questions of law, interpret constitutional and statutory provisions, and determine the meaning or applicability of the terms of an agency action. The reviewing court shall—

(1) compel agency action unlawfully withheld or unreasonably delayed; and
(2) hold unlawful and set aside agency action, findings, and conclusions found to be—
  (A) arbitrary, capricious, an abuse of discretion, or otherwise not in accordance with law;
  (B) contrary to constitutional right, power, privilege, or immunity;
  (C) in excess of statutory jurisdiction, authority, or limitations, or short of statutory right;
  (D) without observance of procedure required by law;
  (E) unsupported by substantial evidence . . . or otherwise reviewed on the record of an agency hearing provided by statute; or
  (F) unwarranted by the facts to the extent that the facts are subject to trial de novo by the reviewing court.

In making the foregoing determinations, the court shall review the whole record or those parts of it cited by a party, and due account shall be taken of the rule of prejudicial error.[28]

Recourse to an administrative agency for resolution of a dispute may be a prerequisite to review of the dispute by a court. Administrative procedures should be allowed to run their full course before recourse is had to the courts. The Washington

Court of Appeals in *Valley View Convalescent Home v. Department of Social Services*, 599 P.2d 1313 (Wash. Ct. App. 1979), held that the Department, in revoking the appellant's license and certification, had failed to follow proper statutory procedure, where the notices of revocation and decertification accompanied the Department's statements of deficiencies, and both notices imposed revocation with no time period for correction. The "Department of Social and Health Services is bound by federal statutes and the rules and regulations promulgated thereunder when the Department accepts federal funds for medical assistance. Social Securities Act, Sec. 1902, 42 U.S.C.A. Sec. 1396a." *Id.* at 1314. The Commonwealth Court held in *Fair Rest Home v. Commonwealth of Pa., Dept. of Health*, 401 A.2d 872 (Pa. Commw. Ct. 1979), that the Department of Health was required to hold a hearing before it ordered revocation of the rest home's license to operate a nursing home. "The Department lapses when in a revocation proceeding it does not give careful consideration to its statutorily mandated responsibility to hear testimony." *Id.* at 873.

Regulations and decisions of administrative agencies that are reviewed by the courts may be upheld, modified, overturned, or reversed and remanded for further proceedings. The owner and operator of a licensed residential care facility brought an action challenging regulations, promulgated by the Department of Human Services through its Office of Long Term Care, governing administration of medicines in residential care facilities. *Department of Human Services v. Berry*, 764 S.W.2d 437 (Ark. 1989). The regulations challenged by the owner state:

> 3. Under no circumstances shall an operator or employee or anyone solicited by an operator or employee be permitted to administer any oral medications, injectable medications, eye drops, ear drops or topical ointments (both prescription and non-prescription drugs).
>
> 4. In addition, any owner and/or operator of a Residential Care Facility who is a licensed nurse who administers any medication to a resident will be in violation of operating an unlicensed nursing home.

Id. at 439. The Circuit Court held that the regulations were invalid and the Department of Human Services appealed. The Supreme Court, reversing the Circuit Court's decision, held that the regulations were reasonable in light of the distinctions between residential care facilities and nursing homes.

> In reviewing the adoption of regulations by an agency under its informal rule making procedures, a court is limited to considering whether the administrative action was arbitrary, capricious, an abuse of discretion or otherwise not in accordance with the law.
>
> * * *
>
> A court will not attempt to substitute its judgment for that of the administrative agency.

* * *

> A rule is not invalid simply because it may work a hardship, create inconveniences, or because an evil intended to be regulated does not exist in a particular case.

Id. at 438. Although the appellee was not victorious in this particular case, there are many instances discussed in the text where those who challenge the decisions of administrative agencies have been successful.

Administrative law is particularly important to those in the health care industry. Long-term care facilities are inundated with a proliferation of administrative rules and regulations affecting every aspect of their operations.

The Administrative Procedures Act provides that each agency must make available to the public, by publication in the Federal Register, the following information:

> §552 Public Information agency rules, opinions, orders, records, and proceedings
>
> * * *
>
> (A) descriptions of its central and field organization and the established places at which, the employees . . . from whom and the methods whereby, the public may obtain information, make submittals or requests, or obtain decisions;
> (B) statements of the general course and method by which its functions are channeled and determined, including the nature and requirements of all formal and informal procedures available.
> (C) rules of procedure, descriptions of forms available or the places at which forms may be obtained, and instructions as to the scope and contents of all papers, reports, or examinations;
> (D) substantive rules of general applicability adopted as authorized by law, and statements of general policy or interpretations of general applicability formulated and adopted by the agency; and
> (E) each amendment, revision, or repeal of the foregoing.[29]

In addition to the numerous federal agencies regulating health care, each state has its own system of administrative law. Long-term care facilities, both public and private, which fail to comply with state law, as with federal law, can be subject to civil penalties.

The following case illustrates how various laws within a state may be in conflict, one with the other. The Supreme Court of California in *Kizer v. County of San Mateo*, 806 P.2d 1353 (Cal. 1991), granted review to determine whether California Government Code Section 818 of the Tort Claims Act prevents the state from imposing civil penalties pursuant to the state's Long-Term Care, Health, Safety and Securities Act. Section 818.2 of the Government Code which provides: "A public entity is not liable for an injury caused by adopting or failing to adopt an enactment or by failing to enforce any law." Under the state's Long-Term Care, Health, Safety and Securities Act, a licensed health care facility is required to comply with statutory requirements. The Act authorizes the California Department of Health Services to inspect health care facilities for compliance with statutes and regulations on patient care and to issue citations and penalties to facilities that do not comply with provisions of the Act. The Court held that the Tort Claims Act prohibiting assessment of punitive damages against a public entity does not prevent the state from imposing statutory civil penalties on a state-licensed, county-operated, long-term health care facility.

As with health care providers, state agencies that fail to comply with federal regulations can be subject to statutory penalties. Evidence supported a statutory penalty of $89,429 against the Colorado Department of Social Services for failing to conduct required inspections to review the care received by Medicaid patients in *Colorado Dept. of Social Services v. DHHS*, 928 F.2d 961 (10th Cir. 1991). Congress had subjected the states to penalties for failure to perform inspections pursuant to 42 U.S.C.A. Sections 1396a(a)(26, 31), 1396 b(g)(1). In order to receive Medicaid funds, a state must submit quarterly reports demonstrating that the state has an effective program of medical review of the care of patients in skilled nursing facilities and in intermediate care facilities. The state's "failure to review even a single patient constitutes a failure to inspect that facility." *Id.* at 965. The state agency's admitted failure to review the care of three Medicaid recipients at a health care facility represented failure to inspect the facility, making the assessment of a statutory penalty against the state proper. *Id.* at 965.

Many of the wide variety of federal administrative departments and agencies which regulate the health care industry are reviewed below.

GOVERNMENT ORGANIZATION

The three branches of the federal government, as illustrated in Figure 1-1, are the legislative, executive, and judicial branches. Figure 1-2 illustrates a typical example of a state government organization. A vital concept in the constitutional framework of government on both the federal and the state levels is the separation of powers. Essentially, this principle provides that no one branch of government is clearly dominant over the other two; however, in the exercise of its functions, each may affect and limit the activities, functions, and powers of the others.

Legislative Branch

The legislative branch of the federal government consists of the Senate and the House of Representatives. On the federal level, legislative powers are vested in the Congress of the United States, which consists of a Senate and House of Representatives.

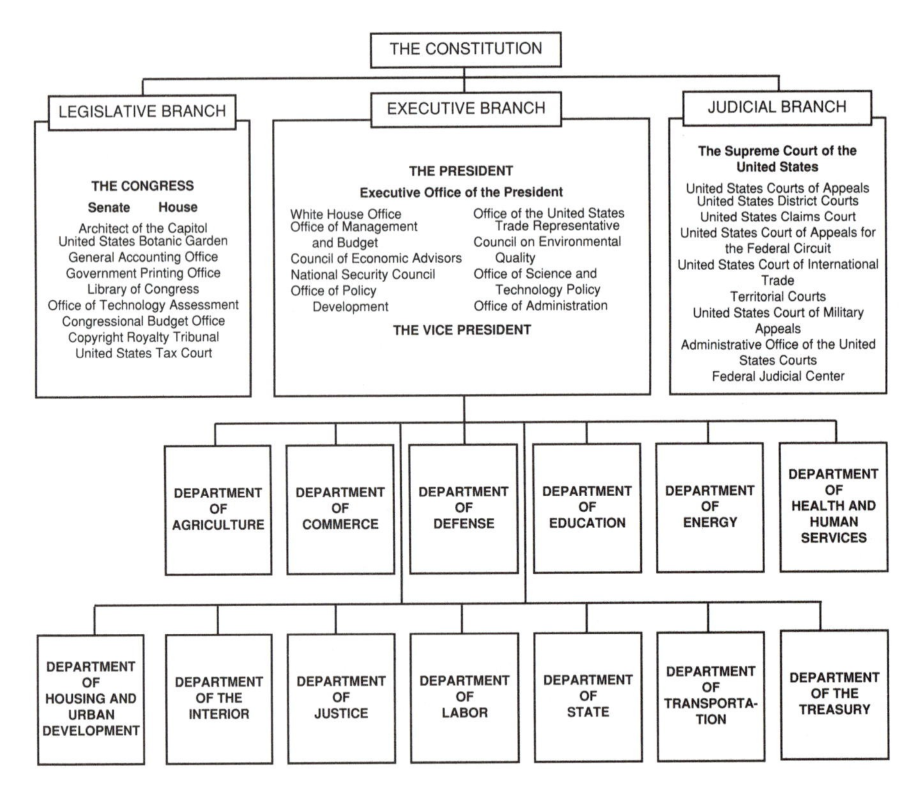

Figure 1-1 The Government of the United States

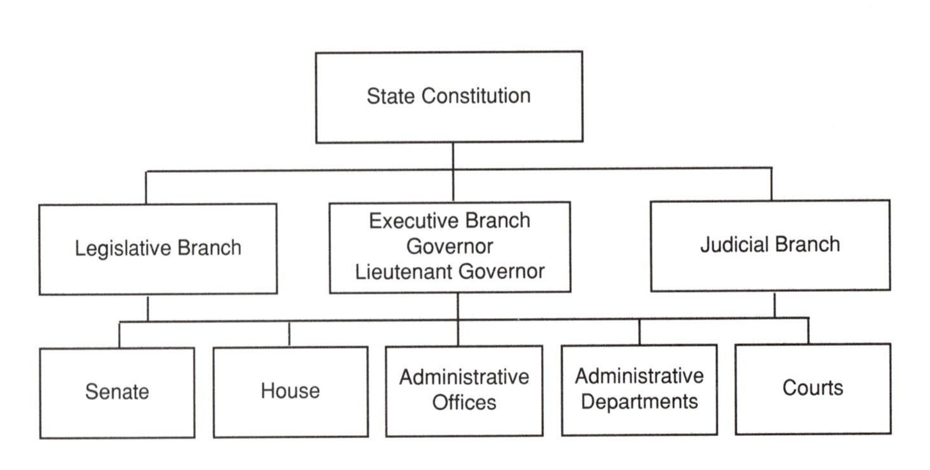

Figure 1-2 State Government Organization

The function of the legislative branch is to enact laws that may amend or repeal existing legislation and to create new legislation. It is the legislature's responsibility to determine the nature and extent of the need for new laws and for changes in existing laws. The work of preparing and considering federal legislation is, for the most part, carried out by committees of both houses of Congress. There are 16 standing committees in the Senate and 22 in the House of Representatives. "The membership of the standing committees of each house is chosen by a vote of the entire body; members of other committees are appointed under the provisions of the measure establishing them."[30]

Legislative proposals are assigned or referred to an appropriate committee for study. The committees conduct investigations and hold hearings where interested persons may present their views regarding proposed legislation. These proceedings provide additional information to assist committee members in their consideration of proposed bills. A bill may be reported out of a committee in its original form, favorably or unfavorably; it may be reported out with recommended amendments; or the bill might be allowed to lie in the committee without action. Some bills eventually reach the full legislative body where, after consideration and debate, they may be either approved or rejected.

The United States Congress and all state legislatures are bicameral (consisting of two houses), except for the Nebraska legislature, which is unicameral. Both houses in a bicameral legislature must pass identical versions of a legislative proposal before the legislation can be brought to the chief executive.

Executive Branch

The primary function of the executive branch of government on the federal and state level is to enforce and administer the law. The chief executive, either the president of the United States or the governor of a state, also has a role in the creation of law through the power to approve or veto legislative proposals.

The United States Constitution provides that "the executive Power shall be vested in a President of the United States of America. He shall hold his Office during the Term of four years, . . . together with the Vice President, chosen for the same term . . . ." The president serves as the administrative head of the executive branch of the federal government, which includes 13 executive departments (see Figure 1-1), as well as a great variety of agencies, both temporary and permanent.

> The Cabinet, a creation of custom and tradition dating back to George Washington's administration, functions at the pleasure of the President. The Cabinet is composed of the 13 executive departments. Its purpose is to advise the President upon any subject on which he requests information (pursuant to Article II, section 2 of the Constitution).[31]

Each department is responsible for a different area of public affairs, and each enforces the law within its area of responsibility. For example, the Department of Health and Human Services administers much of the federal health law enacted by Congress. Most states are also organized on a departmental basis. These departments administer and enforce state law concerning public affairs.

On a state level, the governor serves as the chief executive officer. The responsibilities of a state governor are provided for in the state's constitution. The Massachusetts State Constitution, for example, describes the responsibilities of the governor as including:

- presenting an annual budget to the state legislature
- recommending new legislation
- vetoing legislation
- appointing and removing department heads
- appointing judicial officers
- acting as Commander-in-Chief of the state's military forces (the Massachusetts National Guard).[32]

Judicial Branch

> As I have said in the past, when government bureaus and agencies go awry, which are adjuncts of the legislative or executive branches, the people flee to the third branch, their courts, for solace and justice.[33]
>
> Justice J. Henderson, Supreme Court of South Dakota

The function of the judicial branch of government is adjudication—resolving disputes in accordance with law. As a practical matter, most disputes or controversies that are covered by legal principles or rules are resolved without resort to the courts.

Alexis de Tocqueville, a foreign observer commenting on the primordial place of the law and the legal profession, stated, "scarcely any political question arises in the United States that is not resolved, sooner or later, into a judicial question."[34]

> It is emphatically the province and duty of the judicial branch to say what the law is. Those who apply the rule to particular cases, must of necessity expound and interpret that rule. If two laws conflict with each other, the courts must decide on the operation of each.
>
> So if a law be in opposition to the constitution; if both the law and the constitution apply to a particular case, so that the court must either decide that case conformably to the law, disregarding the constitution; or conformably to the constitution, disregarding the law; the court must deter-

> mine which of these conflicting rules govern the case. This is the very essence of judicial duty.
>
> * * *
>
> . . ., it is apparent, that the framers of the constitution contemplated that instrument, as a rule for the government of courts, as well as of the legislature.
>
> Why otherwise does it direct the judges to take such an oath to support it? *Marbury v. Madison*, 5 U.S. (1 Cranch) 137, 177–180 (1803).

The decision as to which court has jurisdiction—the legal right to hear and rule on a particular case—is determined by such matters as the locality in which each party to a lawsuit resides and the issues of a lawsuit. Each state in the United States provides its own court system, which is created by the state's constitution and/or statutes. The oldest court in the United States, established in 1692, is the Supreme Judicial Court of Massachusetts.[35] Most of the nation's judicial business is reviewed and acted on in state courts. Each state maintains a level of trial courts that have original jurisdiction. This jurisdiction may exclude cases where the monetary value of the claim is below a specified minimum and cases involving probate matters (i.e., wills and estates) and worker's compensation. Different states have designated different names for trial courts (e.g., superior, district, circuit, or supreme courts). Also on the trial-court level are minor courts such as city, small claims, and justice of the peace courts. States such as Massachusetts have consolidated their minor courts into a statewide court system.

There is at least one appellate court in each state. Many states have an intermediate appellate court between the trial courts and the court of last resort. Where this intermediate court is present, there is a provision for appeal to it, with further review in all but select cases. Because of this format, the highest appellate tribunal is seen as the final arbiter in cases that possess importance in themselves or for the particular state's system of jurisprudence. (Figure 1-3 depicts a typical state court system.)

The trial court of the federal system is the United States district court. There are 89 district courts in the 50 states (the larger states having more than one district court) and one in the District of Columbia. The Commonwealth of Puerto Rico also has a district court with jurisdiction corresponding to that of district courts in the various states. Generally only one judge is required to sit and decide a case, although certain cases require up to three judges. The federal district courts hear civil, criminal, admiralty, and bankruptcy cases. The Bankruptcy Amendments and Federal Judgeship Act of 1984 (28 U.S.C. §151) provided that the bankruptcy judges for each judicial district shall constitute a unit of the district court to be known as the bankruptcy court.[36]

The United States courts of appeals (formerly called circuit courts of appeals) are appellate courts for the 11 judicial circuits. Their major purpose is to review cases

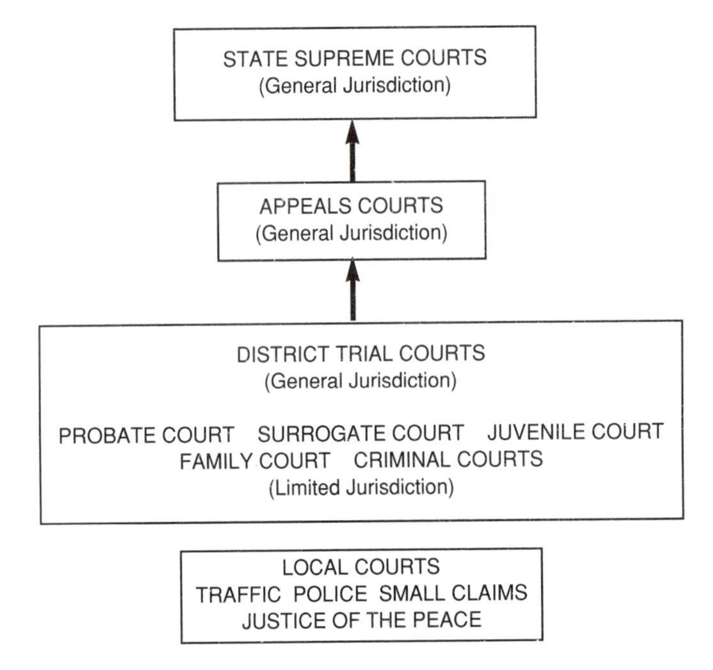

Figure 1-3 Typical State Court System

tried in federal district courts within their respective circuits, but they also possess jurisdiction to review orders of designated administrative agencies and to issue original writs in appropriate cases. The courts of appeals are intermediate appellate courts created to relieve the United States Supreme Court of having to consider all appeals in cases originally decided by the federal trial courts.

The Supreme Court, the nation's highest court, is the only federal court created directly by the Constitution.

> The Judicial Power of the United States, shall be vested in one supreme Court, and in such inferior Courts as the Congress may from time to time ordain and establish. The Judges, both of the supreme and inferior Courts, shall hold their offices during good Behaviour, and shall, at stated Times, receive for their Services, a Compensation, which shall not be diminished during their Continuance in Office.[37]

Eight associate justices and one chief justice sit on the Supreme Court. The Court has limited original jurisdiction over the lower federal courts and the highest state courts. In a few situations an appeal will go directly from a federal or state court to the Supreme Court, but in most cases today review must be sought through the discretionary writ of certiorari, an appeal petition. In addition to the aforementioned courts, there are special federal courts that have jurisdiction over particular subject matters. The United States Court of Claims has jurisdiction over certain claims against the government. The United States Court of Customs and Patent Appeals has appellate jurisdiction over certain customs and patent matters. The United States Customs Court reviews certain administrative decisions by customs officials. Also, there are a United States Tax Court and a United States Court of Military Appeals. (The federal court system is illustrated in Figure 1-4.)

Separation of Powers

The concept of separation of powers—in effect, a system of checks and balances—is illustrated in the relationships among the branches of government in regard to legislation. On the federal level, when a bill creating a statute is enacted by Congress and signed by the president, it becomes law. If the president vetoes a bill, it takes a two-thirds vote of each house of Congress to override the veto. The president can also prevent a bill from becoming law by avoiding any action while Congress is in session. This procedure, known as a pocket veto, can temporarily

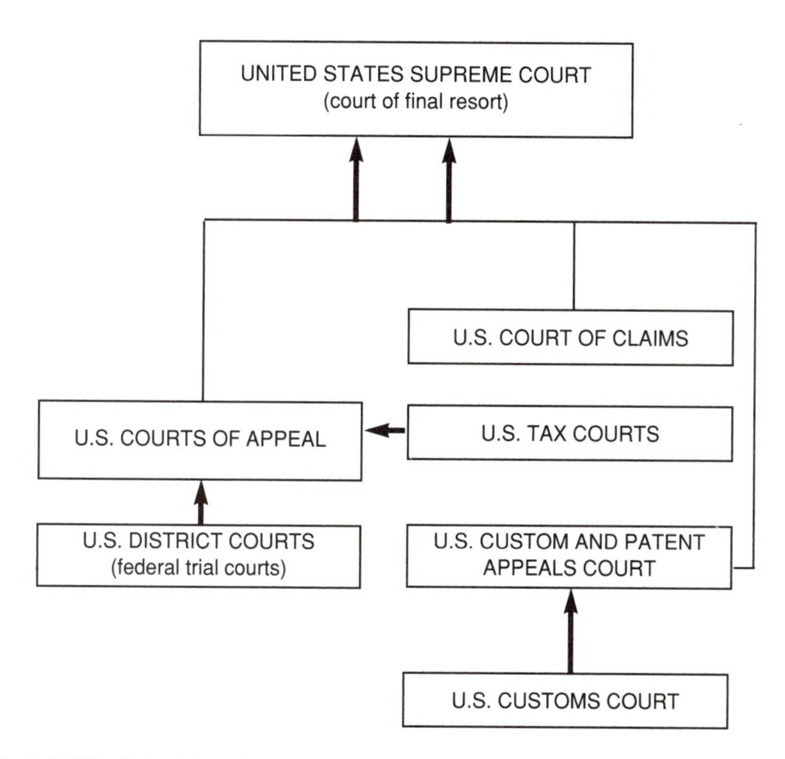

Figure 1-4 The Federal Court System

stop a bill from becoming law and may permanently prevent it from becoming law if later sessions of Congress do not act favorably on it.

A bill that has become law may be declared invalid by the Supreme Court if it decides that the law is in violation of the Constitution. "It is not entirely unworthy of observation, that in declaring what shall be the Supreme law of the land, the constitution itself is first mentioned; and not the laws of the United States generally, but those only made in pursuance to the constitution, have that rank." *Marbury v. Madison* at 180.

Even though a Supreme Court decision is final regarding a specific controversy, Congress and the president may generate new, constitutionally sound legislation to replace a law that has been declared unconstitutional. The procedures for amending the Constitution are complex and often time consuming, but they can serve as a way to offset or override a Supreme Court decision.

ADMINISTRATIVE DEPARTMENTS AND AGENCIES

The following paragraphs review many of the federal administrative agencies and departments that affect the health care industry. In addition to the federal-level departments and agencies described below, a variety of departments and agencies on the state and local levels also address many of those matters addressed on the federal level (e.g., public health, finance, education, welfare, labor, housing, and other needs and concerns of state residents).

Department of Health and Human Services (DHHS)

The Department of Health and Human Services (see Figure 1-5), a cabinet-level department of the executive branch of the federal government, is concerned with people and is most involved with the nation's human concerns. The secretary of DHHS, serving as the department's administrative head, advises the president with regard to health, welfare, and income security plans, policies, and programs. Within the Department of Health and Human Services there are five operating divisions: the Social Security Administration, the Health Care Financing Administration, the Office of Human Development Services, the Public Health Service, and the Family Support Administration. The DHHS is responsible for developing and implementing appropriate administrative regulations for carrying out national health and human services policy objectives. The DHHS is the major source of regulations affecting the health care industry.

The DHHS is responsible for many of the programs designed to meet the needs of senior citizens, including social security benefits (e.g., retirement, survivors, and disability), Supplemental Security Income (which assures a minimum monthly income to needy persons and is administered by local social security offices), Medicare, Medicaid and programs under the Older Americans Act (e.g., in-home

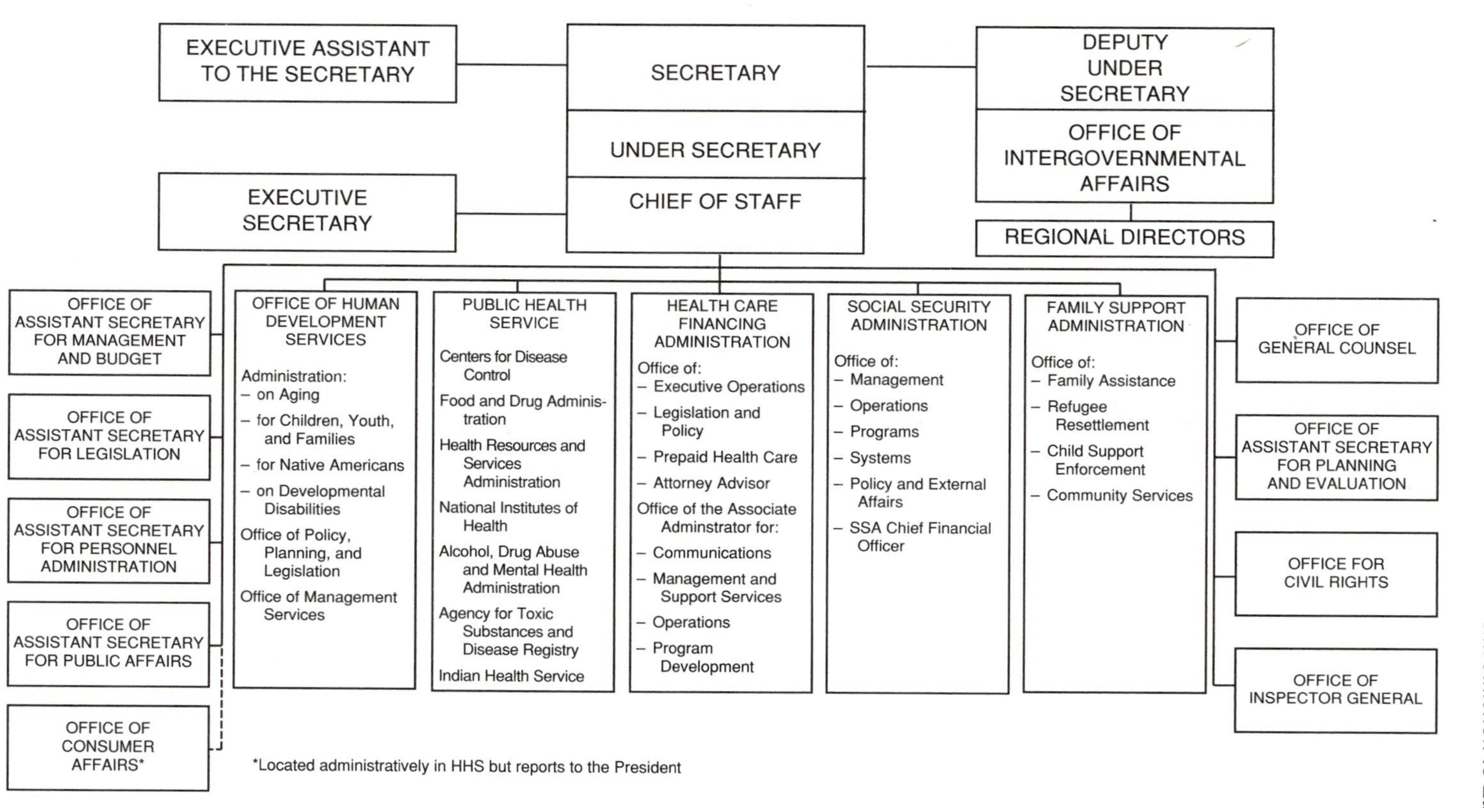

Figure 1-5 Department of Health and Human Services

services, such as home health and home delivered meals, and community services, such as adult day care, transportation, and ombudsman services in long-term care facilities).

Public Health Service (PHS)

The mission of the Public Health Service is to promote the protection of the nation's physical and mental health. The PHS accomplishes its mission by coordinating with the states setting and implementing national health policy and pursuing effective intergovernmental relations; generating and upholding cooperative international health-related agreements, policies and programs; conducting medical and biomedical research; sponsoring and administering programs for the development of health resources, the prevention and control of diseases, and alcohol and drug abuse; providing resources and expertise to the states and other public and private institutions in the planning, direction, and delivery of physical and mental health care services; and enforcing laws to ensure the safety of drugs and protection against impure and unsafe foods, cosmetics, medical devices, and radiation-producing projects.[38]

Within the Public Health Service are smaller agencies responsible for carrying out the purpose of the division and DHHS. The Food and Drug Administration (FDA) is one such agency. The FDA supervises and controls the introduction of drugs, foods, cosmetics, and medical devices into the marketplace and protects society from impure and/or hazardous items. Virtually every consumer product in a supermarket or a drugstore is regulated by the FDA. The FDA engages in the following activities. It

- inspects plants where foods, drugs, cosmetics, or other products are made or stored to make sure good practices are being observed.
- reviews and approves new drug applications and food additive petitions before new drugs or new food additives can be used.
- approves every batch of insulin and antibiotics, and most color additives, before they can be used.
- sets standards for consumer products, such as foods that are made according to a set recipe (peanut butter, for example), and tests products to ensure that they meet government standards.
- is conducting a review of all prescription and nonprescription medicines, biological drugs, and veterinary drugs now on the market to make sure they are safe, effective, and properly labeled.
- develops regulations for proper labeling. For example, the FDA developed new regulations requiring cosmetic ingredient labeling and nutrition labeling on many foods.
- works with the industries it regulates to help them develop better quality-control procedures.

- tests drugs regularly after approval to ascertain whether they meet standards of potency, purity, and quality.
- issues public warnings when hazardous products have been identified.[39]

Health Care Financing Administration (HCFA)

The Health Care Financing Administration is responsible for administering the Medicare and Medicaid programs. HCFA is also responsible for the related medical care quality assurance provisions of both Medicare and Medicaid. Under the Medicare program, HCFA develops and implements policies and procedures and provides guidance related to program recipients, including nursing facilities, hospitals, physicians, and the contractors who process claims such as Blue Cross and Blue Shield. Under the Medicaid program, HCFA provides grants to the states for medical care services for those who are unable to pay. HCFA is also responsible for working with the states under the Medicaid program to develop approaches toward meeting the needs of the indigent.[40]

Social Security Administration

The Social Security Administration oversees the nation's social insurance program. Social security provides retirement income to most citizens over age 65 (persons age 62 may qualify under certain conditions). The program is funded by contributions from both employers and employees. The funds are pooled into special trusts. When the earnings of an employee are reduced or discontinued due to death or disability, social security benefits are paid to assist the employee and his or her family.

Family Support Administration

The Family Support Administration (FSA) serves as adviser to the Secretary of Health and Human Services for children and families; provides leadership and direction to family support programs; recommends actions that improve the coordination of family support programs with other DHHS programs, federal agencies, state and local governments, and private sector organizations; directs and coordinates programs with the Secretary of Labor for employment and training; manages and provides leadership and planning and develops FSA programs; and supervises the use of research and evaluation funds and controls equal employment opportunity programs for FSA.[41]

Office of Human Development Services (HDS)

The Office of Human Development Services provides leadership and direction to programs for the aging; children, youth, and families; Native Americans; those living in rural areas; and handicapped persons. The HDS is responsible for the management and provision of leadership in planning and developing HDS programs; supervision of research; control of equal employment opportunity and civil rights policies and programs for HDS; directing public affairs, regional operations, and correspondence and assignment tracking activities; and recommendations for program improvements.[42]

Administration on Aging (AoA)

The Administration on Aging, established by Congress on October 1, 1965, is the only federal agency devoted exclusively to the concerns and potential of this country's older population.[43] The AoA is located within the Department of Health and Human Services. The Commissioner of the AoA is appointed by the President with the advice and consent of the Senate. The primary goals of the AoA, as envisioned by the Act, are:

- to create and support a national network of state agencies on aging and area agencies on aging covering the entire nation and its territories;
- to develop and oversee responsive systems of services and opportunities to meet the social and human service needs of the elderly in each and every community of this nation; and
- to serve as a visible advocate on behalf of the elderly within the DHHS and with other federal agencies, national organizations, and programs affecting older people.[44]

The AoA is comprised of ten regional offices which assist the states in developing responsive community-based systems of comprehensive and coordinated services throughout the nation. The AoA allocates funds to the states and territorial units based on the 60-plus population in each area. The various states and territorial units then make grants to the 670 area agencies on aging. The AoA also works with many other national, professional and voluntary organizations concerned with long-term care, elder abuse, transportation, caregiver support, etc.

Federal Council on Aging (FCoA)

The Federal Council on Aging, composed of 15 members, is responsible for advising and assisting the president on matters relating to the special needs of older Americans. Funds appropriated for the council are included in the overall appropriations of the Department of Health and Human Services. The council

- reviews and evaluates, on a continuing basis, federal policies regarding the aging and programs and other activities affecting the aging conducted or assisted by all federal departments and agencies for the purpose of appraising their value and their impact on the lives of older Americans;
- serves as a spokesman on behalf of older Americans by making recommendations to the president, to the secretary, to the commissioner, and to the Congress with respect to Federal policies regarding the aging and fed-

erally conducted or assisted programs and other activities relating to or affecting them;

- informs the public about the problems and needs of the aging by collecting and disseminating information, conducting or commissioning studies and publishing the results thereof, and by issuing publications and reports; and
- the Council also provides for public forums for discussing and publicizing the problems and needs of the aging and obtaining information relating thereto, by conducting public hearings, and by conducting or sponsoring conferences, workshops, and other such meetings.[45]

The council is required by law to prepare an annual report for the president regarding FCoA activities, public meetings and recommendations. Copies of the FCoA annual report are distributed to members of Congress, governmental and private agencies, institutions of higher education and others interested in FCoA activities.

Recommendations by the FCoA can have an effect on all federal departments. For example, because of increasing labor shortages, the Federal Council on Aging in its 1988 Annual Report to the President communicated that

> One of the key factors to solving a share of these shortages could be a quality of life for older Americans that included an extended worklife, aided by such programs as ABLE (Ability Based on Long Experience) which coordinates employer and senior employee needs, and the Council feels that tax changes favoring older workers should be considered.
>
> To this end the FCoA sees the Department of Labor playing a larger and more influential role in legislative and administrative decisions affecting older Americans.[46]

National Institute on Aging (NIA)

The National Institute on Aging is one of 13 institutes of the National Institutes of Health (NIH). The NIA is responsible for the "conduct and support of biomedical, social, and behavioral research and training related to the aging process and the diseases and other special problems and needs of the aged."[47] The NIA engages in collaborative activities with other NIH institutes and federal agencies. Research is conducted through interventions and other clinical trials, where appropriate.[48] The priorities of the NIA are as follows:

- Alzheimer's disease and related dementias
- Understanding aging
- Frailty, disability, and rehabilitation

- Health and effective functioning
- Long-term care for older people
- Special older populations
- Training and career development
- International activities (e.g., cross-cultural and cross-national comparative studies involving diverse populations)[49]

Department of Justice

The Department of Justice is responsible for enforcing the laws of the United States. The attorney general is the administrative head of the department, which consists of various offices, divisions (e.g., the Antitrust, Civil, Criminal, Civil Rights, and Tax Divisions), bureaus (e.g., the Federal Bureau of Investigation and the Drug Enforcement Administration), and boards (e.g., the Executive Office for Immigration Review).

Department of Labor

The Department of Labor is the ninth executive department of the executive branch of government. The secretary of labor advises the president on labor policies and issues. The functions of the Department of Labor are to

> . . . foster, promote, and develop the welfare of wage earners of the United States, to improve working conditions, and to advance opportunities for profitable employment. In carrying out this mission, the department administers a variety of federal labor laws guaranteeing workers' rights to safe and healthful working conditions, a minimum hourly wage and overtime pay, freedom from employment discrimination, unemployment insurance, and workers' compensation. The department also protects workers' pension rights; provides for job training programs; helps workers find jobs; works to strengthen free collective bargaining; and keeps track of changes in employment prices and other national economic measurements. As the department seeks to assist all Americans who need and want to work, special efforts are made to meet the unique job market problems of older workers, youths, minority group members, women, the handicapped, and other groups.[50]

Within the Department of Labor are various agencies responsible for carrying out the purpose of the department (e.g., Occupational Safety and Health Administration).

National Labor Relations Board

The National Labor Relations Board (NLRB) is an agency, independent of the Department of Labor, responsible for preventing and remedying unfair labor practices by employers and labor organizations or their agents, and conducting secret ballot elections among employees in appropriate collective bargaining units to determine whether or not they desire to be represented by a labor organization. The NLRB conducts secret ballot elections among employees who have been covered by a union-shop agreement to determine whether or not they wish to revoke their union's authority.

The General Counsel of the NLRB has final authority to investigate charges of unfair labor practices, issue complaints, and prosecute such complaints before the NLRB. There are 33 regional directors, under the direction of the General Counsel, that are responsible for processing representation, unfair labor practice, and jurisdictional dispute cases.[51]

NOTES

1. B. SCHWARTZ, THE LAW IN AMERICA 15 (1974).
2. A.K.R. KIRALFY, POTTER'S HISTORICAL INTRODUCTION TO ENGLISH LAW 9 (1962).
3. 1 J. REEVES, HISTORY OF THE ENGLISH LAW 2 (1814).
4. *Id.*
5. G.W. KEETON, ENGLISH LAW 70 (1974).
6. *Id.* at 3.
7. *Id.*
8. *Id.*
9. *Id.*
10. A.K.R. KIRALFY, *supra* note 2, at 9–10.
11. G.W. KEETON, *supra* note 5, at 70.
12. U.S. DEPARTMENT OF HEALTH AND HUMAN SERVICES, TASK FORCE ON MEDICAL LIABILITY AND MALPRACTICE 3 (1987) [hereinafter TASK FORCE].
13. B. SCHWARTZ, *supra* note 1, at 29.
14. *Id.*
15. *Id.* at 30, 31.
16. L. FRIEDMAN, A HISTORY OF AMERICAN LAW 92 (1985).
17. B. SCHWARTZ, *supra* note 1, at 51.
18. Task Force, *supra* note 12, at 3.
19. *Id.*
20. Zinman, *Study Finds Hospitals 'Harm' Some*, 50(177), Newsday, March 1, 1990 at 17.
21. 5 U.S.C.A. §500 *et. seq.* (1977).
22. An "agency means each authority of the Government of the United States, . . . but does not include—(A) the Congress; the courts of the United States; . . . . " 5 U.S.C.A. §551 (1977).
23. 5 U.S.C.S. §551 (1989) at 69.
24. 5 U.S.C.S. §702 (1989) at 282, 283.
25. 5 U.S.C.S. §703 (1989) at 350.

26. 5 U.S.C.S. §7054 (1989) at 367.

27. 5 U.S.C.S. §705 (1989) at 418.

28. 5 U.S.C.S. §706 (1989) at 430.

29. 5 U.S.C.S. §552 (1989) at 100.

30. OFFICE OF THE FEDERAL REGISTER, NATIONAL ARCHIVES AND RECORDS ADMINISTRATION, THE UNITED STATES GOVERNMENT MANUAL 1988/89 at 29 (1988).

31. *Id.* at 13.

32. YOUR MASSACHUSETTS GOVERNMENT 14, (D. Levitan, 10th ed.1984).

33. *Heritage of Yankton, Inc. v. South Dakota Department of Health*, 432 N.W.2d 68, 77 (S.D. 1988).

34. B. SCHWARTZ, *supra* note 1, at 15.

35. YOUR MASSACHUSETTS GOVERNMENT, *supra* note 32, at 32.

36. THE UNITED STATES GOVERNMENT MANUAL, *supra* note 30, at 71–72.

37. U.S. CONST. art. III, §1.

38. *Id.* at 296.

39. UNITED STATES FOOD AND DRUG ADMINISTRATION, WE WANT YOU TO KNOW ABOUT TODAY'S FDA (1974).

40. *Id.* at 307–308.

41. THE UNITED STATES GOVERNMENT MANUAL, *supra* note 30, at 309–310.

42. *Id.* at 293–294.

43. Department of Health and Human Services, The Administration on Aging, *Fact Sheet*, March 1988, at 1.

44. *Id.*

45. FEDERAL COUNCIL ON THE AGING, ANNUAL REPORT TO THE PRESIDENT 1989, 1–2; *see also*, 42 U.S.C.A. §3015(d).

46. FEDERAL COUNCIL ON THE AGING, ANNUAL REPORT TO THE PRESIDENT 1988, 17.

47. National Institute on Aging, National Institutes of Health, *Fact Sheet*, June 1990, at 1.

48. *Id.*

49. *Id.*

50. *Id.* at 400.

51. *Id.* at 631.

Chapter 2

Tort Law

> Every instance of a man's suffering the penalty of the law, is an instance of the failure of that penalty in effecting its purpose, which is to deter from transgression.
>
> Whately

A tort is a civil wrong, other than a breach of contract, committed against a person or property (real or personal) for which a court provides a remedy in the form of an action for damages. The basic purposes of tort law are to keep peace between individuals by supplying a substitute for vengeance, to find fault for wrongdoing, to deter the wrongdoer (tort-feasor) from committing future torts by assessing damages to be paid to the victim(s) of the wrongdoing, and to encourage adherence to the law. It is interesting to note the conclusion reached by the Harvard Medical Practice Study commissioned by the state of New York after a review of some 30,000 medical records:

> . . . between 2,967 and 3,888 malpractice claims are filed by patients each year in the state. Comparing these figures with their estimate for the number of medical injuries caused by negligence during the same period (27,179), the research group suggested that only one claim makes its way into the tort system for every eight cases of injury caused by medical negligence.
>
> * * *
>
> Moreover, because prior research has shown that only about 50 percent of claimants ever receive compensation, the study team estimates that 16 times as many people actually suffer injuries due to negligence as receive compensation through the tort system.
>
> * * *

> Martin Hatlie of the American Medical Association . . . believes, "the message the tort system is sending to doctors is not so much deterrence, in terms of practicing good medicine, but more just 'drive defensively,' because any patient you may see may be a litigant."[1]

Since an adverse medical outcome generally results in some financial damage, the effect of finding fault by the court is to determine who shall bear the cost of an unfavorable outcome—the provider or the recipient of health care. To avoid cost, the plaintiff must prove the negligence of the provider. Conversely, the provider fights to avoid fault determination. Underlying this adversary proceeding is the assumption that if the provider is forced to bear the cost, it will discourage further acts of negligence by the provider and by other similarly situated providers of health care. However, "professional liability insurance insulates the individual physician's wallet from the actual cost of claims."[2]

There are three basic categories of torts: negligent torts, intentional torts, and torts in which liability is assessed irrespective of fault (e.g., against manufacturers of defective products). Although most incidents that raise issues of liability concern harm allegedly resulting from negligence, a person may also be liable for intentional wrongs. Intentional tortious conduct (conduct implying civil wrong) that may arise in the context of resident care includes assault, battery, false imprisonment, invasion of privacy, and infliction of mental distress. Liability, irrespective of fault, may be imposed in certain situations where the activity, regardless of intentions or negligence, is so dangerous to others that public policy demands absolute responsibility on the part of the tort-feasor.

There are two major differences between intentional and negligent wrongs. The first is intent, which is present in intentional but not in negligent wrongs. For a tort to be considered intentional, not only must the act be intentionally committed, but also the wrongdoer must realize to a substantial certainty that harm would result. The second difference is less obvious. An intentional wrong always involves a willful act that violates another's interests; a negligent wrong may not involve committing an act at all. In certain situations involving negligence, a person may be held liable for not acting in the way that a reasonably prudent person would have acted.

NEGLIGENCE

Negligence is a tort—a civil or personal wrong distinguished from criminal conduct. It is the unintentional commission or omission of an act that a reasonably prudent person would or would not do under given circumstances. It is a form of conduct caused by heedlessness or carelessness that constitutes a departure from the standard of care generally imposed on reasonable members of society. Negligence can occur: (1) where one has considered the consequences of an act and has exercised the best possible judgment; (2) where one fails to guard against a risk that should be appreciated; or (3) where one engages in certain behavior expected to involve unreasonable danger to others.

Degrees of Negligence

There are basically two degrees of negligence.

1. Ordinary negligence—the failure to do what a reasonably prudent person would do, or the doing of that which a reasonably prudent person would not do, under the circumstances of the act or omission in question.
2. Gross negligence—the intentional or wanton omission of care that would be proper to provide or the doing of that which would be improper to do.

Elements of Negligence

The four elements that must be present in order for a plaintiff to recover damages due to negligence are a duty to care, breach of that duty, actual injury, and proximate cause (see Exhibit 2-1). All four elements must be present in order for a plaintiff to recover for damages suffered as a result of a negligent act. When the four elements of negligence are proved, the plaintiff is said to have presented a prima facie case of negligence which will enable him/her to prevail.

The burden of proof in a negligence case is not as great as the "beyond a reasonable doubt" standard borne by a prosecutor in a criminal case. Therefore, if a plaintiff supports his negligence claim with evidence sufficient to outweigh the evidence presented by the defendant, the defendant will be found liable for the negli-

Exhibit 2-1 Elements of Negligence

1. Duty to Care
- An obligation to care
- Failure to conform to required standard of care

2. Breach of Duty
- Failure to adhere to obligation
- Failure to conform to required standard

3. Injury
- Actual damages required
- No injury, no damages

4. Causation
- Injury proximately caused by breach of duty
- Injury must be foreseeable

gent act he committed. He will then be ordered by the court, in accordance with the verdict rendered by the jury or by the court itself, to monetarily compensate the plaintiff for the harm the plaintiff suffered. The purpose of compensatory damages is to put the injured party in the same financial situation he was in before he suffered any harm. In addition to compensatory damages, in some cases punitive damages could be awarded by the court to the plaintiff, for pain and suffering caused by conduct of the defendant that would be considered egregious.

Duty To Use Due Care

The first requirement in establishing negligence is for the plaintiff to prove the existence of a legal relationship between himself/herself and the defendant. "Duty" is defined as a legal obligation of care, performance, or observance imposed upon one to safeguard the rights of others. This duty may arise from a special relationship such as that between a physician and a patient. The existence of this relationship implies that a physician/patient relationship was in effect at the time an alleged injury occurred. The duty to care can arise from a simple telephone conversation. It can arise out of a physician's voluntary act of assuming the care of a resident. Duty can also be established by statute or contract between the plaintiff and defendant. It should be noted that:

> There is no presumption of negligence on the part of the institution merely because of the injury to a patient . . . [A]fter showing it has provided reasonable care for the safety and well-being of its patient under the circumstances presented, a nursing home is not liable for injury caused by an untoward event unless it has breached a contractual agreement to furnish special care beyond that usually furnished which relates to the injury giving rise to the cause sued on.[3]

A concise statement of the duty a nursing facility owes to its residents is found in *Lagrone v. Helman*, 233 Miss. 654, 103 So. 2d 365 (1958), where an action was brought against the operator of the nursing facility for injuries sustained by the resident in a fall. The trial court, which rendered judgment for the defendant, stated in its instructions to the jury, "It was the duty of the defendants to use reasonable care for the safety of the appellant, consistent with her age and physical condition." The plaintiff/appellant appealed the trial court's decision and the Supreme Court of Mississippi affirmed the trial court's decision. The resident was an ambulatory resident in the defendant nursing facility who suffered from cerebral arteriosclerosis, which subjected her to occasional dizzy spells. She had requested medication from a nurse employed by the facility and had followed her to the medicine cabinet. There were two conflicting statements as to what occurred next. The plaintiff claimed that, after obtaining the medicine, the nurse suddenly, carelessly, and negligently whirled around and struck her, knocking her down and causing her to suffer a fracture of her left hip. The facility claimed that the nurse handed the pill to the plaintiff, who dropped it, and in bending over to pick it up, became dizzy and fell to the floor. Although judgment was entered for the nursing facility, had the jury accepted the plaintiff's description of the facts, the result might have been liability for the nursing facility on the basis of respondeat superior.

The children of the deceased nursing facility resident in *McGillivray v. Rapides Iberia Management Enterprises ENT.*, 493 So.2d 819 (La. Ct. App. 1986), brought a wrongful death action against the nursing facility. The resident had died of heart failure after wandering out of the facility in light sleepwear, unattended and in 42-degree weather. The trial court awarded each of the four children $25,000. The court stated:

> . . . the fact that this patient, who was elderly and had serious health problems and had the habit of wandering off and for whom his family has authorized the use of restraints, was able to simply to walk out of [appellant's] facility . . . clothed in light sleep attire on this cold night without anyone seeing him or being aware that he had exited the building, constitutes negligence on the part of the [appellant].

Id. at 823. On appeal by the nursing facility, the court held that the record supported the conclusion that the nursing facility's substandard care factually and legally caused or contributed to the death of the resident.

Some duties are created by statute, as when a statute specifies a particular standard that must be met. Many standards are created by administrative agencies under the provisions of a statute. In general, the violation of a statute or regulation is evidence of negligence.

Duties can be created by an institution through its internal rules and regulations. The courts hold that such internal rules are indicative of the organization's knowledge of the proper procedure to follow and, hence, create a duty. Thus, if an employee of an institution fails to follow an operating rule of that institution, and, as a result, another person is injured, the employee who violated the rule would be considered negligent.

A duty of care may also be created by a nursing facility in its contract for services with the resident or with a third party. Where there is a contractual duty of care and an injury occurs, residents have a choice of theories upon which lawsuits may be pursued—breach of contract or, alternatively, tort. In some jurisdictions, the statute of limitations for breach of contract is longer than for negligence actions. The existence of a contractual duty of care may extend the liability of a nursing facility for several years.

Texas courts recognize that an employer has a duty to hire competent employees, especially where they are engaged in an occupation that could be hazardous to life and limb and requires skilled or experienced persons. The appellant in *Deerings West Nursing Center v. Scott*, 787 S.W.2d 494 (Tex. Ct. App. 1990), was found to have negligently hired an incompetent employee that it knew or should have known was incompetent, thereby causing unreasonable risk of harm to others. An eighty-year-old visitor had gone to Deerings to visit her infirm older brother at 5:30 A.M.

She had a habit of visiting at all hours, even though it was contended that she was asked to restrict her visitation to certain hours. As she walked down the hall, nurse Hopper, a six-foot-four-inch male employee of Deerings, confronted her in order to prevent her from visiting. The visitor stated: "He was so angry and his face just started with—looked like hate to me. He looked like—He looked like, I might have said, crazy man at one time." *Id.* at 497. She stated that upon his approach she had thrown up her hands to protect her face but he hit her on the chin, slapped her down on the concrete floor and got on top of her, pinning her to the floor.

Hopper testified that he was hired "sight unseen" over the telephone by the Director of Nursing for Deerings. Even though the following day he went to the nursing facility to complete an application, he still maintained that he was hired over the phone. In his application he falsely stated that he had a Texas LVN license and that he had not been convicted of a crime. *Id.* at 498. In reality, he had been previously employed by a bar, was not a Texas licensed vocational nurse (LVN), and had committed over 56 criminal offenses of theft and was on probation at the time of his testimony.

The trial court had awarded the plaintiff a judgment of $35,000 for actual damages and $200,000 in punitive damages. The Court of Appeals held that there was evidence supporting findings that the failure of the nursing employee to have a nursing license was the proximate cause of the visitor's damages and that the negligent hiring was a heedless and reckless disregard to the rights of others.

> It is common knowledge that the bleakness and rigors of old age, drugs and the diseases of senility can cause people to become confused . . . and cantankerous. It is predictable that elderly patients will be visited by elderly friends and family. It is reasonable to anticipate that a man of proven moral baseness would be more likely to commit a morally base act on an eighty year old woman. Fifty-six convictions for theft is some evidence of mental aberration. Hopper was employed not only to administer medicine but to contend with the sometimes erratic behavior of the decrepit. The investigative process necessary to the procurement of a Texas nursing license would have precluded the licensing of Hopper. In the hiring of an unlicensed and potentially mentally and morally unfit nurse, it is reasonable to anticipate that an injury would result as a natural and probable consequence of that negligent hiring.

Id. at 496.

The duty of care in this case is clear. The appellant violated the very purpose of Texas licensing statutes by failing to validate whether or not Hopper had a valid license. The appellant then placed him in a position of authority and not only allowed him to dispense drugs but assigned him to a shift as supervisor. This negligence eventually resulted in the inexcusable assault on an elderly woman. The appellant failed to follow even the very basic standard of checking the nurse's credentials.

Standard of Care. When injury has been suffered by a resident, the resident must show that the defendant failed to meet the prevailing standard of care in order for the defendant to be held liable for negligence. The fact that an injury is suffered, without proof that the defendant deviated from the practice of competent members of his or her profession, is not sufficient for imposing liability.

Duty requires that all health care workers conform to a specific standard of care to protect others. A nurse, for example, who assumes the care of a resident has the duty to exercise in the care and treatment of the resident that degree of skill, care, and knowledge ordinarily possessed and exercised by other nurses. A nurse must be reasonable in the exercise of professional judgment as to the care he or she renders, however, reasonable judgment must not represent a departure from the requirements of accepted nursing practice.

> Persons who are known to have mental or physical disabilities, or who are young and inexperienced, are entitled to a degree of care exercised by others proportioned to their incapacity to protect themselves. They are not to be accorded the same treatment as persons of mature years and of sound mentality. No general rule can be articulated, for the standard of care in situations involving victims having these characteristics requires that a determination of what constitutes "reasonable care" be made in each individual case, taking into consideration the victim's known mental and physical condition. Generally the greater the disability, the greater is the degree of care required. The rationale for this principle of law is that natural justice requires that greater consideration and care are due to persons known to be unable to care of themselves than to those who are fully able to do so."[4]

Duty is often difficult to establish. However, "Firmly rooted in the common law lies the concept that although one individual need do nothing to rescue another from peril not of that individual's own making, nevertheless, a person who undertakes to do an act must do it with reasonable care."[5] Once a duty of care has been established, the standard that the person owing the duty must have met to avoid potential liability must be determined.[6]

The standard of care describes what conduct is expected of an individual in a given situation. The general standard of care that must be exercised is that which a reasonably prudent person would do acting under the same or similar circumstances.

> . . . the standard of conduct of a reasonable person may be: (a) established by a legislative enactment or administrative regulation which so provides, (b) adopted by the court from a legislative enactment or an administrative regulation which does not so provide, or (c) established by judicial decision, or, (d) applied to the facts of the case by the trial judge or jury, if there is no such enactment, regulation or decision.[7]

The "reasonably prudent person" concept describes a nonexistent, hypothetical person who is set up as the community ideal of what would be considered reasonable behavior. It is a measuring stick representing the conduct of the average person, in the community, under the circumstances facing the defendant at the time of the alleged negligence. The reasonableness of conduct is judged in light of the circumstances apparent at the time of injury and by reference to various characteristics of the actor, such as age, sex, physical condition, education, knowledge, training, mental capacity, etc. The actual performance of an individual in a given situation will be measured against what a reasonably prudent person would or would not have done. Deviation from the standard of care will constitute negligence if there is a resulting injury.

In determining how a reasonably prudent person should perform in a particular situation, courts may utilize the services of an expert witness to testify regarding the professional standard of care required in the same or similar communities. A resident's expert witness in a malpractice action in *Stogsdill v. Manor Convalescent Home, Inc. and Hiatt, M.D.*, 343 N.E.3d 589, 590 (Ill. 1976), who practiced some 12 miles from the convalescent home at which the defendant physician treated the resident was found to be competent to testify. The defendant had objected on the grounds that the expert never practiced in the county where the malpractice occurred.

> The court overruled this objection on the grounds that locality cannot be construed so narrowly as to be determined by county lines and also took judicial notice of the fact that Buffalo Grove is very near the DuPage County Line, in what he would call the metropolitan area and with the means of communications and text books and so forth nowadays, he believed the "locality" is a very broad one.

Expert testimony is necessary because the jury is not trained or qualified to determine what the reasonably prudent professional's standard of care would be under similar circumstances. Essentially, the expert testifies to aid the judge and the jury by providing a measure for properly assessing the actual conduct required of the professional.

> Expert testimony is required to establish the specific standard of care for professionals, and to assist in the determination of a professional's conformity to the relevant standard, even in bench trials, except where the matter under investigation is so simple, and the lack of skill so obvious, as to be within the range of the ordinary experience and comprehension of even nonprofessional persons.[8]

The courts have been moving away from reliance on a community standard and have applied an "industry" or "national" standard. This trend has developed as a result of a more reasonable belief that the standard of care should not vary according to the locale where an individual receives care. The conduct of health professionals and nursing facilities will be increasingly compared with what is considered reasonable in the industry in view of current professional practice. It would be unreasonable for any one nursing facility and/or health professional to set the standard simply because there is no local basis for comparison.

> . . . in regard to health care professionals, geographical proximity rules are increasingly giving way to a national standard, with the standard in the professional's general locality becoming simply a factor in determining whether the professional has exercised that degree of care expected of the average practitioner in the class to which he/she belongs.[9]

The ever-evolving advances in medicine, mass communications, availability of medical specialists, the development of continuing education programs, and the broadening scope of governmental regulations continue to raise the standard of care required of health professionals, nursing facilities and hospitals. The courts have been increasingly adopting the view that the practice of medicine should be national in scope. Evidence of the standard of care applicable to professional activities may be found in a variety of documents, such as regulations of governmental agencies and standards established by such private organizations as the Joint Commission on Accreditation of Healthcare Organizations. The personnel of a nursing facility, subject to such regulations or standards, are responsible for meeting the standards of care prescribed. A professional's failure to do so provides a basis for finding the professional and the facility liable for negligence.

Although the courts tend to favor a broader standard of care, the community standard can be extremely important in any given situation.

> Assume for a moment that the question is whether a doctor in a remote area of Alaska has placed patients at an unnecessarily high risk by receiving telephone inquiries from nurses in Eskimo villages at even more remote areas and attempting to prescribe by phone. Clearly, such conduct would violate the standard of care in San Francisco, and in San Francisco, would place his patients in an "unnecessarily" high risk situation. For the doctor in Alaska, on the other hand, this method of consultation may be the only possible one, and thus not at all unnecessary or a gross and flagrant violation.[10]

The standard of care required of physicians was established for the first time in Michigan by statute.[11] The Michigan medical malpractice law holds general practitioners accountable for medical treatment that meets the recognized standard of care in the community in which they practice. In effect, the law also holds medical specialists accountable to the recognized standard of care within their specialty. Generally, most states hold professionals and people with special skills, such as physicians, nurses, and dentists, to a standard of care that is reasonable in light of their special abilities and knowledge.

In order for liability to be established, based on a defendant's failure to follow the standard of care outlined by statute, the following elements must be present: (1) The defendant must have been within the specified class of persons outlined in the statute, (2) the plaintiff must have been injured in a way that the statute was designed to prevent, and (3) the plaintiff must show that the injury would not have occurred if the statute had not been violated.

> There are no degrees of care in fixing responsibility for negligence, but the standard is always that care which a prudent person should use under like circumstances. The duty to exercise reasonable care is a standard designed to protect a society's members from unreasonable exposure to potentially injurious hazards; negligence is conduct that falls short of the reasonable care standard. Perfection of conduct is humanly impossible, however, and the law does not exact an unreasonable amount of care from anyone.[12]

Breach of Duty

Once the duty to care has been established, the plaintiff must show that the defendant breached that duty by failing to comply with the accepted standard of care required. Breach of duty is the failure to conform to or the departure from a required duty of care owed to a person. The obligation to perform according to a standard of care may encompass either doing or refraining from doing a particular act. It can be the result of: (1) malfeasance, the execution of an unlawful or improper act (e.g., administering contraindicated medication); (2) misfeasance, the improper performance of an act (e.g., injuring a resident by bathing him/her in scalding hot water); or (3) nonfeasance, the failure to act, when there is a duty to act, as a reasonably prudent person would in similar circumstances (e.g., failing to order diagnostic tests or prescribe medications that should have been ordered or prescribed under the circumstances).

Evidence of a breach of duty can be offered through direct testimony, circumstantial evidence, res ipsa loquitur, etc. The test of breach of duty relies on the reasonably prudent person doctrine: Did the defendant act reasonably under the circumstances?

In *Dunahoo v. Brooks*, 272 Ala. 87, 128 So.2d 485 (1961), the court stated that since the defendant nursing facility operator had been aware of the 94-year-old plaintiff's infirmities and had agreed to provide her nursing care, the nursing facility assumed an obligation to exercise care commensurate with her physical condition. While the plaintiff was getting out of bed one day, she tripped and fell over a light cord that was laying loose on the floor, in an area that the defendant knew the plaintiff frequently used. The cord was plugged into a socket that was on the floor, five inches from the baseboard. The court was impressed with the ease with which the situation could have been corrected. It noted that the cord could have been fastened down with a few nails and the outlet placed on the baseboard instead of almost in the middle of the floor. The court also noted that the defendant had complete charge of the resident.

The nursing facility in *Booty v. Kentwood Manor Nursing Home, Inc.*, 483 So. 2d 634 (La. Ct. App. 1985), was found negligent in permitting a 90-year-old resident to wander outside the facility where he fell and suffered a hip fracture. The resident's physical condition deteriorated and he eventually died. The staff was aware that the resident was confused and had a tendency to stray. On the evening of the accident the resident ". . . on at least two occasions had to be retrieved from outside the building by an orderly." *Id.* at 638. Although a nursing facility's "duty to care" generally does not include having an attendant follow an ambulatory resident around at all times, it is responsible for taking reasonable steps to prevent injury to an ambulatory but mentally confused and physically fragile resident. *Id.* at 635. The nursing facility's alarm system might have alerted the staff of unauthorized resident departures, however, it had been deactivated and the doors propped open for the convenience of the staff. The record demonstrated that inadequate supervision of the resident had been the cause in fact of his departure and that he probably would not have suffered injury but for the nursing facility's "breach of duty" owed to the resident.

In *Roberson v. Provident House*, 559 So. 2d 838 (La. Ct. App. 1990), a resident had brought a personal injury action against the nursing facility claiming that while he was at Provident House a Foley catheter was implanted that caused an infection, bleeding, and impaired urine output. The trial court limited its conclusions to the issue of negligence and concluded that the plaintiff did not carry his burden of proving a breach in the standard of care of the nursing facility. The plaintiff appealed. The appellate court held that there was a lack of expert testimony as to the applicable standard of care, which precluded a finding that the nursing facility had negligently implanted a Foley catheter.

There was a dissenting opinion by Justice Barry. "A careful review of the record reveals that the pleadings were enlarged to include the issue of whether the catheter was inserted without the resident's consent." *Id.* at 843. Roberson objected to the insertion of a catheter and one was inserted over his protests. Such an action constitutes a battery. (See the discussion of battery later in this chapter.) There was testimony that no emergency existed which precipitated the insertion of the catheter. In addition, there was no attempt by the defendants to prove that the resident was of unsound mind. *Id.* at 845.

Injury/Actual Damages

A defendant may be negligent and still not incur liability if no injury or actual damages result to the plaintiff. The presence of damages is essential for a malpractice case because the purpose of legal redress is to obtain some compensation for damages suffered. The term injury includes more than physical harm. Without harm or injury there is no liability. Injury is not limited to physical harm but includes loss of income or reputation, compensation for pain and suffering, etc.

A 26-year-old severely retarded nursing facility resident suffered the ultimate injury, an untimely death, in *Estes Health Care Centers, Inc. v. Bannerman*, 411 So. 2d 109 (Ala. 1982), due to burns suffered in a bath given by a nursing facility attendant. The resident had been placed in a bath on approximately December 22, 1978, and the aide left the room to gather some articles to complete the resident's bath. Upon returning to the bathroom, the aide found the resident in a tub partially filled with hot water. The resident was removed from the tub and it was discovered several hours later that he had blisters over the lower portion of his body. The attending nursing facility physician ordered medical treatments and nutrition. The resident failed to take sufficient amounts of fluid and was transferred to Jackson Hospital, where he died on December 30, 1978. A wrongful death action was brought against the nursing facility. Subsequently, Jackson Hospital and two physicians, one associated with the nursing facility and one with the hospital, were added by amendment as parties defendant. The circuit court entered a jury verdict against the nursing facility and hospital in the amount of $500,000. On appeal by the defendants, the jury verdict was affirmed by the Supreme Court of Alabama.

The patient in *Lucas v. HCMF Corporation*, 384 S.E.2d 92 (Va. 1989), had been transferred to a nursing facility following hospitalization for several ailments including early decubitus ulcers on September 21, 1984. The nursing facility resident was returned to the hospital on October 15, some 24 days later. "At that time the ulcer on her hip had become three large ulcers that reached to the bone and tunneled through the skin to meet one another. The ulcer on her buttocks which had been one inch in diameter had grown to eight inches in diameter and extended to the bone. Additional ulcers had developed on each of her ribs, on her left arm and wrist, and on the left side of her face." *Id.* at 93. The standard of care required in preventing and treating decubitus ulcers required that the resident be mobilized and turned every two hours to prevent deterioration of tissue. The treatment records reflected that the resident ". . . was not turned at all from September 22 through October 1; nor was she turned on October 4, 7, or 12." *Id.* at 93. Failure to periodically turn the resident and move her to a chair had caused deterioration in her condition.

> The occurrence of an injury, standing alone, does not establish negligence for which the law imposes liability, since the injury may be the result of an unavoidable accident, or an Act of God, or some cause so remote to the person sought to be held liable for negligence that he cannot be charged with responsibility for the injury. As it has been said, rules of law and parameters for conduct cannot be premised on mere possibility."[13]

Proximate Cause/Causation

There must be a reasonable, close, and causal connection or relationship between the defendant's negligent conduct and the resulting damages suffered by the plaintiff. The defendant's negligence must be a substantial factor causing the injury. Proximate cause is a term referring to the relationship between a breached duty and the injury. The breach of duty must be the proximate cause of the resulting injury. The mere departure from a proper and recognized procedure is not sufficient to enable a resident to recover damages unless the plaintiff can show that the departure was unreasonable and the proximate cause of the resident's injuries. In *Palmer v. Intermed, Inc.*, 606 S.W.2d 87 (Ark. Ct. App. 1980), a nursing facility operator was sued to recover damages for a hip injury sustained by a resident. The court held that the nursing facility could not be held liable on the ground of alleged violation of a board of health regulation requiring double bed rails "absent a showing of any connection between the violation and the injury." *Id.* at 87. Negligence is not actionable if it cannot be established that it caused injury.

In the case of *Powell v. Parkview Estate Nursing Home*, 240 So. 2d 53 (La. Ct. App. 1970), a suit was brought against the nursing facility for injuries sustained by the plaintiff's 77-year-old mother, who suffered injuries when she fell from her bed. The court held that the employees of the nursing facility were aware of the plaintiff's senile and helpless condition and that this knowledge gave rise to a duty to protect the resident from harm by making sure that her bed rails were raised whenever the resident was in bed. The court further found that at the time of the fall complained of the bed rails were not in position, and that the bed stand used to keep the resident from falling out of bed was also pulled away. The nursing facility was negligent by not observing a reasonable standard of care and taking into consideration the resident's mental and physical condition: the nursing facility's "fault" was the "proximate cause" of the resident's injury.

The administrator of the estate of the deceased resident, Mr. Facey, brought an action against the operators of the rest home in *Facey v. Merkle*, 146 Conn. 129, 148 A.2d 261 (1959), because of fatal injuries suffered by the deceased in a fall down a stairway in the home. The deceased, a seventy-nine-year-old resident, had been discharged from a hospital following a cataract operation. He was then admitted to a private convalescent hospital where he spent six weeks and was then transferred to the defendants' rest home. Mr. Facey had been placed in a room on the second floor that opened to a landing on top of the stairs. The plaintiff and his wife pointed out to the defendant, Mrs. Merkle, the potential danger of Mr. Facey coming out of his room and falling down the stairs. The plaintiffs were assured that a gate would be installed and that Mr. Facey would be supervised. There came a time in the rest home that Mr. Facey soiled his slippers and Mrs. Merkle began to clean them while he went upstairs to get his shoes. Shortly thereafter, the fall occurred. The Superior Court entered a judgment for the administrator of Mr. Facey's estate and the operators of the home appealed. The Supreme Court of Errors held that, "Although the evidence was weak, it cannot be said as a matter of law it was inadequate to support the finding of the jury, as indicated by the verdict, that under all the circumstances it was more probable than not that the decedent's fall at the head of the stairs was proximately caused by the proximity of the doorway to the stairway, as alleged." *Id.* at 264.

> The primary wrong upon which a cause of action for negligence is based consists in the breach of a duty on the part of one person to protect another against injury, the proximate result of which is an injury to the person to whom the duty is owed. These elements of duty, breach, and injury are essentials of actionable negligence, and in fact most judicial definitions

> of the term 'negligence' or 'actionable negligence' are couched in those terms. In the absence of any one of them, no cause of action for negligence will lie.[14]

Foreseeability. Foreseeability, as an element of negligence, may be defined as the reasonable anticipation that harm or injury is likely to result from an act or an omission to act. The test for foreseeability is whether any one of ordinary prudence and intelligence should have anticipated the danger to others caused by his or her negligence. *Clark v. Wagoner*, 452 S.W.2d 437, 440 (Tex. 1970). "The test is not what the wrongdoer believed would occur; it is whether he ought reasonably to have foreseen that the event in question, or some similar event would occur." *Id.* at 440.

If the action of a defendant meets or surpasses the recognized standard of care and injury results, there has been no negligence or carelessness—just an unavoidable accident. There is no expectation that the actor can guard against events that cannot reasonably be foreseen or that are so unlikely to occur that they would be disregarded. For example, in *Haynes v. Hoffman*, 164 Ga. App. 236, 238(3), 296 S.E.2d 216 (1982), the plaintiff had brought a medical malpractice action against the defendant physician for his alleged negligence in prescribing a medication to which the plaintiff suffered an allergic reaction. The trial court returned a verdict in favor of the defendant and the plaintiff appealed. The evidence at trial had revealed that the plaintiff had not disclosed her history of allergies to the physician. The physician testified that, at the time of the physical examination of the plaintiff, she denied having any allergies. The physician testified that he would not have prescribed the drug had he known the plaintiff's complete history. By failing to disclose her allergies to the physician, the plaintiff was contributorily negligent. "Foreseeability" involves guarding against that which is probable and likely to happen, not against that which is only remotely and slightly possible.

If a defendant's actions fail to meet the standard of care, then there has been negligence, and the jury must make two determinations. First, was it foreseeable that harm would occur from the failure to meet the standard of care? Second, was the carelessness or negligence the proximate or immediate cause of the harm or injury to the plaintiff? "The broad test of negligence is what a reasonably prudent person would foresee and would do in the light of this foresight under the circumstances."[15]

The question of foreseeability was an issue in *Ferguson v. Dr. McCarthy's Rest Home*, 335 Mass. 733, 142 N.E.2d 337 (1957). The plaintiff, a resident in the defendant's nursing facility, suffered from paralysis of the left side, but was able to roll towards the left side in bed. The defendant had knowledge of this ability. A radiator which was approximately the same height as the bed was next to the plaintiff's bed on the left side. During the night the plaintiff's left foot came in contact with the radiator and she suffered third degree burns. She had been placed too close to the left side of the bed in an effort to prevent her from rolling out of bed, which had not been properly equipped with bed rails. The court held that this type of accident was "foreseeable" with respect to a person in the plaintiff's condition, particularly since the defendant had knowledge of the plaintiff's condition. The defendant should have either shielded the radiator or not placed the plaintiff next to it.

An 80-year-old nursing home resident brought an action against a nursing facility in *Gunn v. HI-C-Home, Inc.*, 490 P.2d 999 (Or. 1971), for personal injuries she sustained from a fall. The resident had been standing near an outside concrete pool containing a water fountain, operated by a submersible pump, when it was suddenly turned on. The resident became startled and fell, breaking her hip. Although there was conflicting evidence presented, there was considerable evidence indicating that the fountain made a noise when it was turned on. Mrs. Magorian, another resident, who was talking to the plaintiff at the time of the injury testified:

> Q Now did you see anybody else out there while you were talking to Mrs. Gunn?
>
> A Well, not for awhile. We sat there—stood there and talked and all of a sudden Mr. Erickson came out there and he stood there for a minute, and then he went back in and he turned on the water for that lake, that fenced placed where the water was.
>
> Q What happened when the water came on?
>
> A It scared the life out of her.
>
> * * *
>
> Q All right, Mrs. Magorian. Here, let me ask you now: Would you describe the noise to us, please, that it made?
>
> A Well, it was just all of a rumble. You know how water will come out, you know, because it was in—it's kind of a lake there that's fenced around there. And he drained it at night, and then he turned it on in the daytime, see. And he come out there and seen it wasn't on and he went back in, and he never told us what he was going to do, but all of a sudden he turned that water on and it—it was such a rumble and such a noise it just scared her and she fell flat right down there on the concrete.

Id. at 1000, 1001.

The Supreme Court of Washington held that, in light of the resident's age and physical condition, the nursing facility should have reasonably foreseen that turning on the fountain when a resident was standing nearby without any warning would expose the resident to an unreasonable risk of harm because of the startling nature of the noise. The "[q]uestion of negligence is one of foreseeability and the test is whether the ordinary person ought to foresee that his conduct will expose another to an unreasonable risk of harm." *Id.* at 999.

Summary Case

The record in *Caruso v. Pine Manor Nursing Center*, 538 N.E.2d 722 (Ill. App. Ct. 1989), supported a finding that a resident had suffered from dehydration as a result of nursing facility negligence. The defendant appealed from a jury verdict awarding $65,000 in damages to the plaintiff. The trial court increased this amount to $195,000 (three times actual damages) pursuant to Section 3–602 of the Nursing Home Reform Act. Ill. Rev. Stat. ch. 111 1/2, para. 4153–602 (1987). The appellate court held that the trial court's finding that the resident suffered dehydration as a result of the nursing facility's treatment of him was supported by the evidence. The elements of negligence—duty to care, breach of duty, injury, and proximate cause—were shown in this case, as discussed below.

Duty To Care

The nursing facility by statute had a duty to provide its residents with food and water.

> [1} Under the Nursing Home Care Reform Act (the Act), "[T]he owner and licensee [of a nursing home] are liable to a resident for any intentional or negligent act or omission of their agents or employees which injured the resident. Ill. Rev. Stat. 1981, ch. 111 1/2, para. 4153–601)." The Act defines "neglect" as "a failure in a facility to provide adequate medical or personal care or maintenance, which failure results in physical or mental injury to a resident or in the deterioration of the resident's condition." [Ill. Rev. Stat. 1981, ch. 111 1/2, para. 4151–116, 4151–117.] Personal care and maintenance include providing food and water and assistance with meals necessary to sustain a healthy life. Ill. Rev. Stat. 1981, ch. 111 1/2, para. 4151–116, 4151–120.]

Id. at 724.

Breach of Duty

The nursing facility maintained no records of the resident's fluid intake and output. A nurse testified that such a record was a required standard nursing facility procedure that should have been followed for a person in the resident's condition but was not. The resident's condition had deteriorated after a stay at the nursing facility of six and one-half days. Upon leaving the nursing facility and entering a hospital emergency room, the treating physician diagnosed the resident as suffering from severe dehydration caused by an inadequate intake of fluids. The nursing facility offered no alternative explanation for the resident's dehydrated condition and failed to keep a chart of fluid intake and output as required by applicable statute.

Injury

The resident suffered severe dehydration requiring hospital treatment.

Proximate Cause

The evidence presented clearly demonstrated that the proximate cause of the resident's dehydration was the nursing facility's failure to administer proper nourishment to him. It was not unreasonable for the jury to conclude that the resident suffered dehydration and that the nursing facility's treatment of him caused the dehydration.

Case Lessons

Each case presented in this text illustrates real life experiences of plaintiffs and defendants. It is anticipated that the reader will learn from these experiences and apply them to real life situations. The lessons in this particular case are obvious.

1. Every nursing facility resident must receive proper nourishment.
2. The intake and output of fluids should be closely monitored and documented in the medical record.
3. Corrective measures must be taken when fluid input and output signal a medical problem.

CORPORATE NEGLIGENCE

Corporate negligence occurs when a nursing facility fails to perform those duties it owes directly to anyone coming in contact with it. If such a duty is breached and a resident is injured as a result of that breach, the institution can be held culpable under the theory of corporate negligence. There are duties that the corporation itself owes to the general public and to its residents. These duties arise from statutes, regulations, principles of law developed by the courts, and the internal operating rules of the institution. A corporation is treated no differently than an individual. If a corporation has a duty to fulfill and fails to do so, it has the same liability to the injured party as an individual would have.

The benchmark case in the health care field, which has had a major impact on the liability of health care facilities, as well as hospitals and physicians, was decided in 1965. The U.S. Supreme Court denied review of the Illinois case of *Darling v. Charleston Community Memorial Hospital*, 33 Ill. 2d 326, 211 N.E.2d 253 (1965), *cert. denied*, 383 U.S. 946 (1966).

This case involved an 18-year-old college football player who was preparing for a career as a teacher and coach. The patient, a defensive halfback for his college football team, was injured during a play. He was rushed to the emergency room of a small, accredited community hospital where the only physician on emergency room duty that day was Dr. Alexander, a general practitioner. Dr. Alexander had not treated a major leg fracture for three years.

The physician examined the patient and ordered an x-ray that revealed that the tibia and the fibula of the right leg had been fractured. The physician reduced the fracture and applied a plaster cast from a point three or four inches below the groin to the toes. Shortly after the cast had been applied, the patient began to complain continually of pain. The physician split the cast and continued to visit the patient frequently while he remained in the hospital. He did not call in any specialist for consultation because he did not think it was necessary.

After two weeks, the student was transferred to a larger hospital and placed under the care of an orthopedic surgeon. The specialist found a considerable amount of dead tissue in the fractured leg. During a period of two months he removed increasing amounts of tissue in a futile attempt to save the leg until it became necessary to amputate the leg eight inches below the knee. The student's father did not agree to a settlement and filed suit against the physician and the hospital. Although the physician later settled out of court for $40,000, the case continued against the hospital.

The documentary evidence that was relied on to establish the standard of care included (1) the Rules and Regulations of the Illinois Department of Public Health under the Hospital Licensing Act; (2) the Standards for Hospital Accreditation of the Joint Commission on Accreditation of Hospitals; and (3) the Bylaws, Rules and Regulations of Charleston Hospital. These documents were admitted into evidence without objection. No specific evidence was offered that the hospital had failed to conform to the usual and customary practices of hospitals in the community.

The trial court instructed the jury to consider those documents, along with all other evidence, in determining the hospital's liability. Under the circumstances in which the case reached the Illinois Supreme Court, it was held that the verdict against the hospital should be sustained if the evidence supported the verdict on any one or more of the 20 allegations of negligence. The two allegations specified asserted that the hospital was negligent in its failure to provide a sufficient number of trained nurses for bedside care of all patients at all times—in this case, capable of recognizing the progressive gangrenous condition of the plaintiff's right leg—and in the failure of its nurses to bring the condition to the attention of the hospital administration and staff so that adequate consultation could be secured and the condition rectified.

Although these generalities provided the jury with no practical guidance for determining what constitutes reasonable care, they were considered relevant to aid the jury in deciding what was feasible and what the hospital knew or should have known concerning hospital responsibilities for the proper care of a patient. There was no expert testimony characterizing when the professional care rendered by the attending physician should have been reviewed, who should have reviewed it, or whether the case required consultation.

Evidence relating to the hospital's failure to review Dr. Alexander's work, require consultation or examination by specialists, and require proper nursing care was found to be sufficient to support a verdict for the patient. Judgment was eventually returned against the hospital in the amount of $100,000.

The Illinois Supreme Court held that the hospital could not limit its liability as a charitable corporation to the amount of its liability insurance. ". . . [T]he doctrine of charitable immunity can no longer stand . . . a doctrine which limits the liability of charitable corporations to the amount of liability insurance that they see fit to carry permits them to determine whether or not they will be liable for their torts and the amount of that liability, if any." 211 N.E.2d at 260. In effect, the hospital was liable as a corporate entity for the negligent acts of its employees and physicians. Among other things, the Darling case indicates the importance of instituting effective credentialing and continuing medical evaluation and review programs for all members of a facility's professional staff.

A nursing facility is responsible for failing to meet the standard of care required within the facility. A nursing facility is in the best position to protect its residents; it consequently has an independent duty to select and retain competent independent physicians seeking staff privileges. The corporate negligence doctrine imposes on all health care facilities an implied duty to select and retain competent physicians.

INTENTIONAL TORTS

Assault and Battery

It has long been recognized by law that a person possesses a right to be free from aggression and the threat of actual aggression against one's person. The right to expect others to respect the integrity of one's body has roots in both common and statutory law. The distinguishing feature between assault and battery is that assault effectuates an infringement upon the mental security or tranquillity of another while battery constitutes a violation of another's physical integrity.

Assault

An assault is the deliberate threat, coupled with the apparent present ability, to do physical harm to another. No actual contact is necessary. It is the deliberate threat or attempt to injure another or the attempt by one to make bodily contact with another without his or her consent. To commit the tort of assault, two conditions must exist: first, the person attempting to unlawfully touch another must possess the apparent present ability to commit the battery; and second, the person threatened must be aware of or have actual knowledge of an immediate threat of a battery and must fear it.

Battery

A battery is an intentional touching of another's person, in a socially impermissible manner, without that person's consent. It is intentional conduct that violates the physical security of another. The receiver of the battery does not have to be aware that a battery has been committed. The unwanted touching may give rise to a cause of action for any injuries brought about by the touching.

The law provides a remedy to the individual if consent to a touching has not been obtained or if the act goes beyond the consent given. Therefore, the injured person may initiate a lawsuit against the wrongdoer for damages suffered. Punitive damages in *Peete v. Blackwell*, 504 So. 2d 22 (Ala. 1986), in the amount of $10,000 were awarded to a nurse in her action against a physician for assault and battery. Evidence showed that the physician struck the assisting nurse on the arm and cursed at her when the physician ordered her to turn on the suction. Although there were no injuries, $1 in compensatory damages and $10,000 in punitive damages were awarded by the jury.

In the health context, the principle of law concerning battery and the requirement of consent to medical and surgical procedures is critically important. Liability for acts of battery is most common in situations involving lack of or improper consent to medical procedures. It is inevitable that a resident in a nursing facility will be touched by many persons for many reasons. Most procedures involve some touching of a resident. Therefore, they must be authorized by the resident. If they are not authorized, the person performing the procedure could be subject to an action for battery.

It is of no legal importance that a procedure constituting a battery has improved a resident's health. If the resident did not consent to the touching, the resident may be entitled to such damages as can be proved to have resulted from commission of the battery.

Not only must individual staff members be aware of potential assault and battery hazards by fellow employees, as well as themselves, but they also must be alert to potential problems between residents (e.g., problems caused by smoking, racial or religious bias, and emotional conflicts).

A long-term nursing facility has a particular duty to supervise especially closely those residents whose mental condition makes it probable that they will injure themselves or others. The nursing facility in *Sayes v. Pilgrim Manor Nursing Home, Inc.*, 536 So. 2d 705 (La. Ct. App. 1988), was found liable to a police officer who was injured while rescuing a suicidal nursing facility resident. The injuries were found to be the result of the facility's negligent lack of supervision of the resident. The resident was discovered missing from the premises and was reportedly threatening to commit suicide in a nearby sewerage waste reservoir. The fourth police officer to arrive on the scene, believing the suicide to be imminent, dove into the water. He carried the resident to the shore and the resident then experienced an epileptic grand mal seizure. During the ensuing struggle, the police officer suffered a broken elbow. He underwent five operations and eventually had an artificial elbow implanted, which placed severe restrictions on his physical activity. The 41-year-old police officer was forced to resign as Chief of Police and go into early retirement. The defendants appealed the trial court's finding for the plaintiff on the grounds that: (1) the trial court erred in determining that Pilgrim Manor was negligent in its supervision of the resident; (2) the trial court erred in determining that Pilgrim Manor breached a duty to the plaintiff; and (3) the trial court erred in determining that the plaintiff was not contributorily negligent or assumed the risk of the accident. *Id.* at 709. The plaintiff answered the appeal and asked the court to increase the pain and suffering award and the award for loss of future income.

The Court of Appeal held that by accepting a mentally retarded epileptic resident with violent tendencies, the nursing facility had a higher duty to protect the resident and public from harm. By accepting the resident with full knowledge of her condition, the nursing facility was obligated to take extra care, over and above that given other residents, in order to protect her and other residents. Pilgrim Manor presented no evidence that extra care was given to the resident. Evidence showed that she was treated like any other resident who had nominal physical or mental disabilities. The resident's treating physician testified that a person with her problems should not have been given freedom to leave the nursing facility at will. Despite the physician's opinion and the documented serious mental and physical problems of the resident, the director of nursing and the administrator testified that the resident had complete freedom to leave the nursing facility premises, either alone or in the company of other residents. Police officers and firemen cannot be expected to expose themselves to injury from negligent conduct that has occurred on a repeated basis and that could have been prevented. The Court of Appeal found no contributory negligence on the part of the plaintiff. *Id.* at 708. An award of $60,000 for pain and suffering was not considered an abuse of discretion. The judgment of the District Court was amended to increase the plaintiff's award for loss of future earnings from $150,000 to $200,000. *Id.* at 713.

It was alleged in a suit involving a wrongful death action in *May v. Triple C Convalescent Centers*, 578 P.2d 541 (Wash. Ct. App. 1978), that a nursing facility knew or should have known that a certain resident was belligerent and aggressive and might injure other residents by fighting. Thus, it was argued, the nursing facility owed something more than the ordinary duty of reasonable care to another resident who died of injuries suffered in a fight with the belligerent resident. The court rejected this argument, pointing to the absence of evidence to support the contention that the nursing facility knew or should have known that the resident was dangerous.

Since senile psychosis tends to cause irrational behavior, a nursing facility would appear to have a duty to protect residents from the effects of such irrational behavior, whether or not it has actual knowledge of such behavior on the part of a particular resident.

False Imprisonment

False imprisonment is the unlawful restraint of an individual's personal liberty or the unlawful restraining or confining of an individual. The personal right to move freely and without hindrance is basic to our legal system. Any intentional infringement upon this right may constitute false imprisonment. Actual physical force is not necessary to constitute false imprisonment. All that is necessary is that an individual who is physically "confined" to a given area experience a reasonable fear that force, which may be implied by words, threats, or gestures, will be used to detain the individual or to intimidate him or her without legal justification. Excessive force used to restrain a resident may produce liability for both false imprisonment and battery.

In certain cases, preventing a resident from leaving a nursing facility may constitute false imprisonment. For example, detaining a resident until the bills are paid would qualify as false imprisonment.

A resident's insistence on leaving should be noted on the medical record. The resident should also be informed of the possible harm in leaving against medical advice. If a resident ultimately decides to leave the nursing facility against medical advice, he or she should be requested to sign a discharge against advice and release form.

It is important to note that a resident does not actually have to be constrained to be falsely imprisoned. A threat of restraint that a resident may reasonably expect to be carried out may be enough to constitute false imprisonment. In order to recover for damages, a plaintiff must be aware of the confinement and have no reasonable means of escape. Availability of a reasonable means of escape may bar recovery. To lock a door when another is reasonably available to pass through is not imprisonment. However, if the only other door provides a way of escape that is dangerous, the law may consider it an unreasonable way of escape and, therefore, false imprisonment may be a cause of action. Whether or not false imprisonment has taken place will be a matter for the courts to decide. No actual damage need be shown in order for liability to be imposed.

In *Big Town Nursing Home, Inc. v. Newman*, 461 S.W.2d 195 (Tex. Ct. App. 1970), the court held that there was sufficient evidence to support a finding that a 67-year-old man had been falsely imprisoned in a nursing facility, in which he was kept against his will for 51 days. Three days after he was taken to the facility by his nephew, the man had attempted to leave; however, he was caught by the facility's employees and forcibly returned. He was placed in a wing with persons who were addicted to drugs and alcohol and those who were mentally disturbed. He asked during the ensuing weeks that he be permitted to leave and attempted to leave five or six times. He was eventually confined to a restraint chair. He was not allowed to utilize the telephone and his clothes had been taken from him. Describing the actions of the nursing facility staff as being in utter disregard of the resident's legal rights, inasmuch as there was no court order for his commitment and the agreement for his admission stated that he was not to be kept against his will, the court stated that the staff acted recklessly, willfully, and maliciously by unlawfully detaining him.

Where legal justification is absent, the arrest or imprisonment is false and the person denied free movement will be permitted to seek a remedy at law for any injury. There are occasions and circumstances when a person must be confined and the arrest or imprisonment is proper. Criminals are incarcerated; as are sometimes the mentally ill, who may present a danger to themselves or others; long-term care residents are sometimes restrained to prevent falls; children are retained after school for disciplinary reasons; each of these are examples of limitations imposed on the right of another to be freely mobile. In these examples, the right to move about freely has been violated, but the infringement occurs for reasons which are justifiable under the law.

The plaintiff in *Celestine v. United States*, 841 F.2d 851 (8th Cir. 1988), brought an action alleging battery and false imprisonment because security guards had placed him in restraints. The plaintiff-appellant sought psychiatric care at a Veterans Administration (VA) hospital and became physically violent while waiting to be seen by a physician. The VA security guards found it necessary to place the individual in restraints until he could be examined by a psychiatrist. The United States Court of Appeals for the Eighth Circuit held that the record supported a finding that the hospital was justified in placing the patient under restraint. Under Missouri law, no false imprisonment or battery occurred in view of the common law principle that a person believed to be mentally ill could be lawfully restrained if such was considered necessary to prevent immediate injury to that person or others.

Restraints

Restraints are generally utilized to control behavior when residents are disoriented or may cause harm to themselves (e.g., from falling, contaminating wounds, or pulling out hypodermics) or to others. The use of restraints raises many questions of a resident's rights in the areas of autonomy, freedom of movement, and the accompanying health problems that can result from continued immobility. In general, a resident has a right to be free from any physical restraints that are imposed or psychoactive drugs that are administered for purposes of discipline or convenience, and that are not required to treat a resident's medical symptoms.

A study of skilled nursing facilities in Connecticut concluded that "restraint use involves a choice between safety and independence. Unfortunately, the decision is made with an almost complete lack of data concerning the effectiveness of restraints on reducing injury or improving behavior."[16] Although the motivations for using restraints appear sound, there has been a tendency toward overuse. The fear of litigation over injuries sustained because of the failure to apply restraints further compounds the problem of overuse. As a result, regulations governing the use of restraints under the Omnibus Budget Reconciliation Act of 1987 (OBRA 87) make it clear that restraints are to be applied as a last resort rather than as a first option in the control of a resident's behavior. Since prescription drugs are sometimes used to restrain behavior, these regulations represent the first time that prescription drugs must by law "be justified by indications documented in the medical chart."[17]

The quality of life of nursing facility residents can be significantly improved through the scrupulous application of physical restraints and medication by developing appropriate clinical guidelines for their use. "Care plans should plan not only for care while the resident is restrained but should show effort to find alternative treatments to restraints, or there should be documentation in the medical record that no alternative is appropriate."[18]

A survey of 113 nursing homes in New York State was conducted by the Hospital Association of New York State to identify nursing homes that were implementing policies aimed at eliminating or reducing the use of restraints.[19]

> Of the 113 facility survey respondents, 20 reported having implemented new policies aimed at eliminating the use of restraints entirely. Although none of the facilities had accomplished this goal, several programs were well under way. In addition 74 facilities were in the process of developing new policies aimed at reducing if not eliminating reliance on restraints, or were in the early stages of reducing their use of restraints.[20]

The proper and limited use of restraints will lead to better facility-resident relations, improve the quality of life for residents, and help to deter liability for improper application. Principles that should be followed in implementing a program for the effective use of restraints include the following:

- written policies that conform to federal and state guidelines (e.g., a policy that prescribes that the least restrictive device will be utilized to maintain the safety of the resident, a policy requiring the periodic review of residents under restraint, and a policy requiring physician orders for restraints)
- procedures for implementing facility policies (e.g., alternatives to follow before restraining a resident may include family counseling to encourage increased visitations, environmental change, activity therapies, and resident counseling)
- periodic review of policies and procedures, with revision as necessary
- assignment of an individual in the facility to train staff in the use of restraints
- education and orientation programs for the staff, to be conducted inside and outside the facility
- education programs for residents and their families
- a sound appraisal of each resident's needs
- informed consent from the resident, and when and where appropriate from the legal guardian (see Appendix B)
- the application of the least restrictive restraints
- constant monitoring of the resident to determine
    1. need for restraints
    2. injury to the resident
    3. complaints by the resident
- documentation
    1. the need for restraints
    2. consents for the application of restraints
    3. resident monitoring
    4. reappraisals of the continuing need for restraints on the resident's medical record

Defamation of Character

Defamation of character consists of oral or written communication to someone other than the person defamed that tends to hold that person's reputation up to scorn and ridicule in the eyes of a substantial number of respectable people in the community. Libel results from the written word and slander from the spoken word. Libel can be presented in the form of signs, photographs, letters, cartoons, etc. To be an actionable wrong, defamation must be communicated to a third person. Defamatory statements communicated only to the injured party are not grounds for an action.

Libel

A libel suit was brought against the Miami Herald Publishing Company more than two years after its publication of an editorial cartoon depicting a nursing facility in a distasteful manner. *Keller v. Miami Herald Publishing Co.,* 778 F.2d 711 (11th Cir. 1985). The cartoon was described in the following manner:

> On October 29, 1980, The Herald published an editorial cartoon which depicted three men in a dilapidated room. On the back wall was written "Krest View Nursing Home," and on the side wall there was a board which read "Closed by Order of the State of Florida." The room itself was in a state of total disrepair. There were holes in the floor and ceiling, leaking water pipes, and exposed wiring. The men in the room were dressed in outfits resembling those commonly appearing in caricatures of gangsters. Each man carried a sack with a dollar sign on it. One of the men was larger than the other two and was more in the forefront of the picture. One of the others addressed him. The caption read: "Don't Worry, Boss, We Can Always Reopen It As a Haunted House for the Kiddies."

Id. at 713. The court held that the newspaper's editorial cartoon depicting persons resembling gangsters in a dilapidated building, identified as a particular nursing facility that had been closed by state order, was an expression of pure opinion and thus was protected by the First Amendment against the libel suit alleging that the cartoon defamed the owner of the facility.

It is interesting that the court in *Wisconsin Association of Nursing Homes*, 285 N.W.2d 891 (Wis. Ct. App. 1979), would not compel the newspapers to accept and print an advertisement in the exact form submitted by the Wisconsin Association of Nursing Homes and various individual homes.

> Plaintiffs allege in their complaint that the defendants published a series of "investigative reports" in the Milwaukee Journal which dealt with the quality of care and services in several nursing homes. Plaintiffs further characterized the conclusions of the article as being false and

> erroneous. As a result, the plaintiffs prepared a full page advertisement which purported to respond to, and refute the allegations set out in the above mentioned "reports." The defendant newspaper refused to publish the advertisement in the form presented, and referred the question of possibly libelous matter to the attention of plaintiffs' attorneys.

Id. at 893. The Court held that it was within the newspaper's journalistic discretion to reject the advertisement on the ground that it contained possibly libelous material. "[T]he clear weight of authority has not sanctioned any enforceable right of access to the press. In sum, a court can no more dictate what a privately owned newspaper can print than what it cannot print." *Id.* at 894.

> Unlike broadcasting, the publication of a newspaper is not a government conferred privilege. As we have said, the press and the government have had a history of disassociation.
>
> We can find nothing in the United States Constitution, any federal statute, or any controlling precedent that allows us to compel a private newspaper to publish advertisement without editorial control merely because such advertisements are not legally obscene or unlawful.[21]

The appellee in *Stevens v. Morris Communications Corp.*, 317 S.E.2d 652 (Ga. Ct. App. 1984), alleged that a newspaper article, which identified her as a representative of a convalescent center at a city counsel meeting, had defamed her by implying her responsibility for the convalescent center's problems of maintenance and disrepair. The court held that the appellee was not defamed by the article. Using the reasonable person test, the court found that it was highly unlikely that a reasonable person could have read the newspaper article as being defamatory.

Libel "on its face" is actionable without proof of special damage. In certain cases, a court will presume that the words caused injury to the person's reputation. The four generally recognized exceptions where no proof of actual harm to reputation is required in order to recover damages are (1) accusing someone of a crime; (2) accusing someone of having a loathsome disease; (3) using words that affect a person's profession or business; and (4) calling a woman unchaste. Professionals are legally protected against libel when complying with a law that requires the reporting of venereal or other diseases, which could be considered loathsome.

Slander

There are few slander lawsuits because of the difficulty in proving defamation, the small awards, and the high legal fees. The Georgia case of *Carry v. Laugh*, 111 Ga. App. 813, 143 S.E.2d 489 (1965), involved a nurse who brought a defamation action, charging that a physician had slandered her in the course of a consultation concerning the commitment of her husband to a mental institution. The nurse requested damages for mental pain, shock, fright, humiliation, and embarrassment.

The nurse alleged that if the physician's statement were made known to the public, her job and reputation would be adversely affected. The court held that the physician's statement concerning the nurse did not constitute slander because the physician was not referring to the nurse in a professional capacity.

With slander, the person bringing suit generally must prove special damages; however, when any allegedly defamatory words refer to a person in a professional capacity, the professional need not show that the words caused damage. It is presumed that any slanderous reference to someone's professional capacity is damaging; the plaintiff therefore has no need to prove damages. In this case, however, since the court held that the physician's statement did not refer to the nurse in her professional capacity, the plaintiff had to demonstrate damages in order to recover. The plaintiff was unable to show damages.

Professionals who are called incompetent in front of others have a right to sue to defend their reputation. However, it is difficult to prove that an individual comment was injurious. If the person making an injurious comment cannot prove the comment is true, that person can be held liable for damages. Therefore, health professionals should avoid making disparaging remarks about other health professionals.

Defenses to a Defamation Action

Essentially, there are two defenses to a defamation action: truth and privilege. When a person has said something that is damaging to another person's reputation, the person making the statement will not be liable for defamation if it can be shown that the statement was true. A privileged communication is one that might be defamatory under different circumstances, but is not defamatory under the circumstances in which it was made because of a higher duty with which the person making the communication is charged. For example, many states have statutes providing immunity to doctors and health care institutions in connection with peer review proceedings. The person making the communication must do so in good faith, on the proper occasion, in the proper manner, and to persons who have a legitimate reason to receive the information.

There are two types of privilege that may provide a defense to an action for defamation. Absolute privilege attaches to statements made during judicial and legislative proceedings as well as to confidential communications between spouses. Qualified privilege, on the other hand, which attaches to statements such as those made as a result of a legal or moral duty to speak in the interests of third persons, may provide a successful defense only when such statements are made in the absence of malice. If it can be shown that a statement was made as a result of some hatred, ill will, or spite on the part of the speaker, the law will not permit that speaker to hide behind the shield of privilege and avoid liability for defamation.

The defense of privilege is illustrated in the case of *Judge v. Rockford Memorial Hospital*, 17 Ill. App. 2d 365, 150 N.E.2d 202 (1958). There, a nurse brought an action for libel based on a letter written to a nurses' professional registry by the director of nurses at the hospital to which the nurse had been assigned by the registry. In the letter, the director of nurses stated that the hospital did not wish to have the nurse's services available to them because of certain losses of narcotics during times when this particular nurse was on duty. The court refused the nurse recovery. Since the director of nurses had a legal duty to make the communication in the interests of society, the director's letter constituted a privileged communication. Therefore, the court held that the letter did not constitute libel because it was privileged.

Public figures have more difficulty in pursuing defamation litigation than the average individual. One who occupies a position of considerable public responsibility is considered a public figure for the purposes of the law of defamation and is generally more vulnerable to public scrutiny. Legal action against a defendant generally will be denied in the absence of any showing of actual malice in connection with alleged defamatory references to a plaintiff. "Actual" malice applies only in cases involving public figures and encompasses knowledge of falsity or recklessness as to truth.

Fraud

Fraud is defined as willful and intentional misrepresentation that could cause harm or loss to a person or property. Intentional misrepresentation can give rise to an action for deceit. A nursing facility that knowingly makes a false statement that it has no foundation for believing to be true, and that makes it anyway to the detriment of a resident, can be held liable for misrepresentation.

Invasion of Privacy

Residents have a right to personal privacy and a right to the confidentiality of their personal and clinical records. Under OBRA, these rights include

(1) Personal privacy includes accommodations, medical treatment, written and telephone communications, personal care, visits, and meetings of family and resident groups, but this does not require the facility to provide a private room;
(2) Except as provided in paragraph (e)(3) of this section, the resident may approve or refuse the release of personal and clinical records to any individual outside the facility;
(3) The resident's right to refuse release of personal and clinical records does not apply when—
  (i) The resident is transferred to another health care institution; or
  (ii) Record release is required by law or by third-party payment contract.[22]

Invasion of privacy is a wrong that invades the right of a person to personal privacy. Absolute privacy has to be tempered with reality in the medical or nursing care of any resident, and this fact is recognized by the courts. However, negligent disregard for residents' rights of privacy is intolerable and legally actionable, particularly when residents are unable to adequately protect themselves because of unconsciousness or immobility. Unfortunately, familiarity with the long-term care environment tends to diminish the conscious concern that personnel should have for the protection of the privacy of residents.

The right of privacy is recognized by the law as the right to be left alone—the right to be free from unwarranted publicity and exposure to public view, as well as the right to live one's life without having one's name, picture, or private affairs made public against one's will. Nursing facilities and health professionals may become liable for invasion of privacy if, for example, they divulge information from a resident's medical record to improper sources or if they commit unwarranted intrusions into a resident's personal affairs.

The information on a resident's chart is confidential and should not be disclosed without the resident's permission. Those who come into possession of the most intimate personal information about residents have both a legal and an ethical duty not to reveal confidential communications. The legal duty arises because the law recognizes a right to privacy. To protect this right, there is a corresponding duty to obey. The ethical duty is broader and applies at all times.

There are occasions when there is a legal obligation or duty to disclose information. The reporting of communicable diseases, gunshot wounds, child abuse, and other matters is required by law.

The liberty extended to the publication of personal matters, names, or photographs varies. Many public figures will not be heard to complain if their lives are given publicity, and ordinary citizens who voluntarily adopt a newsworthy course of conduct have no grounds for complaint if the activity is reported along with their names and pictures. Generally, the subject of a newsworthy occurrence cannot complain if his or her identity is exposed and exploited by unwarranted publication.

The news media should be accommodated within the limitations placed on such communications by the nursing facility's administration and by applicable statutes and regulations pertaining to the release of information. In any event, a resident's right of privacy must be protected. Public relations officers and other health care professionals should restrict interviews and releases to avoid any injury to the reputation of a resident.

The press should not be given detailed statements about the physical condition of a resident. Health care professionals are not in a position to comment concerning the occurrence that led to a resident's admission. Comments concerning a resident's physical condition should come from the physician. Since such matters do involve protected information, disclosure should be with the resident's permission.

Intentional Infliction of Mental Distress

The intentional or reckless infliction of mental distress is characterized by conduct that is so outrageous that it goes beyond the bounds tolerated by a decent society. It is a civil wrong for which a tort-feasor can be held liable for damages. Mental distress includes mental suffering resulting from painful emotions, such as grief, public humiliation, despair, shame, wounded pride, etc. Liability for the wrongful infliction of mental distress may be based on either intentional or negligent misconduct. Recovery is generally permitted even in the absence of physical harm.

An action, in *Greer v. Medders*, 336 S.E.2d 329 (1985), was brought by a patient and his wife against a physician for the intentional infliction of emotional distress. The superior court entered summary judgment for the physician, and the plaintiff appealed. The defendant physician was covering for the attending doctor who was on vacation. The patient, Mr. Greer, was in the hospital and had not seen the covering physician for several days, so he called the physician's office to complain. The physician later entered the patient's room, in an agitated manner, and became verbally abusive in the presence of Mrs. Greer and a nurse. He said to the patient: "Let me tell you one damn thing, don't nobody call over to my office raising hell with my secretary . . . I don't have to be here every damn day checking on you because I check with physical therapy . . . I don't have to be your damn doctor." *Id.* at 329. When the physician left the room, Mrs. Greer began to cry, and Mr. Greer experienced episodes of uncontrollable shaking for which he had psychiatric treatment. The Court of Appeals of Georgia held that the physician's abusive language willfully caused emotional upset and precluded summary judgment for the defendant.

A plaintiff may recover damages if he or she can show that the defendant intended to inflict mental distress, knew, or should have known that his or her actions would give rise to it.

PRODUCTS LIABILITY

Products liability is the liability of a manufacturer, seller, or supplier of chattels to a buyer or other third party for injuries sustained due to a defect in a product. An injured party may proceed with a lawsuit against a seller, manufacturer, or supplier on three legal theories: negligence, breach of warranty (express or implied), and strict liability.

Negligence, as applied to products liability, requires the plaintiff to establish duty, breach, injury, and causation. The manufacturer of a product is not liable for injuries suffered by a patient if they are the result of negligent use by the user. Product users must conform to the safety standards provided by the manufacturers of supplies and equipment. Failure to follow proper safety instructions can prevent recovery in a negligence suit if injury results from improper use.

Manufacturers are liable for injuries that result from the unsafe design of their products. In order to reduce the risks of liability, they generally provide detailed safety instructions to the users of their products. It can be assumed that failure to provide such instructions could be considered negligence on the part of the manufacturer.

NOTES

1. The Robert Wood Johnson Research Foundation, *The Tort System for Medical Malpractice: How Well Does It Work, What Are the Alternatives?*, ABRIDGE 2, Spring 1991.

2. *Id.* at 2.

3. Murphy v. Allstate Insurance Company, 295 So. 2d 29, 34–35 (La. Ct. App. 1974).

4. 57A AM. JUR. 2D §199(1989).

5. 57A AM. JUR. 2D §208(1989).

6. 57A AM. JUR. 2D §143(1989).

7. 57A AM. JUR. 2D §148(1989).

8. 57A AM. JUR. 2D §193(1989).

9. *Id.*

10. Greene v. Bowen, 639 F. Supp. 544, 561 (E.D. Cal. 1986).

11. Hospital Week, January 6, 1978, at 1.

12. 57A AM. JUR. 2D §26 (1989).

13. 57A AM. JUR. 2D §78 (1989).

14. 57A AM. JUR. 2D §80 (1989).

15. 57A AM. JUR. 2D §134 (1989).

16. Tinetti, Liu, Marottoli, & Ginter, *Mechanical Restraint Use Among Residents of Skilled Nursing Facilities*, 265(4) JAMA 471 (1991).

17. Garrard, *Evaluation of Neuroleptic Drug Use by Nursing Home Elderly under Proposed Medicare and Medicaid Regulations*, 265(4) JAMA 463 (1991).

18. 42 C.F.R. §488.15 (1990).

19. HOSPITAL ASSOCIATION OF NEW YORK STATE, RESTRAINTS AND THE FRAIL ELDERLY PATIENT 23 (1990).

20. *Id.*

21. Associates & Aldrich Co. v. Times Mirror Co., 440 F.2d 133, 136 (9th Cir. 1971).

22. 42 C.F.R. §483.10 (1990).

Chapter 3

Criminal Aspects of Long-Term Care

> Laws are made to restrain and punish the wicked; the wise and good do not need them as a guide, but only as a shield against rapine and oppression; they can live civily and orderly, though there were no law in the world.
>
> John Milton (1608-1674)

Criminal law is society's expression of the limits of acceptable human and institutional behavior. A crime is any social harm defined and made punishable by law.[1] The objectives of criminal law are to maintain public order and safety, protect the individual, utilize punishment as a deterrent to crime, and rehabilitate the criminal for return to society.

Crimes are generally classified as misdemeanors or felonies. The difference between a misdemeanor and a felony revolves around the severity of the crime. A misdemeanor is an offense punishable by less than one year in jail and/or a fine (e.g., petty larceny and driving while intoxicated). A felony is a much more serious crime generally punishable by imprisonment in a state or federal penitentiary for more than one year (e.g., rape, murder).

Peculiar to the health care facility setting is the fact that residents are helpless and at the mercy of others. Such facilities are far too often places where the morally weak and mentally deficient prey on the physically and sometimes mentally helpless. The very institutions that are designed to help residents recover and feel safe can provide the setting for criminal conduct.

This chapter presents the procedural aspects of criminal law, as well as a variety of criminal cases that have occurred in the health care industry. The cases reviewed are by no means exhaustive for a particular health care institution or profession. The purpose of this chapter is to provide students and health care professionals with an elementary review of the criminal law as it applies to health care.

ARREST

Prosecutions for crimes generally begin with the arrest of a defendant by a police officer or with the filing of a formal action in a court of law and the issuance of an arrest warrant or summons. Upon arrest, the defendant is taken to the appropriate law enforcement agency for processing, which includes paperwork and finger printing. Accusatory statements, such as misdemeanor complaints and felony complaints, are also prepared by the police. Detectives are assigned to cases when necessary to gather evidence, interview persons suspected of committing a crime and witnesses to a crime, and assist in preparing a case for possible trial. After processing has been completed, a person is either detained or released on bond.

A felony complaint commences a criminal proceeding; however, an individual may be tried for a felony after indictment by a grand jury unless the defendant waives presentment to the grand jury and pleads guilty by way of a superior court information. Felony cases are presented to a grand jury by a district attorney or an assistant district attorney. The grand jury is presented with the prosecution's evidence and then charged that they may indict the target if they find reasonable cause to believe from the evidence presented to them that all of the elements of a particular crime are present. The grand jury may request that witnesses be subpoenaed to testify. A defendant may choose to testify and offer information if he or she wishes. Actions of a grand jury are handed up to a judge, after which the defendant will be notified to appear to be arraigned for the crimes charged in the indictment.

ARRAIGNMENT

The arraignment is a formal reading of the accusatory instrument and includes the setting of bail. The accused should appear with counsel or have counsel appointed by the court if he or she cannot afford his or her own. After the charges are read, the defendant pleads guilty or not guilty. A not guilty plea is normally offered on a felony. Upon a plea of not guilty, arrangements will be made by the defense attorney and the prosecutor regarding bail. Following arraignment of the defendant, the judge will set a date for the defendant to return to court. Between the time of arraignment and the next court date, the defense attorney and the prosecutor will confer about the charges and evidence in the possession of the prosecutor. At that time, the defense will offer any mitigating circumstances it believes will cause the prosecutor to lessen or drop the charges.

CONFERENCE

Both felony and misdemeanor cases are taken to conference, and plea bargaining commences with the goal of an agreed-on disposition. If no disposition can be reached, the case is adjourned, motions are made, and further plea bargaining takes place. Generally after several adjournments, a case is assigned to a trial court.

THE PROSECUTOR

The role of the prosecutor in the criminal justice system is well defined in *Berger v. United States*, 295 U.S. 88 (1935).

> The United States Attorney is the representative not of an ordinary party to a controversy, but of a sovereignty whose obligation to govern impartially is as compelling as its obligation to govern at all; and whose interest, therefore, in a criminal prosecution is not that it shall win a case, but that justice will be done. As such, he is in a peculiar and very definite sense the servant of the law, the twofold aim of which is that guilt shall not escape or innocence suffer.

The potential of the prosecutor's office is not always fully realized in many jurisdictions. In many cities the combination of the prosecutor's staggering caseload and small staff of assistants prevent sufficient attention being given to each case.[2]

THE DEFENSE ATTORNEY

The defense attorney generally sits in the proverbial hot seat, being perceived as the "bad guy." While everyone seems to understand the attorney's function in protecting the rights of those represented, the defense attorney is often not very popular.

> There is a substantial difference in the problem of representing the "run-of-the-mill" criminal defendant and one whose alleged crimes have aroused great public outcry. The difficulties in providing representation for the ordinary criminal defendant are simple compared with the difficulties of obtaining counsel for one who is charged with a crime which by its nature or circumstances incites strong public condemnation.[3]

THE CRIMINAL TRIAL

The processes of a criminal trial are similar to that of a civil trial and include jury selection, opening statements, presentation of witnesses and other evidence, summations, instructions to the jury by the judge, jury deliberations, verdict, and opportunity for appeal to a higher court.

Many areas of criminal law can have an impact upon health care employees. The following paragraphs discuss some of the more common areas where health care employees have been confronted with criminal charges.

DRUGS

Drug abuse has been described as the number one problem facing the United States today. It is no surprise that health care facilities and health professionals are affected by the theft of drugs, drug abuse, and the illegal sale of drugs. There appears to be no end to the stream of cases entering the nation's courtrooms.

CRIMINAL NEGLIGENCE

Criminal negligence is the reckless disregard for the safety of others. It is the willful indifference to an injury that could follow an act.

The defendants in *State v. Brenner*, 486 So. 2d 101 (La. 1986), were charged with cruelty to the infirm. The defendants brought a challenge stating that the criminal statutes under which they were charged were constitutionally vague. According to the court, Louisiana Revised Statutes §14.12 defines criminal negligence as follows:

> Criminal negligence exists when, although neither specific nor general criminal intent is present, there is such disregard of the interest of others that the offender's conduct amounts to a gross deviation below the standard of care expected to be maintained by a reasonably careful man under like circumstances.

Brenner Id. at 103. Criminal negligence requires:

> . . . a gross deviation below the standard of care expected to be maintained by a reasonably careful man under like circumstances . . . . It calls for substantially more than the ordinary lack of care which may be the basis of tort liability, and furnishes a more explicit statement of that lack of care which has been variously characterized in criminal statutes as "gross negligence" and "recklessness."

Id.

In the bill of particulars, the state alleged that the administrator of the nursing facility neglected and/or mistreated residents by failing to assure that: the nursing facility was maintained in a sanitary manner; necessary health services were performed; the staff was properly trained; there were adequate medical supplies and sufficient staff; records were properly maintained; and the residents were adequately fed, watered, and cared for. There were allegations that the director of nursing neglected and/or mistreated the residents and also failed to properly train the staff at the nursing facility in correct nursing procedures. The controller was alleged to have failed to purchase adequate medical supplies for proper treatment. The admissions director allegedly failed to exercise proper judgment regarding admissions procedures and the physical therapist allegedly failed to provide adequate physical therapy services. The defendants asserted that the term "neglect" was unconstitutionally vague. The Supreme Court of Louisiana, on appeal by the defendants from two lower courts, held that the phrases "intentional or criminally negligent mistreatment or neglect" and "unjustifiable pain and suffering" were not vague and that they were sufficiently clear in meaning to afford a person of ordinary understanding fair notice of the conduct that was prohibited. *Id.* at 101, 104.

FALSIFICATION OF RECORDS

Falsification of records (e.g., medical and business) is grounds for criminal indictment. Civil recovery for damages suffered as a result of falsification of records is available to those damaged by such actions.

FRAUD

A two-year probe of proprietary nursing homes in New York City completed in 1960 by Louis I. Kaplan, Commissioner of Investigations, painted a gloomy picture of the industry. The report that resulted from the probe included the following observations:

- Many operators were attracted by the opportunity to make substantial returns on capital investments and were neither socially motivated nor professionally equipped for the undertaking.
- Public regulation, because of the profit incentive, had to become more vigorous if the public interest was to be served.

* * *

- Nursing home operators had committed crimes by filing false reports and false instruments. Many freely admitted to Kaplan's investigators that they had committed such crimes. "Just about everyone admitted to filing false documents," said one of the investigators.[4]

Although no prosecution resulted from the investigation, it did influence changes in the city's nursing home code that later served as a model for changes in the state's nursing home code. Passage of Article 28 in New York State, as well as Medicare and Medicaid regulations in 1965, increased scrutiny of the nursing home industry. In 1975, the Governor of New York State appointed a Special Prosecutor to investigate nursing homes and vendors to the industry.[5] "The activities of the OSP (Office of the Special Prosecutor) quickly attracted federal attention. Section 17 of the Medicare-

Medicaid Fraud and Abuse Bill of 1977 uses it as a model for developing legislation to encourage other states to create long-term fraud control units."[6] The Health Care Financing Administration (HCFA) was established by the Secretary of Health and Human Services on March 8, 1977. HCFA places under one administration the oversight of the Medicare and Medicaid programs and related federal medical care quality control staffs. Medicare and Medicaid are the major programs directed by HCFA.[7]

Office of Inspector General (OIG)

The Office of Inspector General was established at the Department of Health and Human Services (HHS) by Congress in 1976 to identify and eliminate fraud, abuse, and waste in HHS programs and to promote efficiency and economy in departmental operations. It carries out this mission through a nationwide network of audits, investigations, and inspections. To help reduce fraud in the Medicare and Medicaid programs, the Office of Inspector General actively investigates violations of the Medicare and Medicaid anti-kickback statute, 42 U.S.C. Section 1320a-7b(b). This statute is very broad and among other things, it penalizes anyone who knowingly and willfully solicits, receives, offers or pays anything of value as an inducement in return for

(1) referring an individual to a person for the furnishing or arranging for the furnishing of any item or service payable under the Medicare or Medicaid program, or
(2) purchasing, leasing, or ordering or arranging for or recommending purchasing, leasing, or ordering any good, facility, service, or item payable under the Medicare or Medicaid program.[8]

Violators are subject to criminal penalties or exclusion from participation in the Medicare and Medicaid programs.[9]

A major study on resident abuse in nursing homes was conducted by the Office of Evaluations and Inspections, one of three major offices within the OIG. The study involved 232 interviews with representatives from federal, state and national organizations that either are involved in receiving, investigating and/or resolving nursing home abuse complaints; or are knowledgeable and concerned about nursing homes and resident issues. Major findings of the study revealed the following:

- Nearly all respondents indicate abuse is a problem in nursing homes.
- Respondents differ, however, regarding the severity of the problem. A majority of the State oversight agencies and resident advocates for nursing homes perceive abuse as a serious problem, while many nursing home administrators and industry representatives perceive the problem as minor.
- Physical neglect, verbal and emotional neglect, and verbal or emotional abuse are perceived as the most prevalent forms of abuse.

- Nursing home staff, medical personnel, other patients, and family or visitors all contribute to abuse. However, aides and orderlies are the primary abusers for all categories of abuse except medical neglect.
- Respondents believe nursing home staff lack training to handle some stressful situations.
- Most respondents believe staff certification and training will help to deter resident abuse.
- Administrative or management factors also contribute to nursing home resident abuse (e.g., inadequate supervision of staff, high staff turnover, low staff to resident ratios).[10]

As a result of this study, it was recommended that (1) ongoing training programs be conducted for nurses' aides, with nursing homes documenting staff training and understanding of abuse and reporting responsibilities; (2) new residents to nursing homes be informed about the differences between living in a nursing home environment and their own homes, possible problems that they may encounter, and ways to deal with such problems; (3) HCFA support research concerning long-term care policies that promote staff stability and provide for adequate staff-to-patient ratios necessary to control stress and abuse; and (4) the Administration on Aging collect and disseminate information about nursing home practices which avoid stress and abuse, and promote staff stability and adequate supervision.[11] HCFA was in agreement with these recommendations and believes that implementation of the Omnibus Budget Reconciliation Act of 1989 (OBRA 89) and the Social Security Act will fulfill the recommendations in the report.[12]

Joint Ventures

The heavy dependence on government funding and related programs, such as Medicare and Medicaid, and the continuous shrinkage occurring in such revenues have forced some health care providers to seek alternative sources of revenue. Competition has contributed to the need to seek alternative revenue sources. The traditional corporate structures for nursing facilities may no longer be appropriate to accommodate both normal long-term care activities and those additional activities that may need to be undertaken to provide alternative sources of revenue.

The Office of the Inspector General has become aware of a proliferation of arrangements known as "joint ventures" between those in a position to refer business and those providing items or services for which Medicare or Medicaid pays. Joint venture arrangements have involved such services as diagnostic testing and such items as durable medical equipment.[13]

Joint ventures with certain features could be construed as business arrangements that violate the anti-kickback statute. Questionable features of joint ventures that have been identified by the inspector general include: (1) investors who are chosen because they are in a position to make referrals, and (2) physicians expected to make a large number of referrals who are offered a greater investment opportunity in the joint venture than those anticipated to make fewer referrals.[14]

Department of Justice—Fraud Section

The Fraud Section of the Department of Justice directs and coordinates the federal effort against fraud and white collar crime, focusing primarily upon frauds against government programs and procurement, transnational and multi-district fraud, the securities and commodity exchanges, banking practices, and consumer victimization. It prosecutes fraud cases of national significance or great complexity.[15]

Those who dare to make a fast dollar through fraudulent activities must pay a price. "A conviction of a crime based on medicare or medicaid fraud in connection with nursing home operations has been held to be a conviction of an industry-related felony within the meaning of a statute providing for the revocation of a nursing home operating certificate on the holder's conviction of an industry-related felony."[16] Health professionals must be aware of criminal liability common to their profession. The following cases describe several areas where health professionals have been involved in criminal fraud.

Billing Fraud—Pharmacist

The pharmacist in *State v. Heath*, 513 So. 2d 493, (La. Ct. App. 1987), was convicted on three counts of Medicaid fraud where the pharmacist had submitted claims for reimbursement on brand name medications rather than on the less expensive generic drugs that were actually dispensed. A licensed pharmacist and former employee of the defendant had contacted the Medicaid Fraud Unit of the Louisiana Attorney General's office and reported the defendant's conduct in substituting generic drugs for brand name drugs. As a result of the complaint, a "call out" was conducted by the Medicaid Fraud Unit.

> In a recipient call out, the Medicaid Fraud Unit sends letters to Medicaid recipients in the general area of the pharmacy involved and asks them to bring all their prescription drugs to the welfare office on a specific date. The call out revealed that some of the prescription vials issued by the aforesaid pharmacies contained generic drugs while the labels indicated that they should contain brand name drugs.

Id. at 495.

The court of appeals in *State v. Beatty*, 308 S.E.2d 65 (N.C. Ct. App. 1983), upheld the superior court's finding that the evidence submitted against a defendant pharmacist was sufficient to sustain a conviction for Medicaid fraud. The state was billed for medications that had never been dispensed, for more medications than some patients received, and in some instances for the more expensive trade name drugs when cheaper generic drugs had been dispensed.

Billing for Services Not Furnished

The physician in *State v. Cargille*, 507 So. 2d 1254 (La. Ct. App. 1987), was found to have submitted false information for the purpose of obtaining greater compensation than was otherwise permitted under the Medicaid program. Sufficient evidence had been presented to sustain a conviction of Medicaid fraud. The physician had argued that he felt justified for multiple billings for single office visits because of the actual amount of time that he saw a patient. He believed that his method of reimbursement was more equitable than was that of Medicaid.

Falsification of Records by Nursing Home Stockholder

The principal stockholder of a nursing home corporation in *Chapman v. United States, Department of Health and Human Services*, 821 F.2d 523 (10th Cir. 1987), was convicted of making 19 false line item cost entries in reports to the Kansas Medicaid agency. The United States Court of Appeals found that the Department of Health and Human Services did not act unreasonably when it imposed a $2,000 penalty for each of the 19 false Medicaid claims and proposed an additional settlement of $118,136 even though the state had already recovered the $21,115 in excessive reimbursement by setoff. The court found that, "the penalty reflects a fair amount of leniency on the part of the Inspector General and the ALJ." *Id.* at 530.

> On the aggravating side of the balance, the record shows that Chapman acted deliberately to submit false data to the Kansas Medicaid agency so that nursing homes owned by him would be reimbursed for goods and services they did not provide. Further, when an audit was scheduled that threatened to reveal the false claims, Chapman had false invoices prepared and checks issued, but not signed, in an effort to cover up the discrepancies that the state audit would reveal.

Id. at 529.

Kickback Arrangements

Kickbacks are criminal acts punishable under federal and state laws. Kickback arrangements with suppliers generally occur under one of the following three arrangements:

> First, arrangements could be made for inflated billings, in which cases invoices exceeded the actual price of the goods purchased. The operator could then receive a cash kickback and proceed to submit the inflated bills in his Medicaid cost reports. Second, arrangements could be made with a supplier for phony billings; that is, the operator could pay bills for nonexistent goods or services and then receive an under-the-table cash kickback. Finally, phony items could be submitted along with regular invoices, with the same method of sharing the spoils.[17]

Revocation of a physician's license in *In the Matter of Alaimo v. Ambach*, 457 N.Y.S.2d 955 (N.Y. App. Div. 1982), was not considered to be an excessive sanction for his conviction of perjury when he denied that he was receiving kickbacks from suppliers to his three nursing homes. The physician had falsely denied under oath to a grand jury that he had received cash rebates from vendors, when in fact he had received approximately $800 from a pharmacist between December 15, 1974 and January 15, 1975. *Id.* at 956.

Ambulance Service Kickback

A city official was convicted in a federal district court for conspiring to commit Medicare fraud. Some defendants were also convicted of making illegal payments. Bay State Ambulance and Hospital Rental Service, Inc., a privately owned ambulance company, had given cash and two automobiles to an official of a city-owned hospital. The gifts were given as an inducement to the city official for his recommendation that Bay State be awarded the Quincy City Hospital ambulance service contract, for which Bay State received some Medicare funds as reimbursement. The defendants appealed, and the U.S. Court of Appeals for the First Circuit held that the evidence was sufficient to sustain a conviction. *United States v. Bay State Ambulance & Hospital Rental Services, Inc.*, 874 F.2d 20 (1st Cir. 1989).

MURDER

The tragedy of murder in institutions that are dedicated to the healing of the sick has been an all too frequent occurrence. A recent case involved Richard Angelo, a registered nurse on the cardiac/intensive care unit at a Long Island, New York, hospital, who was found guilty of second-degree murder on December 14, 1989, for injecting two patients with the drug Pavulon. Further, he was found guilty of the lesser charges of manslaughter and criminally negligent homicide in the deaths of two other patients. Angelo had committed the murders in a bizarre scheme to revive the patients in order to be perceived as a hero. The attorney for the estate of one of the alleged victims filed a wrongful death suit against Angelo and the hospital a day before the verdict was rendered by the jury.[18]

In another case, *Hargrave v. Landon*, 584 F. Supp. 302 (E.D. Va. 1984), a nurses's aide was convicted of murder in the first degree when he was found to have injected an elderly patient with a fatal dose of the drug lidocaine. He was sentenced to life imprisonment by the circuit court. The nurse's aide appealed the judgment of the circuit court, alleging that his due process rights were violated during the trial, in that:

1. The trial court failed to grant his motion for change of venue.
2. Because of a "carnival atmosphere" surrounding the trial, the trial court should have, but did not, sequester the jury sua sponte.
3. The trial court improperly admitted evidence of other crimes.
4. The evidence was insufficient as a matter of law to sustain the conviction.

Id. at 305.

The court held that the nurse's aide failed to establish that he was denied an impartial jury due to adverse pretrial publicity, especially since the tenor of newspaper articles prior to his trial were primarily informative and factual and the articles treated the story objectively. The evidence was found to have been sufficient to support his conviction for murder.

OPERATING WITHOUT AN OPERATING CERTIFICATE

The Supreme Court, Appellate Division, in *Bielecki v. Perales,* 543 N.Y.S.2d 496 (N.Y. App. Div. 1989), held that substantial evidence supported a finding that an "adult care facility" was being operated without an operating certificate in violation of the Social Services Law. The imposition of a fine in the amount of $1,000 for each day during which the facility was in operation was found to be appropriate.

RESIDENT ABUSE

Resident abuse is the mistreatment or neglect of nursing home residents. Abuse can take many forms. It can be physical, psychological, medical, financial, etc. It is not always easy to identify, since injuries can often be attributed to other causes. Residents often fail to report incidents of abuse because they fear both retaliation and not being believed, as well as because of the difficulty in proving such charges.

> Hospital patients are not dependent upon the facility operator in the same manner as a resident in a nursing home. Persons are usually hospitalized for only brief periods of time, whereas nursing home residents may be dependent upon the facility operator for a period of years. Thus, the potential for long-term abuse and neglect is far greater for nursing home residents than it is for hospital patients.[19]

The plaintiffs in *In re Estate of Smith v. O'Halloran*, 557 F. Supp. 289 (D. Colo. 1983), instituted a lawsuit in an effort to improve deplorable conditions at many nursing homes. The court concluded that:

> The evidentiary record also supports a general finding that all is not well in the nation's nursing homes and that the enormous expenditures of public funds and the earnest efforts of public officials and public employees have not produced an equivalent return in benefits. That failure of expectations has produced frustration and anger among those who are aware of the realities of life in some nursing homes which provide so little service that they could be characterized as orphanages for the aged.

Id. at 293.

The abuse to which nursing facilities and their residents are susceptible are well known and documented by the Senate Subcommittee on Long-Term Care.

> Nursing home patients present particular problems because of several factors: (1) their advanced age (average 82); (2) their failing health (average four disabilities); (3) their mental disabilities (55 percent are mentally impaired); (4) their reduced mobility (less than half can walk); (5) their sensory impairment (loss of hearing, vision or smell); (6) their reduced tolerance to heat, smoke and gases; and (7) their greater susceptibility to shock.[20]

One of the subcommittee's findings revealed that nursing home residents frequently suffer from neglect or are the targets of intentional abuse.[21] With only four to nineteen percent of those entering a nursing home departing alive,[22] it is a tragedy that the elderly must be exposed to physical and mental abuses.

Abuse of nursing home residents in the past gave impetus to the strengthening of resident rights under OBRA. "The resident has the right to be free from verbal, sexual, physical, or mental abuse, corporal punishment, and involuntary seclusion."[23] Although resident rights have been significantly strengthened, resident abuse continues to be in the headlines. For example, the headline "Nurse's Aide Jailed for Punching Patient" topped a story about a nurse's aide who was jailed for punching a 91-year-old senile man in the nose. The aide had been previously convicted of resident abuse.[24] In response to the seriousness of the ongoing problem, the National Association of Attorney Generals and the National Association of Medicaid Fraud Control Units have developed model state legislation to prohibit patient and resident abuse. They are strongly urging both its adoption and the prosecution of abuse cases.[25]

A report by the Chairman of the Subcommittee on Health and Long-Term Care of the House Select Committee on Aging reached the following conclusions:

- Abuse of the elderly is increasing nationally. About 5 percent or 1 out of 20 older Americans may be victims of abuse from moderate to severe. It is estimated that 1.5 million older Americans are victims of abuse each year.

- Elderly abuse is more likely to be reported than child abuse. While one out of three child abuse cases are reported, only one out of every eight elder abuse cases are reported.
- A majority of states (43 including the District of Columbia) have enacted state statutes or adult protective services laws to require the mandatory reporting of elder abuse.
- Absent the passage of legislation providing assistance to the states, the states are severely hampered in channelling monies into this area. Some states, such as Louisiana, have simply stopped providing elder abuse protective services because of financial constraints.
- Physical violence, including negligence, and financial abuse appear to be the most common forms of abuse, followed by abrogation of basic constitutional rights and psychological abuse.
- Most instances of elder abuse are recurring events rather than one time occurrences.
- Victims are often 75 years of age or older and women are more likely to be abused than men.
- Older people are often ashamed to admit their children or loved ones abuse them or they may fear reprisals if they complain.
- Many middle-aged family members, finally ready to enjoy time to themselves, are resentful of a frail and dependent elderly parent.
- The majority of the abusers are relatives.[26]

Policy recommendations of the Subcommittee on Health and Long-Term Care include:

- A need for a coordinated national effort to confront the issue of elder abuse. The federal government should assist the states in dealing with this problem.
- Amendments to the Older Americans Act provided for a program of elder abuse identification and prevention as well as increased authorities for ombudsmen. These programs, however, were never fully funded. Congress should fund these programs.
- Provide long-term care services in the home to the chronically ill, elderly, disabled, and children.
- States should consider enacting mandatory reporting legislation.
- Congress should authorize the state Medicaid Fraud Control Units to investigate and prosecute all resident abuse and neglect complaints involving violations of state criminal laws for residents of nursing homes and board and care homes.[27]

Residents have a right to be free from abuse and the unnecessary use of restraints. To help ensure these rights, surveyors of nursing facilities have been instructed to watch for signs of resident abuse during long-term care surveys. OBRA provides that:

The facility must develop and implement written policies and procedures that prohibit mistreatment, neglect or abuse of residents.

(1) The facility must—

(i) Not use verbal, mental, sexual, or physical abuse, including corporal punishment, or involuntary seclusion; and

(ii) Not employ individuals who have been convicted of abusing, neglecting or mistreating individuals.

(2) The facility must ensure that all alleged violations involving mistreatment, neglect or abuse, including injuries of unknown source, are reported immediately to the administrator of the facility or to other officials in accordance with State law through established procedures.

(3) The facility must have evidence that all alleged violations are thoroughly investigated, and must prevent further potential abuse while the investigation is in progress.

(4) The results of all investigations must be reported to the administrator or his designated representative or to other officials in accordance with State law within 5 working days of the incident, and if the alleged violation is verified, appropriate corrective action is taken.[28]

They will be looking for:

- The number of residents that are physically restrained.
- The type of restraints being used.
- Whether or not they are applied correctly.
- The apparent physical and mental condition of those residents restrained.
- Whether restraints are released every two hours and whether at least ten minutes of exercise is provided for the resident.
- Whether the staff responds to requests for water, assistance to the bathroom, etc., from a resident who is restrained, and the interval of time between the request and the response.
- How often restrained residents are observed by the staff.
- The effect of restraints on residents and signs of over-medication.
- The frequency of over-medication.
- Signs of mental and physical abuse of residents.
- Any signs of harassment, humiliation, or threats from staff or residents.
- Whether residents are comfortable with the staff.
- The numbers of residents with bruises or other injuries. (Since the skin of the elderly bruises easily, abuse or injury should not be automatically assumed.)
- Resident to resident interactions and staff response to any physical or mental abuse of one resident by another.
- Evidence of resident neglect or residents left in urine or feces without cleaning.[29]

Residents are expected to feel comfortable to voice complaints about how they are treated. Failure of residents to speak freely may be an indication of abuse.

Case Reviews

The following cases of abuse are indicative of the magnitude of the problem.

Abuse and Revocation of License

The operator of a nursing facility appealed an order by the Department of Public Welfare revoking his license because of resident abuse in *Nepa v. Commonwealth Department of Public Welfare*, 551 A.2d 354 (Pa. Commw. Ct. 1988). Substantial evidence supported the department's finding. Three former employees testified that the nursing facility operator had abused residents in the following incidents:

- He unbuckled the belt of one of the residents, causing his pants to drop, and then grabbed a second resident, forcing them to kiss. (Petitioner's excuse for this behavior was to shame the resident because of his masturbating in public.)
- On two occasions he forced a resident to remove toilet paper from a commode after she had urinated and defecated in it. (Denying that there was fecal matter in the commode, petitioner's excuse was that this was his way of trying to stop the resident from filling the commode with toilet paper.)
- He verbally abused a resident who was experiencing difficulty in breathing and accused him of being a fake as he attempted to feed him liquids.

Id. at 355. The nursing facility operator claimed that the findings of fact were not based on substantial evidence, and that even if they were the incidents did not amount to abuse under the code. He attempted to discredit the witnesses with allegations from a resident and another employee that one of the former employees jumped into bed with a resident, another had taken a picture of a male resident while in the shower and had placed a baby bottle and humiliating sign around the neck of another resident. The court was not impressed. Although these incidents, if true, were reprehensible, they were collateral matters that had no bearing on the witnesses' reputation for truthfulness and therefore could not be utilized for impeachment purposes. *Id.* at 356, 357. The court held that there was substantial evidence supporting the department's decision and the activities committed by the operator were sufficient to support revocation of his license.

> We believe Petitioner's treatment of these residents as found by the hearing examiner to be truly disturbing. These residents were elderly and/or mentally incapacitated and wholly dependent on Petitioner while residing in his home. As residents, they are entitled to maintain their dignity and be cared for with respect, concern, and passion.

> Petitioner testified that he did not have adequate training to deal with the patients he received who suffered from mental problems. Petitioner's lack of training in this area is absolutely no excuse for the reprehensible manner in which he treated various residents. Accordingly, DPW's order revoking Petitioner's license to operate a personal care home is affirmed.

Id. at 357.

Abusive Search

The nurse in *People v. Coe*, 501 N.Y.S.2d 997 (Sup. Ct. 1986), was charged with a willful violation of the Public Health Law in connection with an allegedly abusive search of an 86-year-old resident at a geriatric center and with the falsification of business records in the first degree. The resident, Mr. Gersh, had heart disease and difficulty in expressing himself verbally. Another resident claimed that two five dollar bills were missing. Nurse Coe assumed that it was Mr. Gersh because he had been known to take things in the past. The nurse proceeded to search Mr. Gersh, who resisted. A security guard was summoned, and another search was undertaken. When Mr. Gersh again resisted, the security guard slammed a chair down in front of him and pinned his arms while the defendant nurse searched his pockets, failing to retrieve the two five dollar bills. Five minutes later, Mr. Gersh collapsed in a chair gasping for air. Nurse Coe administered CPR, but was unsuccessful, and he expired.

Nurse Coe was charged with violation of Section 175.10 of the Penal Law for falsifying records, because of the defendant's "omission" of the facts relating to the search of Mr. Gersh. These facts were considered relevant and should have been included in the nurse's notes in order to make the note regarding this incident more accurate. "The first sentence states, 'Observed resident was extremely confused and talks incoherently. Suddenly became unresponsive . . .' This statement is simply false. It could only be true if some reference to the search and the loud noise was included." *Id.* at 1001. A motion was made to dismiss the indictment at the end of the trial.

The court held that the search became an act of physical abuse and mistreatment, the evidence was sufficient to warrant a finding of guilt on both charges, and the fact that searches took place quite frequently did not excuse an otherwise illegal procedure.

> It may well be that this incident reached the attention of the criminal justice system only because, in the end, a man had died. In those instances which are equally violative of residents' rights and equally contrary to standards of common decency but which do not result in visible harm to a patient, the acts are nevertheless illegal and subject to prosecution. A criminal act is not legitimized by the fact that others have, with impunity, engaged in that act.

Id. at 1001.

Physical Abuse

The revocation of a personal care home license was found to be proper in *Miller Home, Inc. v. Commonwealth, Department of Public Welfare*, 556 A.2d 1 (Pa. Comw. Ct. 1989), because of repeated medication violations and resident abuse. Evidence was presented that the son of the personal care home's manager was hired as a staff member after having acted as a substitute, even though he had had physical altercations with residents of the home. On one occasion, the manager's son had punched a female resident resulting in her hospitalization for broken bones around the eye, and on other prior occasions, he had been involved in less physical altercations that required police intervention on two occasions. *Id.* at 2.

In *Brinson v. Axelrod*, 499 N.Y.S.2d 24 (N.Y. App. Div. 1986), the court found that the record contained substantial evidence supporting a finding that a nurse's aide had abused an elderly resident by causing injuries to his face and hand. A $450 penalty imposed on the nurse's aide was found to be reasonable.

A nursing facility orderly challenged a determination by the Commissioner of the State Department of Health finding him guilty of resident abuse in *Reid v. Axelrod*, 559 N.Y.S.2d 417 (N.Y. App. Div. 1990). The orderly maintained that the resident struck him with his cane and that he merely pushed the cane away to avoid being struck a second time. A co-employee testified that the orderly struck the resident in the chest after being hit with the cane. The court held that the determination was supported by substantial evidence and that the three-year delay in conducting the hearing did not warrant dismissal of the petition charging the orderly with resident abuse. Public policy requires that residents must be protected from abusive health care workers.

The resident in *Stiffelman v. Abrams*, 655 S.W.2d 522 (Mo. 1983), died from

> . . . 'blows, kicks, kneeings, or bodily throwings intentionally, viciously, and murderously dealt him from among the facility's staff over a period of approximately two to three weeks prior to his death'; that the 'beatings were repeated and were received by the decedent at ninety years of age and in a frail, defenseless, and dependent condition'; that the beatings so administered to the decedent were 'physically and mentally tortuous; that he was caused by them to live out his final days in agony and terror; and that his physical injuries included thirteen fractures to his ribs, subpleural hemorrhaging, and marked lesions to his chest, flanks, abdomen, legs, arms, and hands; that during and following the period of the beatings the decedent lay at the facility for days unattended and unaided as to the deterioration and grave suffering he was undergoing.'

Id. at 526. The executors of the estate had brought suit against the operator and individual and corporate owners of the facility for damages for personal injuries resulting in the death of the resident. The executors were requesting under Count I, $1.5 million in survival damages because of the physical and mental pain and suffering of the decedent, as well as $3 million for punitive damages, and under Count

II, $1,504,084.84 in contractual breaches of the resident's admission contract with the facility. The executors claimed that certain standards of care and personal rights contained in the contract were violated. *Id.* at 526, 527. The trial court sustained the nursing facility's motion for dismissal of the case on the grounds that the plaintiffs failed to state a claim upon which relief could be granted. On appeal, the judgment of the trial court was reversed with respect to Count I and the dismissal of Count II was sustained. The case was remanded requiring the executors to proceed under appropriate statutory authority and not under contract.

Forcible Administration of Medications

The medical employee in *Matter of Axelrod*, 560 N.Y.S.2d 573 (N.Y. App. Div. 1990), sought review of a determination by the Commissioner of Health that she was guilty of resident abuse. Evidence showed that the employee, after a resident refused medication, "held the patient's chin and poured the medication down her throat." *Id.* at 573. There was no indication or convincing evidence that an emergency existed that would have required the forced administration of the medication. The court held that substantial evidence supported the Commissioner's finding that the employee had been guilty of resident abuse.

> The Commissioner properly found that the notation in the record that 'staff are asked to, please, make every effort to make sure that she [the patient] takes them [her medication]' does not authorize the forcible administration of medication. This is particularly so when the notation was not made by a medical doctor authorized to prescribe medication and when the written policy of the facility, was that the head nurse was to be notified if a patient refused medication.

Id. at 573, 574.

Intimidation of Abusive Resident

A difficult and abusive 80-year-old resident of a Veterans Home in *Beasley v. State Personnel Board,* 178 Cal. Rptr. 564 (Cal. Ct. App. 1981), slapped the face of an aide who was assisting him. The resident, referring to his inability to have sex, said that he might as well have it cut off. The aide responded by indicating that if he did not behave she might accommodate him. A nursing supervisor who passed by at that moment noted that a nursing assistant and a hospital aide who were standing nearby laughed and did nothing to intervene. The aide was fired and the other two employees were suspended for ten days. "After the State Board upheld the overkill, the three employees went by mandate to the superior court where Beasley's dismissal was ruled too severe . . . ." *Id.* at 565. The trial court found that action against the nursing assistant and hospital aide, though harsh, was within discretion. On appeal, the court held that the aide's comments did not constitute misconduct and the Veterans Home nursing assistant and hospital aide did not commit actionable conduct by "sort of laughing." When this incident was viewed "in its context and in light of the whole record," it did not support the state personnel board's finding that the aide's attitude toward patients was poor. *Id.* at 566.

Allegations of Abuse Not Supported by the Evidence

Complaints of resident abuse cannot always be substantiated as was the case in *Mullen v. Axelrod*, 549 N.E.2d 144 (N.Y. 1989). The petitioner, Mr. Mullen, alleged that he was near death as a result of the abuse, mistreatment, and neglect he suffered in the nursing facility. Mr. Mullen claimed that the facility failed to properly care for an ankle injury he sustained. The petitioner developed gangrene, which eventually resulted in amputation of his leg. He filed a complaint with the State Department of Health alleging abuse, mistreatment, and neglect. Following investigation, the Department of Health informed the petitioner of its determination that there was "insufficient credible evidence to sustain a violation of the Public Health Law." *Id.* at 145.

Improper Care and a Plea of Nolo Contendere

A nursing facility had been charged with engaging in conduct wantonly endangering a resident by failing to provide necessary and proper care in *Commonwealth v. Hillhaven Corp.*, 687 S.W.2d 545 (Ky. Ct. App. 1984). At a pretrial hearing the facility asked to have a plea of "nolo contendere" accepted and acknowledged and its willingness to pay a maximum fine of $10,000. The court accepted the plea and the commonwealth appealed. Examples of the facility's poor care to the resident included ". . . the failure to provide adequate skin care, nutrition, sanitary care, laboratory work, and medications." *Id.* at 546. The Court of Appeals held that Kentucky courts have no inherent discretionary power to accept a plea of nolo contendere and that all pleas in such matters must be either "guilty" or "not guilty."

PETTY THEFT

Nursing facilities must be alert to the potential ongoing threat of theft by unscrupulous employees, physicians, residents, visitors, and trespassers. The theft of supplies and equipment is substantial and can cost nursing facilities millions of dollars a year.

The physician in *Eufemio v. University of the State of New York*, 516 N.Y.S.2d 129 (N.Y. App. Div. 1987), was convicted in Maryland for the crime of petty theft that arose out of financial irregularities at a nursing facility owned by the physician. The physician moved to New York before the Maryland Commission of Medical Discipline could impose a penalty on him because of his conviction. The New York State Commissioner of Education's determination that the physician's license to practice medicine should be suspended for three years was upheld by a New York court.

Criminal charges of theft were imposed because of misapplication of property in *State v. Pleasant Hill Health Facility, Inc.*, 496 A.2d 306 (Me. 1985). The facility had commingled the residents' personal funds (social security checks and personal allowances) in a corporate account. There were times that the residents' funds remained in the corporate account for three to six months, before being transferred to the residents' account, during which time the combined funds were used to pay corporate expenses. The facility had described their relationship with the residents as debtor-creditor and not a trust relationship. The facility claimed that the funds were always available to residents and they were never denied a request for their funds. The Supreme Judicial Court of Maine held that the facility's handling of the residents' funds was not a debtor-creditor relationship but a trust relationship. "Pleasant Hill's commingling of patients' personal need funds with corporate funds and use of the combined funds to pay corporate expenses constituted dealing with the money as its own and a violation of the corporation's trust agreement." *Id.* at 308. The facility argued that it ultimately transferred all of the residents' personal funds from a transfer account to the residents' account. The court concluded that violation occurred at the moment the residents' personal funds were deposited without segregating them from the corporation's own funds. *Id.* at 308.

SEXUAL IMPROPRIETIES

A significant number of cases address health professionals who have been involved in sexual relationships with their patients. Such cases are being litigated, in many instances, in both civil and criminal arenas. Health professionals finding themselves in such unprofessional relationships must seek help for themselves as well as refer their patients to other appropriate professionals. In addition to being subject to civil and criminal litigation, health professionals are also subject to having their licenses revoked.

CONCLUSION

It is a sad commentary on today's society that criminal activity takes place in health care facilities around the country. Health care providers must be vigilant in seeking out and putting into place safeguards to insure the health and safety of their patients and caregivers.

NOTES

1. R.M. Perkins, Criminal Law and Procedure 2 (1972).
2. J. Kaplan, Criminal Justice: Introductory Cases and Materials 228 (1973).
3. *Id.* at 259.
4. D.B. Smith, Long-Term Care in Transition, 91–92 (1981).

5. *Id.* at 92–97.

6. *Id.* at 97.

7. Office of the Federal Register, National Archives and Records Administration, The United States Government Manual 1988/89, at 307 (1988).

8. Office of Inspector General, Department of Health and Human Services, Special Fraud Alert, Joint Venture Arrangements 1(1) (1989).

9. *Id.*

10. Office of Inspector General, Office of Inspections and Evaluations, Resident Abuse in Nursing Homes, Pub. No. OEI-06-88-00360 (1990), at ii–iii.

11. *Id.* at iii.

12. *Id.* at 22.

13. *Id.*

14. *Id.* at 2(2).

15. The United States Government Manual, *supra* note 7, at 375.

16. 53 A.L.R. 4th 689 (1987).

17. *D.B. Smith, supra* note 4, at 102.

18. Colwell, *The Verdict of Angelo*, Newsday, 50(103), Dec. 15, 1989, at 3.

19. Harris v. Manor Healthcare Corp., 49 N.E.2d 1374 (Ill. 1986).

20. Senate Subcommittee on Long-Term Care of the Special Committee on Aging, 94th Cong., 2d Sess., Failure in Public Policy, Supporting Paper No. 7 (1976).

21. *Id.* at 165–173.

22. *Nursing Home Access: Making the Patient Bill of Rights Work*, 54 J. Urb. L. 473, 474 (1977).

23. 42 C.F.R. §483.13 (1989).

24. *Nurse's Aide Jailed for Punching Patient*, The Baltimore Sun, 307(38), sec. D, June 29, 1990, at 2.

25. Boggs, *OBRA Requirements Spotlight Resident/Provider Rights Issues*, Legal Currents 16, 21 (May 1990).

26. Senate Subcomm. on Health and Long-Term Care, Elder Abuse: A Decade of Shame and Inaction, Comm. Pub. No. 752 (1990) at x–xiv.

27. *Id.* at xiv–xv.

28. 42 C.F.R. §483.13 (1989).

29. 42 C.F.R. §488.115 (1989).

Chapter 4

Civil Procedure and Trial Practice

For many students and health care practitioners, this book will be their only formal introduction to the legal aspects of long-term care. This chapter in particular is valuable to both students and long-term care practitioners in understanding the law and its application in the courtroom.

Today, trial by jury plays an important role in civil actions in the United States. Although many of the procedures leading up to and followed during a trial are discussed in this chapter, it should be noted that civil procedure and trial practice are governed by each state's statutory requirements. Cases on a federal level are governed by federal statutory requirements. (See Exhibit 4-1 for an overview of the chapter.)

PLEADINGS

The pleadings of a case (including the summons, complaint, answer, and counterclaims—all the allegations of each party to a lawsuit) are filed with the court. The pleadings may raise questions of both law and fact. If only questions of law are involved, the judge will decide the case on the pleadings alone. If questions of fact are involved, there must be a trial to determine those facts.

Summons and Complaint

The parties to a controversy are the "plaintiff" and the "defendant." The plaintiff is the person who institutes an action by filing a complaint; the defendant is the person against whom a suit is brought. Many cases have multiple plaintiffs and defendants. An action is commenced by filing an order with a court clerk to issue a writ or "summons."

Although the procedures for beginning an action vary according to jurisdiction, there are procedural common denominators. All jurisdictions require service of

Exhibit 4-1 Overview of Trial Procedures

Pleadings

- Summons and Complaint served to defendant.
- Demurrer—Preliminary objection to complaint by defendant.
- Answer—Defendant's response to the complaint.
- Counterclaim—Issued by defendant against the plaintiff.
- Bill of Particulars—A request for more details of the complaint issued.

Discovery/Examination Before Trial

- Process of investigating the facts of a case before trial.
- Parties to a lawsuit have a right to discovery regarding facts of case prior to trial including examination of witnesses and any evidence that might be presented at trial.

Pretrial Proceedings

- Motion to Dismiss because of insufficient evidence to go forward.
- Motion for Summary Judgment because there are no triable facts.

Notice of Trial/Trial Date Set

Memorandum of Law/Trial Briefs

- Optional document prepared for judge by opposing parties.
- Outlines case for judge by summarizing issues, presenting arguments and case citations.

The Trial

- The Judge—determines questions of law.
- Jury Selection— The jury decides on the factual issues of the case.
- Subpoenas for witnesses and documents issued.
- Opening statements—By the plaintiff's and defendant's attorneys.
- Plaintiff presents case—"Burden of Proof" upon the plaintiff to persuade the jury as to the truth of the case.
- Examination of Witnesses and presentation of Evidence.
- Defense attorney presents argument.

Closing Statements

Judge's Charge to the Jury

Jury Deliberations and Decision

Appeals

Execution of Judgment

process on the defendant (usually through a summons) and a return to the court of that process by the person who served it. Where a summons is not required to be issued directly by a court, an attorney, as an officer of the court, may prepare and cause a summons to be served without direct notice to or approval of a court. Notice to a court occurs when an attorney files a summons and complaint in a court, thereby indicating to the court that an action has been commenced.

The first pleading filed with the court in a negligence action is the "complaint." The essential elements contained in a complaint are: (1) a short statement of the grounds upon which the court's jurisdiction depends (the court's authority to hear the case); (2) a statement of the claim demonstrating that the pleader is entitled to relief; and (3) a demand for judgment for the relief to which the plaintiff deems himself or herself entitled. All of these elements apply to any counterclaim, cross-claim or third party claim. The complaint identifies the parties to a suit, states a cause of action, and includes a demand for damages. It is filed by the plaintiff and is the first statement of a case by the plaintiff against the defendant. In some jurisdictions, a complaint must accompany a summons (an announcement to the defendant that a case has been commenced).

The complaint can be served on the defendant either with the summons or within a prescribed time after the summons has been served. Specific formalities must be observed in the service of a summons so that appropriate jurisdiction over a defendant is obtained. Such formalities dictate the manner in which a summons is to be delivered, the time period within which service must be effected, and the geographic limitations within which service must be made. For example, a summons to commence an action in a local municipal court would generally require service within the particular municipality in order for the court to obtain jurisdiction. Where such service is not possible, the action may have to be brought in a different court.

In the preliminary motions the defendant cites possible errors that would defeat the plaintiff's case. For example, the defendant may object that a summons or a complaint was improperly served, that the action was brought in the wrong county, or that there was something technically incorrect about the complaint. The court may then permit the plaintiff to file a new or amended complaint. However, in some instances the defects in the plaintiff's case may be so significant that the case is dismissed.

Demurrer

Upon receiving a copy of the plaintiff's complaint, the defendant can file preliminary objections before answering the complaint.

Answer

Following service of a complaint, a response is required from the defendant in a document called the "answer." In the answer, the defendant responds to each of the allegations contained in the complaint by stating his or her defenses, and by admitting to or denying each of the plaintiff's allegations. If the defendant fails to answer the complaint within the prescribed time, the plaintiff can seek judgment by default against the defendant. However, in certain instances a default judgment will be vacated if the defendant can demonstrate an acceptable excuse for failing to answer. Even if a plaintiff has been granted judgment by default, he or she could be required to present the basis for damages at a hearing before a court. A defaulting defendant may be entitled to oppose the evidence presented by the plaintiff at such a hearing, at least to the extent of the damages claimed.

Personal appearance of the defendant to respond to a complaint is not necessary. The defendant's attorney, in order to prevent default, responds to the complaint with an answer. The defense attorney attempts to show through evidence that the defendant is not responsible for the negligent act. The answer generally consists of a denial of the charges made and specifies a defense or argument justifying the position taken. The defense may show that the claim is unfounded for such reasons as the following: (1) the period within which a suit must be instituted has run out, (2) there is contributory negligence on the part of the plaintiff, (3) any obligation has been paid, (4) a general release was presented to the defendant, or (5) the contract was illegal and therefore canceled by mutual agreement. The original answer to the complaint is filed with the court having jurisdiction over the case, and a copy of the answer is forwarded to the plaintiff's attorney.

Counterclaim

In some cases the defendant may have a claim against the plaintiff and may therefore file a counterclaim. For example, the plaintiff may have sued a nursing facility for personal injuries and property damage caused by the negligent operation of a facility's ambulance. The nursing facility may file a counterclaim on the ground that its driver was careful and that it was the plaintiff who was negligent and is liable to the facility for damage to the ambulance.

Bill of Particulars

Since a complaint may provide very little information regarding the claim, the defense attorney may request a bill of particulars, which limits the scope and generality of the pleadings. This document requests more specific and detailed information than is provided in the complaint. If a counterclaim has been filed, the plaintiff's attorney may request a bill of particulars from the defense attorney. More specifically, a bill of particulars for a malpractice suit may request the following from the plaintiff's attorney:

- Specify the date and time of day when the alleged malpractice occurred. Does the malpractice claim include

1. misdiagnosis or failure to diagnose correctly;
2. failure to perform a test or diagnostic procedure;
3. failure to medicate, treat, or operate;
4. a contraindicated test given or a contraindicated test or surgical procedure performed; and/or
5. administration of a medicine or treatment or performance of a test or surgical procedure in a manner contrary to accepted standards of medical practice?

- Specify where the alleged malpractice occurred.
- Specify how the occurrence of the malpractice is claimed.
- Specify all the commissions and/or omissions constituting the malpractice claimed.
- List all injuries claimed to have been caused by the defendant's alleged malpractice.
- List any witnesses to the alleged malpractice.
- State the length of time the plaintiff was confined to bed.
- State the weekly earnings of the plaintiff.
- State the name and address of the employer.

A death action rider may also be attached if the malpractice allegedly caused death. The rider may request such information as

- the length of time the decedent experienced pain
- the date, time, and place of death, and
- a statement setting forth the cause of death

DISCOVERY/EXAMINATION BEFORE TRIAL

Discovery is the process of investigating the facts of a case prior to trial. The objectives of discovery are to: (1) obtain evidence that might not be obtainable at the time of trial; (2) isolate and narrow the issues for trial; (3) gather knowledge of the existence of additional evidence which may be admissible at trial; and (4) obtain leads to enable the discovering party to gather further evidence. The discovery process is available to promote more just trials by preventing unfair surprise. "Discovery rules were to prevent trial by ambush. To deny a party the right to know absolutely at some meaningful time before trial the names and addresses of all witnesses the opposing side proposes to call in its case-in-chief is an insult to this principle."[1]

Discovery may be obtained on any matter that is not privileged and that is relevant to the subject matter involved in the pending action. The parties to a lawsuit have the right to discovery and to examine witnesses before trial. Examination before trial (EBT) is one of several discovery techniques utilized to enable the parties of a lawsuit to learn more regarding the nature and substance of each other's case. An EBT consists of oral testimony under oath and includes cross-examination. A deposition, taken at an EBT, is the testimony of a witness that has been recorded in a written form. Testimony given at a deposition becomes part of the permanent record of the case. Each question and answer is transcribed by a court stenographer and may be used at the subsequent trial. Truthfulness and consistency are important because answers that differ from those given at trial will be used to erode the credibility of the witness.

Either party may obtain a court order permitting the examination and copying of books and records, such as medical records, as well as the inspection of buildings and equipment. A court order may also be obtained allowing the physical or mental examination of a party when the party's condition is important to the case.

In certain instances, it may be desirable to record a witness's testimony outside the court before the time of trial. In such a case, one party, after giving proper notice to the opposing party and to the prospective missing witness, may require a witness to appear before a person authorized to administer oaths in order to answer questions and submit to cross-examination. The testimony is recorded and filed with the court and is entered in evidence as the testimony of the missing witness. This procedure may be used when a witness is aged or infirm or too ill to testify at the time of trial.

Preparation of Witnesses

The manner in which a witness handles questioning at a deposition or trial is often as important as the facts of the case. Each witness should be well-prepared prior to testifying. Preparation should include a review of all pertinent records. The following are some helpful guidelines for a witness undergoing examination in a trial or a court hearing:

- Review those records (e.g., medical records and other business records) on which you might be questioned.
- Do not be antagonistic in answering the questions. The jury may already be somewhat sympathetic toward a particular party to the lawsuit; your antagonism may only serve to reinforce such an impression.
- Be organized in your thinking and recollection of the facts regarding the incident.
- Answer only the questions asked.
- Explain your testimony in simple, succinct terminology.
- Do not over-dramatize the facts you are relating.
- Do not allow yourself to become overpowered by the cross-examiner.
- Be polite, sincere, and courteous at all times.
- Dress appropriately, and be neatly groomed.

- Pay close attention to any objections your attorney may have as to the line of questioning being conducted by the opposing counsel.
- Be sure to have reviewed any oral deposition that you may have participated in during EBT.
- Be straightforward with the examiner. Any answers designed to cover up or cloud an issue or fact will, if discovered, serve only to discredit any previous testimony you may have given.
- Do not show any visible signs of displeasure regarding any testimony with which you are in disagreement.
- Be sure to have questions that you did not hear repeated and questions that you did not understand rephrased.
- If you are not sure of an answer, indicate that you are not sure or that you just don't know the answer.

MOTIONS

The procedural steps that occur before trial are specifically classified as pretrial proceedings. After the pleadings have been completed, many states permit either party to move for a judgment on the pleadings. When this motion is made, the court will examine the entire case and decide whether to enter judgment according to the merits of the case as indicated in the pleadings. In some states the moving party is permitted to introduce sworn statements showing that a claim or defense is false or a sham. This procedure cannot be utilized when there is substantial dispute concerning the facts presented by the affidavits.

In many states a pretrial conference will be ordered at the judge's initiative or upon the request of one of the parties to the lawsuit. The pretrial conference is an informal discussion during which the judge and the attorneys eliminate matters not in dispute, agree on the issues, and settle procedural matters relating to the trial. Although the purpose of the pretrial conference is not to compel the parties to settle the case, it often happens that cases are settled at this point.

Dismissal

A defendant may make a motion to dismiss a case, alleging that the plaintiff's complaint, even if believed, does not set forth a claim or cause of action recognized by law. A motion to dismiss can be made before, during, or after trial. Motions made before a trial may be made on the basis that the court lacks jurisdiction, that the case is barred by the statute of limitations, that another case is pending involving the same issues, and other similar matters. A motion during trial may be made after the plaintiff has presented his or her case on the ground that the court has heard the plaintiff's case and the defendant is entitled to a favorable judgment as a matter of law. In the case of a motion made by the defendant at the close of the plaintiff's case, the defendant will normally claim that the plaintiff has failed to present a prima facie case—that is, that the plaintiff has failed to establish the minimum elements necessary to justify a verdict even if no contrary evidence is presented by the defendant. After the trial has been completed, either party may move for a directed verdict on the ground that he or she is entitled to such verdict as a matter of law.

A plaintiff has the right to appeal a lower court's decision to an appellate court if a defendant's motion for dismissal is granted. If the court rules against the defendant's motion for dismissal, as well as any other preliminary objections and motions the defendant may have made, the defendant will then be required to file an answer to the plaintiff's complaint.

Summary Judgment

Either party to a suit may believe that there are no triable issues of fact and only issues of law to be decided. In such event, either party may make a motion for summary judgment. This motion asks the court to rule that there are no facts in dispute and that the rights of the parties can be determined as a matter of law, on the basis of submitted documents, without the need for a trial. Although the courts are reluctant to look favorably on motions for summary judgments, they will grant them if the circumstances of a particular case warrant it.

> A motion for summary judgment is a means for the efficient disposition of a cause of action where there is no genuine issue of material fact and the moving party is entitled to judgment as a matter of law.
>
> * * *
>
> Of course courts should exercise caution in deciding issues involving policy considerations.
>
> * * *
>
> However, excessive caution would undercut the purpose of a motion for summary judgment, which provides a means for piercing the allegations of the pleadings to determine whether there are issues requiring disposition at trial.
>
> * * *
>
> If after drawing all inferences of doubt against the movant, a court finds that there is no genuine basis of material fact, it should enter summary judgment.[2]

NOTICE OF TRIAL

The examination before trial may reveal sufficient facts that would discourage the plaintiff from continuing the case, or it may encourage one or both parties to settle out of court. Once a decision to go forward is reached, the case is placed on the court calendar. Postponement of the trial may be secured with the consent of both parties and the consent of the court. A case may not be indefinitely postponed without being dismissed by the court. Where one party is ready to proceed and another party seeks a postponement, a valid excuse must be shown. An example of a valid excuse is that the attorney for the party seeking the postponement is actually engaged in another case. Should a defendant fail to appear at trial, the judge can pass judgment against the defendant by default. A case can also be dismissed if the plaintiff fails to appear at trial.

MEMORANDUM OF LAW

A memorandum of law (or trial brief) is prepared for the court by each attorney. It presents the nature of the case, cites case decisions to substantiate arguments, and aids the court regarding points of law. Trial briefs are prepared by both the plaintiff's and the defendant's attorneys. A trial brief is not required, but it is a recommended strategy. It provides the court with a basic understanding of the position of the party submitting the brief before the commencement of the trial. It also focuses the court's attention on specific legal points that may influence the court in ruling on objections and on the admissibility of evidence in the course of the trial.

THE COURT

A case is heard in the court that has jurisdiction over the subject of controversy. The judge decides questions of law and is responsible for ensuring that a trial is conducted properly in an impartial atmosphere and is fair to both parties of a lawsuit. He or she determines what constitutes the general standard of conduct required for the exercise of due care. The judge informs the jury of what the defendant's conduct should have been, thereby making a determination of the existence of a legal duty.

The judge plays the dominant role in a trial. He or she decides whether evidence is admissible, charges the jury (defines the jurors' responsibility in relation to existing law), and may, in fact, take a case away from the jury (by directed verdict or judgment notwithstanding the verdict) where he or she feels that there are no issues for the jury to consider or that the jury has erred in its decision. This right on the part of the judge with respect to the role of the jury, in fact, narrows the jury's responsibility with regard to the facts of the case. The judge maintains order throughout the suit, determines issues of procedure, and is generally responsible for the conduct of the trial.

THE JURY

The right to a trial by jury is a constitutional right in certain cases. Not all cases entitle the parties to a jury trial as a matter of right. For example, in many jurisdictions, a case in equity (a case seeking a specific course of conduct rather than monetary damages) may not entitle the parties to a trial by a jury. An example of an equity case would be one that seeks a declaration as to the title to real property.

An individual may waive the right to a jury trial. If this right is waived, the judge acts as judge and jury and becomes the trier of facts as well as issues of law.

Members of the jury are selected from a jury list. They are summoned to court by a paper known as the jury process. Impartiality is a prerequisite of all jurors. The number of jurors who sit at trial is 12 in common law. If there are fewer than 12, the number must be established by statute. Doctors, druggists, nurses, and lawyers are generally excused from sitting on a jury.

Counsel for both parties of a lawsuit question each prospective jury member for impartiality, bias, and prejudicial thinking. This process is referred to as the "voir dire," the examination of jurors. Once members of the jury are selected, they are sworn in to try the case. The jury makes a determination of the facts that have occurred, evaluating whether or not the plaintiff's damages were caused by the defendant's negligence and whether or not the defendant exercised due care. The jury must pay close attention to the evidence presented by both sides and decide on a verdict. The verdict must be based on the theory of wrongdoing. The jury makes a determination of the particular standard of conduct required in all cases where the judgment of reasonable people might differ. The jury also determines the extent of damages, if any, and the degree to which the plaintiff's conduct may have contributed to his or her injury, thereby mitigating the responsibility of the defendant (contributory negligence).

SUBPOENAS

A subpoena is a legal order requiring the appearance of a person or documents before a court or administrative body. Subpoenas may be issued by lawyers, judges, and certain law enforcement and administrative officials, depending on the jurisdiction. Subpoenas generally include

- reference number
- names of plaintiff and defendant
- date, time, and place to appear
- name, address, and telephone number of opposing attorney
- documents requested if a subpoena is for records

Some jurisdictions require the service of a subpoena at a specified time in advance of the requested appearance (e.g., 24 hours). In other jurisdictions, no such time limitation exists. A subpoena can be served by a court clerk, sheriff, attorney, process server, or other person as provided by state statute.

A subpoena ad testificandum orders the appearance of a person at a trial or other investigative proceeding to give testimony. Witnesses have a duty to appear and may suffer a penalty for contempt of court should they fail to appear. They may not deny knowledge of a subpoena if they simply refused to accept it. A "bench warrant," ordering the appearance of a witness in court, may be issued by the court if a witness fails to answer a subpoena. Failure to appear may be excused if extenuating circumstances exist. Witnesses are paid nominal fees for time and travel whether they testify or not. Payment can be requested in advance. A subpoena must allow a reasonable amount of time to travel.

A subpoena for records, known as a subpoena duces tecum, is a written command to bring records, documents, or other evidence described in the subpoena to a trial or other investigative proceeding. The subpoena is served on one able to produce such records. Disobedience in answering a subpoena duces tecum is considered contempt of court and carries a penalty of a fine or imprisonment. The custodian of a record may require a record fee and mileage fee prior to appearance in court. The court in *Hernandez v. Lutheran Medical Center*, 478 N.Y.S.2d 697 (N.Y. App. Div. 1984), held that a $1 per page charge for copies of medical records was reasonable within the meaning of the Public Health Law, which authorizes patients or their representatives to obtain copies of a medical record upon payment of a reasonable charge.

OPENING STATEMENTS

The plaintiff's attorney attempts to prove the wrongdoing of the defendant by presenting credible evidence favorable to his or her client. The opening statement by the plaintiff's attorney provides in capsule form the facts of the case, what he or she intends to prove by means of a summary of the evidence to be presented, and a description of the damages to his or her client. In some jurisdictions a list of witnesses, containing what the lawyers hope to obtain from each witness's testimony, is given to the judge and to the opposition prior to commencement of the trial. Included on this list are the names, addresses, and occupations of each witness. The order of the names indicates the order in which each witness will be called to the stand.

The defense attorney makes his or her opening statement indicating the position of the defendant and the points of the plaintiff's case he or she intends to refute. The defense attorney explains the facts as they apply to the case for the defendant.

BURDEN OF PROOF

The party seeking compensation for injuries suffered because of the negligence of another must prove that there actually was such negligence. The burden of proof in a civil lawsuit is the obligation of the plaintiff to persuade the jury regarding the truth of his or her case.

A "preponderance of the credible evidence" must be presented in order for a plaintiff to recover. "Credible evidence" is evidence that in the light of reason and common sense is worthy of belief. A "preponderance of credible evidence" requires that the prevailing side of the case carry more weight than the evidence on the opposing side. If one would envision the "scales of justice," with the evidence presented by the plaintiff on one scale and that presented by the defendant on the opposite scale, the side tipping the scale in their favor will win the suit. If the evidence is evenly balanced between the plaintiff and the defendant, the required burden of proof will not have been met and the plaintiff will not prevail.

The burden of proof in a criminal case requires that the evidence presented against the defendant must be "beyond a reasonable doubt." Note the terminology—"reasonable" doubt—not "all" doubt. In the civil suit, the evidence presented need only tip the scales of justice.

The burden of proof requires that the plaintiff's attorney show that the defendant violated a legal duty by not following an acceptable standard of care and that the plaintiff suffered injury because of the defendant's breach. If the evidence presented does not support the allegations made, the case is dismissed. Where a plaintiff, who has the burden of proof, fails to sustain such burden, the case may be dismissed despite the failure of the defendant to present any evidence to the contrary on his or her behalf. The burden of proof in some states shifts from the plaintiff to the defendant when it is obvious that the injury would not have occurred unless there was negligence.

The burden of proving negligence requires that the plaintiff show by evidence that outweighs the evidence offered by the opposing party that each and every component of negligence is present. This rule is well illustrated in the following case, in which the plaintiff failed to prove a major element of any negligence action—the standard of care to be imposed upon the facility. In *Montgomery v. American Nursing Centers, Inc.*, 349 N.E.2d 516 (Ill. Ct. App. 1976), a resident fell and injured herself in a nursing facility while recuperating from a fractured hip. An incident report prepared by the home indicated that the woman thereafter complained of knee and hip pain. The attending physician, not having read the report, treated her knee, but not her hip, since she complained of no such pain during the examination. Two weeks later during a follow-up examination, the physician observed symptoms of a possible hip injury and ordered x-rays, which disclosed a hip fracture. The resident sued the nursing facility for negligence and the physician for malpractice. In her complaint the resident alleged that the nursing facility had been negligent in failing to supervise her adequately and in failing to report her condition fully to the attending physician. The trial court entered judgment against the nursing facility, but a directed verdict for the physician. The resident appealed.

The appeals court noted that residents generally have the burden of proving, through the use of expert testimony, the proper standard of care that is to be imposed upon physicians and health care facilities in medical malpractice cases. The appeals court noted an absence of expert testimony as to the proper standard of care required. Since the resident failed to satisfy the burden of proof, the appeals court upheld the trial court's verdict for the physician.

The burden of proof in a criminal case lies with the prosecution. Proof of guilt "beyond a reasonable doubt" is required to convict a criminal defendant—a higher standard than that used in a civil case (which is a fair preponderance of the credible evidence presented).

Violation of a Statute

Violation of a statute may constitute direct evidence of negligence, or it simply may voice a duty that is owed to a particular class of persons who are protected by the statute, ordinance or regulation. For example, a nursing facility regulation that specifies a certain nurse–resident ratio requires compliance by the facility. The same regulation should be seen as an expression of the duty imposed upon the home to provide adequate nursing services to residents. The residents are, therefore, a class of persons identified within the regulation who are to have the benefits of the protection to be gained by having a predetermined minimum standard nurse–resident ratio. Such ratios were taken into account in *Nichols v. Greenacres Rest Home*, 245 So. 2d 544, 545 (La. Ct. App. 1971), where it was shown that the nursing facility was in full compliance with all the requirements for the minimum standards for nursing facilities in Louisiana. On the date of the accident, the rest home had 64 residents, with a total of 19 employees providing 150 hours of nursing care for each 24-hour period. According to applicable standards, only 128 hours of nursing care was actually necessary for compliance.

Violation of Internal Policy and Procedures

Internal policy and procedures or rules of conduct of a nursing facility are set for the day-to-day operation of the institution. A violation of a facility's policy and procedures can give rise to evidence for negligence.

Res Ipsa Loquitur

Res ipsa loquitur ("the thing speaks for itself" or "circumstances speak for themselves") is the legal doctrine that shifts the burden of proof from the plaintiff to the defendant. It is an evidentiary device that allows the plaintiff to make a case legally adequate to go to the jury on the basis of well-defined circumstantial evidence. This does not mean that the plaintiff has fully proven the defendant's negligence. It merely shifts the burden of going forward to the defendant—who must argue to dismiss the circumstantial evidence presented as "speaking for itself."

An inference of negligence is permitted from the mere occurrence of an injury when the defendant owed a duty and possessed the sole power of preventing the injury by exercise of reasonable care. For example, the presence of severe burns on a resident's body after being bathed by an employee raises the question of negligence without the need for expert testimony. Negligence is considered so obvious that expert testimony is not necessary. It lies within a layman's realm of knowledge that people do not generally suffer burns from a bath. That alone is sufficient to require a defendant to come forward with a rebuttal. The three elements necessary to shift the burden of proof under the doctrine of res ipsa loquitur are as follows:

1. The event would not normally have occurred in the absence of negligence.
2. The defendant must have had exclusive control over the instrumentality that caused the injury.
3. The plaintiff must not have contributed to the injury.

Negligence can commonly be inferred where individuals suffer burns from hot water bottles, heat lamps, steam vaporizers, chemicals, and bedside lamps and where physicians fail to order x-rays to diagnose possible fractures.

An action was brought against the nursing facility in *Franklin v. Collins Chapel Correctional Hospital*, 696 S.W.2d 16 (Tenn. Ct. App. 1985), to recover damages for the wrongful death of an 82-year-old resident. The resident was admitted to the nursing facility with senility, high blood pressure, and incontinence. Extensive thermal burns were discovered soon after the resident was bathed by an attendant. The complaint sought to invoke the doctrine of res ipsa loquitur because the injuries suffered by the resident do not occur in a nursing facility in the absence of negligence, and the deceased was in the defendant's "sole care, custody and control." *Id.* at 18. The plaintiffs alleged, among other things:

- The decedent was placed in scalding hot water sufficient to cause second and third degree burns.
- The resident was in the care, custody, and control of the defendants.
- The defendants failed to secure prompt medical treatment for the resident.
- The defendant failed to maintain proper water temperatures.
- The defendant failed to discover the burns within a reasonable time after they had been sustained by the resident.
- The defendant failed to exercise reasonable and ordinary care under the circumstances.

The trial court entered a judgment for the nursing facility pursuant to a jury verdict, and the administrators of the estate appealed. The appeals court held that proof that the nursing facility had exclusive control over the bath wherein burns were allegedly suffered and that the burns would not normally occur absent negligence entitled the administrators to a jury instruction on the doctrine of res ipsa loquitur. The case was reversed and remanded for a new trial.

> The general rule for all cases of circumstantial evidence, both ordinary negligence cases and res ipsa loquitur cases, is that, to make out his case, plaintiff does not have to eliminate all other possible causes or inferences than that of defendant's negligence, and it is enough for him if the evidence for him makes such negligence more probable than any other cause.[3]

EVIDENCE

Evidence consists of the facts proved or disproved during a lawsuit. The law of evidence is a body of rules under which facts are proved. The rules of evidence govern the admission of items of proof in a lawsuit. A fact can be proven by either circumstantial or direct evidence. Evidence must be competent, relevant, and material to be admitted at trial.

Direct Evidence

Direct evidence is proof offered through direct testimony. It is the jury's function to receive testimony presented by witnesses and to draw conclusions in the determination of facts.

Examination of Witnesses

Following conclusion of the opening statements, the judge calls for the plaintiff's witnesses. An officer of the court administers an oath to each witness, and direct examination begins. Information must be obtained from each witness in the form of questions by the attorney, not by the attorney's recitation of the story to the witness. On cross-examination by the defense, an attempt will be made to challenge or discredit the plaintiff's witness. Redirect examination by the plaintiff's attorney can follow the cross examination, if so desired. The plaintiff's attorney may at this time wish to have his or her witness review an important point the jury may have forgotten during cross examination. The plaintiff's attorney may ask the same witness more questions in an effort to overcome the effect of the cross-examination. Recross examination by the defense may take place if necessary for the defense of the defendant.

A sampling of preliminary questions that a physician might expect to be asked on a personal injury case, for example, may take the following form:

1. Name, residence, prior residences?
2. Where did you attend medical school?
3. Are you licensed in this state?
4. Where did you serve your internship?

5. Where did you serve your residency?
6. Is your practice general or special?
7. Are you board certified in one or more specialities?
8. How does a physician obtain board certification?
9. Are you presently practicing medicine?
10. How long have you been in practice?
11. During your___________years of practice have you had occasion to treat a good number of personal injury cases?
12. On or about___________did you have occasion to see__________on a professional basis?
13. Where? Describe his/her condition at the time.
14. What, if anything, did you do on that occasion?
15. Have you been the attending physician since that date?
16. Describe the nature of the examination which you made on_________and from time to time since then.
17. Did you see him/her daily, several times a day at first, when he/she was in the nursing facility?
18. Did you continue to see him/her? How often?
19. What, generally, did your treatment consist of?
20. From your examination and treatment of___________did you determine what injuries were sustained?
21. As a result of your examination, did you find it necessary to seek consultation from another physician or specialist?
22. Did there come a time when you found it necessary to transfer the resident to another facility?

The credibility of a witness may be impeached if prior statements are inconsistent with later statements and if there is bias in favor of a party or prejudice against a party to a lawsuit. Either attorney to a lawsuit may ask the judge for permission to recall a witness.

After all the witnesses of the plaintiff have taken the stand, the defense may call its witnesses and the process of direct, cross, redirect, and recross examination is repeated until the defense rests.

Expert Witness

There are certain types of litigation that require witnesses with specialized knowledge to aid a jury in fact finding. The expert witness assists the jury when the issues to be resolved in the case are outside of the experience of the average juror. Expert testimony, as well as scientific data, is utilized to assist in establishing the standard of care required in any given situation. Expert witnesses may be used to assist a plaintiff in proving the wrongful act of a defendant or to assist a defendant in refuting such evidence. In addition, expert testimony may be used to show the extent of the plaintiff's damages or to show the lack of such damages.

The law recognizes that a jury is composed of ordinary men and women and that some fact finding will involve subjects beyond their knowledge. When a jury cannot otherwise obtain sufficient facts from which to draw conclusions, an expert witness who has special knowledge, skill, experience, or training can be called on to submit an opinion. Laymen are quite able to render opinions about a great variety of general subjects, but for technical questions the opinion of an expert is necessary. At the time of testifying, each expert's training, experience, and special qualifications will be explained to the jury. The experts will be asked to give an opinion concerning hypothetical questions based on the facts of the case. Should the testimony of two experts conflict, the jury will determine which expert opinion to accept.

Demonstrative Evidence

Demonstrative or "real" evidence is evidence furnished by things themselves. It is considered the most trustworthy and preferred type of evidence. It consists of tangible objects to which testimony refers, such as medical instruments and broken infusion needles, that can be requested by a jury. Demonstrative evidence is admissible in court if it is relevant, has probative value, and serves the interest of justice. It is not admissible if it is intended to prejudice, mislead, confuse, offend, inflame, or arouse the sympathy or passion of the jury or to be indecent. Other forms of demonstrative evidence include photographs, motion pictures, x-ray films, drawings, human bodies as exhibits, pathology slides, fetal monitoring strips, infection committee reports, medical staff bylaws, rules and regulations, nursing manuals, policy and procedure manuals, census data, staffing patterns, etc. The plaintiff's attorney utilizes all pertinent evidence to reconstruct chronologically the care and treatment rendered.

When presenting photographs as a form of evidence, the photographer or a reliable witness who is familiar with the object photographed must state that the picture is an accurate representation and a fair likeness of the object portrayed. The photograph must not exaggerate a client's physical condition or show coloring of injuries that is prejudicial. Photographs can be valuable legal evidence when they illustrate graphically the nature and extent of a medical injury. Motion pictures are also valuable evidence. They are helpful in re-enacting a crime. The same principles that apply to photographs apply to motion pictures. Motion pictures must not be fraudulently portrayed by destroying continuity (by either cutting or rearranging). Videotape, a modern form of recording events, is admissible in court, assuming appropriate authentication of the matter being taped, the time of the taping, and the manner in which such taping took place.

X-ray films are considered pictures of the interior of the object portrayed and are admitted under the same requirements as photographs and motion pictures. The attorney must show competent evidence that the x-rays taken are the object or body part under consideration—that the x-ray was made in a recognized manner, taken by a competent technician, and interpreted by a competent physician trained to read x-rays. The value of x-rays lies in the fact that they illustrate fractures, foreign objects, etc.

The plaintiff's injuries are admissible as an exhibit if the physical condition of the body is material. The human body is considered the best evidence of the nature and extent of the plaintiff's injury. If there is no controversy about either the nature or the extent of the injury, such evidence can be considered prejudicial material to which the defendant's attorney should object.

Demonstrations are permitted in some instances to illustrate the extent of injuries. The resident in *Hendricks v. Sanford*, 337 P.2d 974 (Or. 1959), had developed serious bed sores on her back. The defendant objected to the offer of the plaintiff to display her back to the jury. The court found that the plaintiff's injuries, which had healed, were completely relevant as evidence. Even though the injuries had healed and a skin graft had been performed, a declivity of about three-and-a-half inches in diameter and about the depth of a shallow ashtray was still discernible on the plaintiff's back. *Id.* at 976.

> Where an issue as to personal injuries is involved, an injured person may be permitted to exhibit to the jury the wound or injury, or the member or portion of his body upon which such wound or injury was inflicted, and if relevant, the exhibition is allowable in the discretion of the court where there is no reason to expect that the sympathy of the jury will be excited.

Id. at 975.

Documentary Evidence

Documentary evidence is written evidence that is capable of making a truthful statement, such as drug manufacturer inserts, autopsy reports, birth certificates, and medical records. Documentary evidence must satisfy the jury as to authenticity. Proof of authenticity is not necessary if genuineness is accepted by the opposing party. In some instances, concerning wills, for example, witnesses are necessary. In the case of documentation, the original of a document must be produced unless it can be demonstrated that the original has been lost or destroyed, in which case a properly authenticated copy may be substituted.

A sampling of preliminary questions that a witness might be asked upon entering a nursing facility record into evidence include the following:

1. Please state your name.
2. Where are you employed?
3. What is your position in the facility?
4. What is your official title?
5. Did you receive a subpoena duces tecum for certain facility records?
6. Did you bring those records with you?

7. Can you identify these facility records?
8. Did you retrieve the records yourself?
9. Are these the complete records?
10. Are these the original records or copies of the originals?
11. How were these records prepared?
12. Are these records maintained under your care, custody, and control?
13. Were these records made in the regular course of business?
14. Was the record made at the time the act, condition, or event occurred or transpired?
15. Is this facility record regularly kept or maintained?

A manufacturer's drug insert or manual describing the use of equipment is admissible. In *Mueller v. Mueller*, 221 N.W.2d 39 (S.D. 1974), a physician was sued by a patient who charged that as a result of the administration of cortisone over an extended period, she had needlessly suffered a deterioration of bone structure and ultimately a collapsed hip. The jury decided that the physician's prolonged use of cortisone was negligent, and the physician appealed. The appeals court held that the manufacturer's recommendations are not only admissible, but also essential in determining a physician's possible lack of proper care.

In another case, *Mulligan v. Lederle Laboratories*, 786 F.2d 859 (8th Cir. 1986), the plaintiff, a medical laboratory technician, brought an action against the drug manufacturer as the result of the side effects of the drug Varidase. The plaintiff developed several chronic health problems including mouth sores, microscopic hematuria, and red cell cast, indicating kidney disease. The trial court awarded $50,000 in compensatory damages and $100,000 in punitive damages for the drug manufacturer's failure to warn of the side effects of the drug Varidase. On appeal by the manufacturer, the appeals court held that the products liability action was not barred by a three-year statute of limitations contained in an Arkansas products liability act and that the evidence was sufficient to award punitive damages. Evidence presented at trial indicated that a number of side effects were associated with the drug.

Judicial Notice Rule

The judicial notice rule prescribes that well-known facts (for example, that fractures need prompt attention and that two x-rays of the same patient may show different results) need not be proven, but rather, they are recognized by the trial judge. If a fact can be disputed, the rule does not apply.

Hearsay Evidence

Hearsay evidence is evidence that is based on what another has said or done and is not the result of the personal knowledge of the witness. Hearsay consists of written or oral statements. Where a witness testifies to the utterance of a statement made outside of court, and the statement is offered in court for the truth of the facts that are contained in the statement, this is hearsay and therefore objectionable. The court in *Costal Health Services, Inc. v. Rozier*, 335 S.E.2d 712 (Ga. Ct. App. 1985), held that a "written report" by an ombudsman (who did not testify at trial), concerning injuries and treatment of an 85-year-old patient, was inadmissible as evidence. It contained hearsay accounts of conversations as well as impressions, opinions, and conclusions regarding the nursing facility's negligence when a patient had wandered into another patient's room and was injured by that resident. However, the court found that the "testimony about one patient's own account of his violent past, made to the nursing home personnel upon his admission, certainly was admissible as original evidence, not as proof of the actual prior incidents, but to show the defendant's notice of the possibility of violent behavior on the part of that patient." *Id.* at 714.

If a statement is offered not as proof of the facts asserted in the statement, but rather only to show that the statement was made, then the statement can come into evidence. For example, if it is relevant that a conversation took place, then the testimony relating to the conversation may be entered as evidence. The purpose of that testimony would be to establish that a conversation took place, not to prove what was said during the course of the conversation.

Because of the ability to successfully challenge hearsay evidence, which rests on the credibility of the witness as well as on the competency and veracity of other persons not before the court, it is admitted as evidence in a trial only under very strict rules.

There are many exceptions to the hearsay rule, which allow testimony that ordinarily would not be admitted. Included in the list of exceptions are admissions made by one of the parties to the action, threats made by a victim, dying declarations, statements to refresh a witness's recollection if he or she is unable to remember the facts he or she once knew, business records, medical records, and other official records (e.g., certified copies of birth and death records). "Where hearsay evidence is admitted without objection, its probative value is for the jury to determine."[4] The above list of exceptions to hearsay evidence is by no means all-inclusive and, therefore, state statutes should be consulted.

Medical Books

Medical books are considered hearsay since the authors are not available for cross examination. Although medical books are not admissible as evidence, a physician may testify as how he or she formed his or her opinion and what part textbooks played in forming that opinion. During cross examination, medical experts may be asked to comment on statements from medical books that contradict their testimony.

DEFENSES AGAINST RECOVERY

Once a plaintiff's case has been established, the defendant may put forward a defense against the claim for damages. The defendant's case is presented to discredit the plaintiff's cause of action and prevent recovery of damages.

This section deals with the defenses available to defendants in a negligence suit. These are principles of law that may relieve a defendant from liability.

Contributory Negligence

Contributory negligence may be defined as any lack of ordinary care on the part of the person injured that, combined with the negligent act of another, caused the injury and without which the injury would not have occurred. A person is contributorily negligent when that person does not exercise reasonable care for his or her own safety. As a general proposition, if a person has knowledge of a dangerous situation and disregards the danger, the person is contributorily negligent. Actual knowledge of the danger of injury is not necessary in order for a person to be contributorily negligent. It is sufficient if a reasonable person should have been aware of the existence of the danger. "Generally a relaxed standard of care is required in the contributory negligence situation by persons who are subject to the infirmities of old age." *Garner v. Crawford*, 288 So. 2d 886 at 888 (La. Ct. App. 1973).

The court in *Powell v. Parkview Estate Nursing Home, Inc.*, 240 So. 2d 53 (La. Ct. App. 1970), found that where a resident is unable to physically and mentally care for herself "it logically follows she could not be held to the same degree of accountability as a normally healthy person." *Id.* at 57. The 77-year-old resident, who had been bedridden for a year or more and weighed less than 100 pounds, fell from her bed at 10:30 P.M. The nurse who found her placed her back in bed and raised the siderails. The nurse noted on the resident's chart that she apparently did not sustain any serious injuries, although she did suffer from abrasions and cuts on her face. The nurse also noted that the resident "does not complain of pain—hard to determine." *Id.* at 55. The night nurse was asked to observe the resident and told that if anything came up to notify the administrator of the nursing facility. The following morning a registered nurse determined that the resident's left leg was broken above the ankle and summoned the doctor. From the testimony presented from witnesses and the nursing facility records entered into evidence, the trial judge concluded that the siderails were down at the time of the accident. In addition, the night table, which was usually placed close to the resident's bed to prevent her from falling, was not in position. Judgment was rendered for the plaintiff. On appeal, the court held that the defendant's employees were aware that the resident was senile and almost helpless and that both rails should have been raised or the table placed against the bed on the side where the rail was down to prevent the very accident that did occur. The "evidence establishes defendant's employees failed to exercise the care required of them under the law in this instance, and this failure constitutes fault . . . ." *Id.* at 57. The defendant's argument that the resident was contributorily negligent requires that the defendant prove that the resident conducted herself in such a way as to constitute negligence. This, the defendant failed to do.

When the issue of contributory negligence is raised, the defendant claims that the conduct of the injured person is below the standard of care reasonably prudent persons would exercise for their own safety. In some jurisdictions, contributory negligence, no matter how slight, is sufficient to defeat a plaintiff's claim. The two elements necessary to establish contributory negligence are (1) that the plaintiff's conduct fell below the required standard of personal care, and (2) that there is a connection between the plaintiff's careless conduct and the plaintiff's injury. Thus, the defendant contends that some, if not all, liability is attributable to the plaintiff's own actions. The defendant, in order to establish a defense of contributory negligence, must show that the plaintiff's negligence was an active and efficient contributing cause of the injury. "For contributory negligence to defeat the claim of the plaintiff, there must not only be negligent conduct by the plaintiff but also a direct and proximate causal relationship between the negligent act and the injury the plaintiff received." *Bird v. Pritchard*, 33 Ohio App. 2d 31, 291 N.E.2d 771 (1973).

The patient, Mr. Cammatte, in *Jenkins v. Bogalusa Community Medical Center*, 340 So. 2d 1065 (La. Ct. App. 1976), was admitted to Bogalusa Community Medical Center on September 11, 1970, for the treatment of a severe gouty arthritic condition. He had been advised not to get out of bed without first ringing for assistance. On the morning of September 16, 1970, he got out of bed without ringing for assistance and went to a bathroom across the hall. As he returned to his room, he fell and fractured his hip. Mr. Cammatte was transferred to Touro Infirmary in New Orleans where he underwent hip surgery and expired on October 5, 1970, during recuperation, due to an apparent pulmonary embolism. The trial court entered judgment for the defendants, and the plaintiffs appealed. The appeals court found that the patient was in full possession of his faculties at the time he fell and fractured his hip. The accident was the result of the patient's knowing failure to follow instructions not to get out of bed without ringing for assistance. The injury in this case was not the result of any breach of the institution's duty to exercise due care.

The rationale for contributory negligence is based on the principle that all persons must be both careful and responsible for their acts. A plaintiff is required to conform to the broad standard of conduct of the reasonable person. The plaintiff's negligence will be determined and governed by the same tests and rules as the negligence of the defendant.

Assumption of the Risk

Assumption of the risk means knowing that a danger exists and voluntarily accepting the risk by taking a chance in exposing oneself to it, knowing that harm might occur. Assumption of the risk may be implicitly assumed, as in alcohol consumption, or expressly assumed, as in relation to warnings found on cigarette packaging.

This defense provides that the plaintiff has expressly given consent in advance, relieving the defendant of an obligation of conduct toward the plaintiff and taking the chances of injury from a known risk arising from the defendant's conduct. For example, one who agrees to care for a resident with a communicable disease and then contracts the disease would not be entitled to recover from the resident for damages suffered. In taking the job, the individual agreed to assume the risk of infection, thereby releasing the resident from all legal obligations.

The following two requirements must be established in order for a defendant to be successful in an assumption of the risk defense: (1) The plaintiff must know and understand the risk that is being incurred, and (2) the choice to incur the risk must be free and voluntary.

Comparative Negligence

A defense of comparative negligence provides that the degree of negligence or carelessness of each party to a lawsuit must be established by the finder of fact, and that each party is then responsible for his or her proportional share of any damages awarded. For example, where a plaintiff suffers injuries of $10,000 from an accident and where the plaintiff is found 20 percent negligent and the defendant 80 percent negligent, the defendant would be required to pay $8,000 to the plaintiff. Thus, with comparative negligence the plaintiff can collect for 80 percent of the injuries, whereas an application of contributory negligence would deprive the plaintiff of any money judgment. This doctrine relieves the plaintiff from the hardship of losing an entire claim when a defendant has been successful in establishing that the plaintiff has contributed to his or her own injuries. A defense that provides that the plaintiff will forfeit an entire claim if he or she has been contributorily negligent is considered too harsh a result in jurisdictions that recognize comparative negligence.

In most states today, contributory negligence will not defeat a plaintiff's claim, but may reduce the amount of damages. A patient's negligence was permitted as a defense to lessen the damages and to reflect her personal contribution to her injury in *Heller v. Medine*, 377 N.Y.S.2d 100 (N.Y. App. Div. 1975). The patient had brought a malpractice action against a physician, alleging improper treatment of a herpes infection following cataract surgery on the right eye. The physician alleged that the plaintiff contributed to her own injury by failing to make two follow-up visits. The trial court entered a verdict in favor of the physician. On appeal, the appellate court held that the patient's failure to follow the physician's instructions did not defeat the action where the alleged improper professional treatment occurred prior to the patient's own negligence. Damages were reduced to the degree that the plaintiff's negligence increased the extent of the injury.

There are a variety of comparative negligence systems adopted by different states, such as, the "pure" system, the "50 percent" system, and several modified systems. In a "pure" system, the plaintiff is permitted to recover an amount for damages reduced by the percentage of his or her fault, even if the plaintiff's share negligence exceeds 50 percent. Under the "50 percent" system, the plaintiff is permitted to recover an amount for damages reduced by his or her fault, provided the plaintiff's share of negligence (depending on the exact wording of the statute) does not exceed 50 percent. Under the modified systems, most states provide that the plaintiff may not recover damages if the plaintiff's percentage of negligence is equal to that of the defendant. In other states, the plaintiff may not recover damages if his or her percentage of negligence exceeds that of the defendant.[5]

Good Samaritan Laws

Most states have enacted good samaritan laws, which relieve physicians, nurses, dentists, and other health professionals, and in some instances laymen, from liability in certain emergency situations. Good samaritan legislation encourages health professionals to render assistance at the scene of emergencies. By offering immunity, the laws attempt to overcome the widespread notion that physicians, nurses, and others who render assistance in emergencies are likely to be held liable for negligence.

State legislatures have enacted good samaritan statutes for a variety of legal, ethical, and moral reasons. It is a generally accepted legal principle that there is no legal duty to assist a stranger in a time of distress. However, if one person has caused distress to another, there is a legal duty to assist. This principle extends to physicians. They are not legally bound to answer the call of strangers who are dying and might be saved; however, it is a generally recognized moral duty to help a person in distress.

Minnesota state law provides for fines of up to $100 for persons who fail to aid others in emergency situations. The law in this instance provides that "reasonable assistance" should be given (i.e., obtain or attempt to obtain aid from medical and/or law enforcement personnel). The law protects an individual from liability unless he or she is reckless or intentionally cruel when rendering aid. If an individual at the scene of an emergency would have to place himself or herself or another in danger by assisting, each would be exempt from providing assistance.

Each good samaritan statute provides a standard of care that delineates the scope of immunity for those persons eligible under the law. The standards vary widely from state to state and are sometimes ambiguous. In most states the scope of immunity is generally qualified by the statement that the person giving aid must act "in good faith." Some statutes require that a physician or the person rendering care must act with "due care," without "gross negligence," or without "willful or wanton" misconduct.

Despite problems of interpretation, it is clear that the purpose of the statutes is to encourage volunteer medical assistance in emergency situations. The language that grants immunity also supports the conclusion that the doctor, nurse, or layman who is covered by the act will be protected from liability for ordinary negligence in rendering assistance in an emergency.

Under most statutes, immunity is granted only during an emergency or when rendering emergency care. The concept of emergency usually refers to a combination of unforeseen circumstances that require spontaneous action to avoid impending danger. Some states have sought to be more precise regarding what constitutes an emergency or accident. According to the Alaska statute, the emergency circumstances must suggest that the giving of aid is the only alternative to death or serious bodily injury.

Most statutes require that emergency services be rendered without payment or expectation of payment. Apparently this provision was inserted to emphasize that the actions of a good samaritan must be voluntary. In order to be legally immune under the good samaritan laws, a physician or nurse must render help voluntarily and without expectation of later pay.

Statute of Limitations

The statute of limitations refers to legislatively imposed conditions that restrict the period of time after the occurrence of an injury during which a legal action must be commenced. Should a cause of action be initiated later than the period of time prescribed, the case cannot proceed. Whether a suit for personal injury can be brought against a defendant often depends on whether the suit was commenced within a time specified by the applicable statute of limitations. The statutory period begins when an injury occurs, although in some cases (usually involving foreign objects left in the body during surgery) the statutory period commences when the injured person discovers or should have discovered the injury.

Many technical rules are associated with statutes of limitations. Statutes in each state specify that malpractice suits and other personal injury suits must be brought within fixed periods of time. The fact that an injured person is a minor or is otherwise under a legal disability may, under the laws of many states, extend the period within which an action for injury may be brought. Computation of the period when the statute begins in a particular state may be based on any of the following factors: (1) the date that the physician terminated treatment, (2) the time of the wrongful act, (3) the time when the patient should have reasonably discovered the injury, (4) the date that the injury is actually discovered, and (5) the date when the contract between the patient and the physician ended.

> The five-year limitation on bringing medical malpractice cases is unconstitutional, the Supreme Court has ruled. The ruling stemming in part from cases dealing with serial killer Donald Harvey—struck down a protection long claimed by medical professionals and hospitals against negligence suits. Mr. Harvey is linked to deaths that occurred 20 years ago while he was working at a local hospital.[6]

The running of the statute will not begin if fraud (the deliberate concealment from a patient of facts that might present a cause of action for damages) is involved. The cause of action begins at the time fraud is discovered.

Ignorance of Fact and Unintentional Wrongs

Ignorance of the law is not a defense; otherwise, the ignorant would be rewarded simply by pleading ignorance. The fact that a negligent act is unintentional is no defense.

> Ignorance of the law excuses no man; not that all men know the law, but because it is an excuse every man will plead, and no man can tell how to confute him.
>
> John Selden (1584–1654)

Intervening Cause

Intervening cause refers to an act of an independent agency that destroys the causal connection between the negligent act of a defendant and the wrongful injury; if the independent act, not the original wrongful act, is the proximate cause of injury, damages are not recoverable.

In *Cohran v. Harper*, 154 S.E.2d 461 (Ga. Ct. App. 1967), the patient sued a physician, charging him with malpractice for an alleged staph infection she received from a hypodermic needle used by the physician's nurse. The nurse gave the patient an injection that resulted in osteomyelitis. The grounds of negligence included an allegation that the physician failed to properly sterilize the hypodermic needle that was used to administer a certain dose of penicillin. The evidence showed, without dispute, that a prepackaged sterilized needle and syringe were used in accordance with proper and accepted medical practice. The physician was not liable. There was inadequate proof that either the physician or his nurse was negligent. The court said that even if there was evidence that the needle was contaminated and that the patient's ailment was caused thereby, there was no evidence that either the physician or his nurse or anyone in his office knew, or by the exercise of ordinary care could have discovered, that the prepackaged needle and syringe were so contaminated. The defense of intervening cause would have been an adequate defense against recovery of damages if it had been established that the needle was contaminated when packaged.

Sovereign Immunity

Sovereign immunity refers to the common law doctrine by which federal and state governments have historically been immune from liability for harm suffered from the tortious conduct of employees. Sovereign immunity has for the most part been abolished by both federal and state governments. Congress enacted the Federal Tort Claims Act (FTCA), which provides redress for those who have been negligently injured by employees of the federal government acting within their scope of employment. Immunity from intentional torts, claims arising from combat, etc., are exceptions to the FTCA.

In *Wooten v. United States*, 574 F. Supp. 200 (W.D. Tenn. 1982), the Veterans Administration Hospital of Memphis, Tennessee, was held negligent for injuries sustained by an 83-year-old heart patient who was found lying outside his room in a hallway of the hospital. This action was brought under the FTCA. The patient had suffered severe head injuries that required surgery. Damages in the amount of $80,000 were awarded the plaintiff. The court held that the evidence was sufficient to raise a duty on the part of hospital personnel attending the patient to use reasonable care to protect him from getting out of bed and injuring himself. This duty was breached, and the patient was injured. The proximate cause of the patient's injuries was related to the hospital's failure to put up the patient's bedrails and its failure to remind him to call a nurse if he needed help. Evidence offered in this case indicated that the Veterans Administration hospital did not meet the standards of care rendered in other large Memphis hospitals.

Independent Contractor

An independent contractor is an individual who agrees to undertake work without being under the direct control or direction of another and is personally responsible for his or her negligent acts. This doctrine has been used by health care facilities as a defense to avoid liability caused by a physician's negligence. The mere existence of an independent contractual relationship is not sufficient to remove a facility from liability for the acts of certain of its professional personnel where the independent contractor status is not readily known to the injured party.

Whether or not a physician is an employee or an independent contractor is of primary importance in determining liability for damages. A nursing facility is generally not liable for injuries resulting from negligent acts or omissions of independent physicians. There is no liability on the theory of respondeat superior where a physician is an independent contractor so long as the physician is not an employee of the facility, is not compensated, maintains a private practice, and is directly chosen by his or her patients.

CLOSING STATEMENTS

The judge, following completion of the plaintiff's case and the defendant's defense, calls for closing statements. The defense proceeds first, then the plaintiff. Closing statements provide lawyers an opportunity to summarize for the jury and the court what they have proven. They may point out faults in their opponent's case and emphasize points they wish the jury to remember.

If there appears to be only a question of law at the end of a case, a motion can be made for a directed verdict. A motion of this nature must be decided by the court. The court will grant the motion if there is no question of fact to be decided by the jury. The directed verdict may also be made on the ground that the plaintiff has failed to present sufficient facts to prove his or her case or that the evidence fails to establish a legal basis for a verdict in the plaintiff's favor.

Following the attorneys' summations, the court charges the jury before the jurors recess to deliberate. Since the jury determines issues of fact, it is necessary for the court to instruct the jury with regard to the applicable law. This is done by means of a charge. The charge defines the responsibility of the jury, describes the applicable law, and advises the jury of the alternatives available to it.

When a charge given by the court is not clear enough on a particular point or when it does not cover various issues in the case, it is the obligation of the attorneys for both sides to request clarification of the charge. When the jury retires to deliberate, the members are reminded not to discuss the case except among themselves.

It should be noted that if a verdict is against the weight of the evidence, a judge may dismiss the case, order a new trial, or set his or her own verdict. At the time judgment is rendered, the losing party has an opportunity to motion for a new trial. If the new trial is granted, the entire process is repeated; if not, the judgment becomes final, subject to a review of the trial record by an appellate court.

JUDGE'S CHARGE TO THE JURY

Upon completion of the closing statements by the plaintiff(s) and the defendant(s), the judge charges the jury as to the applicable law to be applied in the case. As an example, statements from the trial judge's oral charge to the jurors in *Estes Health Care Centers, Inc. v. Bannerman*, 411 So. 2d 109 (Ala. 1982), where a nursing facility resident expired following transfer to a hospital after suffering burns in a bath, included:

> The complaint alleges the defendant Jackson Hospital, that the defendant undertook to provide hospital and nursing care to the deceased, and that the defendant negligently failed to provide proper hospital and nursing care to the plaintiff's intestate.
>
> * * *
>
> The defendants in response to these allegations . . . have each separately entered pleas of the general issue or general denial. Under the law, a plea of the general issue has the effect of placing the burden of proof on the plaintiffs to reasonably satisfy you from the evidence, the truth of those things claimed by them in the bill of the complaint. The defendants carry no burden of proof.
>
> * * *
>
> As to the defendant Jackson Hospital, the duty arises in that in rendering services to a patient, a hospital must use that degree of care, skill, and diligence used by hospitals generally in the community under similar circumstances.

* * *

> Negligence is not actionable unless the negligence is the proximate cause of the injury. The law defines proximate cause as that cause which is the natural and probable sequence of events and without the intervention of any new or independent cause, produces the injury, and without which such injury would not have occurred. For an act to constitute actionable negligence, there must not only be some casual connection between the negligent act complained of and the injury suffered, but connection must be by natural and unbroken sequence, without intervening sufficient causes, so that but for the negligence of the defendant, the injury would not have occurred.

* * *

> If one is guilty of negligence which concurs or combines with the negligence of another, and the two combine to produce injury, each negligent person is liable for the resulting injury. And the negligence of each will be deemed the proximate cause of the injury. Concurrent causes may be defined as two or more causes which run together and act contemporaneously to produce a given result or to inflict an injury. This does not mean that the causes of the acts producing the injury must necessarily occur simultaneously, but they must be active simultaneously to efficiently and proximately produce a result.

* * *

> In an action against two or more defendants for injury allegedly caused by combined or concurring negligence of the defendants, it is not necessary to show negligence of all the defendants in order for recovery to be had against one or more to be negligent. If you are reasonably satisfied from the evidence in this case that all the defendants are negligent and that their negligence concurred and combined to proximately cause the injury complained by the plaintiffs, then each defendant is liable to the plaintiffs.

Id. at 114, 115.

DAMAGES

Damages are fixed by the jury and are either nominal, compensatory, or punitive. Nominal damages are awarded as a mere token in recognition that wrong has been committed when the actual amount of compensation is insignificant. Compensatory damages are estimated reparation in money for detriment or injury sustained (including loss of earnings, medical costs, and loss of financial support). Punitive damages are additional money awards authorized when an injury is caused by gross carelessness or disregard for the safety of others. Punitive damages are awarded over and above that which is intended to compensate the plaintiff for economic losses resulting from the injury. Punitive damages cover such items as physical disability, mental anguish, loss of a spouse's services, physical suffering, injury to one's reputation, and loss of companionship.

Schedule of Damages

Plaintiffs seek recovery from a great variety of damages. The following are typical:

- personal injuries sustained by the plaintiff
- permanent physical disabilities sustained by the plaintiff
- permanent mental disabilities sustained by the plaintiff
- past and future physical and mental pain and suffering sustained and to be sustained by the plaintiff
- loss of enjoyment of life by the plaintiff
- loss of consortium where spouse is injured in the accident
- loss of child's services where minor child is injured in the accident
- medical and other health expenses reasonably paid or incurred, or reasonably certain to be incurred in the future by the plaintiff
- past and future loss of earnings sustained and to be sustained by the plaintiff
- permanent diminution in the plaintiff's earning capacity[7]

A plethora of negligence cases have been litigated throughout the nation. The following cases illustrate types of damages that are sought by plaintiffs.

Punitive damages were referred to as "that mighty engine of deterrence" in *Johnson v. Terry*, No. 537-907 (Wis. Cir. Ct. Mar. 18, 1983).

The court in *Henry v. Deen*, 310 S.E.2d 326 (N.C. 1984), held that allegations of gross and wanton negligence incidental to wrongful death in the plaintiff's complaint gave sufficient notice of a claim against the treating physician and physician's assistant for punitive damages. The original complaint, which alleged that the treating physician, the physician's assistant, and the consulting physician agreed to create and did create false and misleading entries in the patient's medical record, was sufficient to allege a civil conspiracy. The decision of the lower court was reversed, and the case was remanded for further proceedings.

In *Estes Health Care Centers*, discussed above, the court stated that, "While human life is incapable of translation into a compensatory measurement, the amount of an award of punitive damages may be measured by the gravity of the wrong done, the punishment called for by the act of the wrongdoer, and the need to deter similar wrongs in order to preserve human life." 411 So. 2d at 113.

The former resident of an adult care facility in *May v. Marcus*, 429 N.Y.S.2d 241 (N.Y. App. Div. 1980), was entitled to $760 in punitive damages from the owners of the facility for their intentional withholding of part of the resident's state pension and old age survivor's and disability income funds. This was a court test of a state statute governing personal allowance funds that allows punitive damages upon a showing only of intentional withholding of the funds, and not requiring any finding of bad faith and malice. *Id.* at 242.

In *Payton Health Care Facilities, Inc. v. Estate of Campbell*, 497 So. 2d 1233 (Fla. Dist. Ct. App. 1986), a punitive damage award in the amount of $1.7 million for the wrongful death of a patient from infected decubitus ulcers was justified. The treating physician had agreed to a settlement prior to trial in the amount of $50,000. The deceased, a stroke victim, had been admitted to the Lakeland Health Care Center for nursing and medical care. While at the center the patient developed several severe skin ulcers that eventually necessitated hospitalization in Lakeland General Hospital. The patient's condition had deteriorated to such a state that further treatment was inadequate to prolong his life. Expert testimony had been presented that indicated that the standard of care received by the patient while at the nursing facility was an "outrageous" deviation from acceptable standards of care. There was sufficient evidence of the willful and wanton disregard for rights of others to permit an award of punitive damages against the companies who owned and managed the nursing facility. The cause of death was determined to be bacteremia with sepsis, due to extensive infected necrotic decubitus ulcers, that the patient developed at the nursing facility. *Id.* at 1234.

A nursing facility resident in *Mort v. Unicare Health Facilities, Inc.*, 537 So. 2d 203 (Fla. Dist. Ct. App. 1989), appealed from an order denying her motion for assessment and award for attorney's fees. The issue was whether or not the appellee's offer of judgment, omitting any reference to attorney's fees, precluded a subsequent award of statutorily authorized fees. The lower court denied the motion. On appeal by the resident, the court held that the resident was entitled to an award for attorney fees.

Provisions of an Illinois Nursing Home Care Act permitting recovery of treble damages for negligent conduct were found to be valid in *Harris v. Manor Healthcare Corp.*, 489 N.E.2d 1374 (Ill. 1986). The resident had brought an action against the owner of a nursing facility, alleging that as a result of improper care and treatment by the staff, a decubitus ulcer on her left leg became infected, which resulted in amputation of her leg. The Supreme Court of Illinois found that the plaintiff was entitled to recover either punitive damages or treble damages, but not both.

Joint and Several Liability

The doctrine of joint and several liability permits the plaintiff to bring suit against all persons who share responsibility for his or her injury. The doctrine allows the plaintiff to recover monetary damages from any one or all of the defendants. Any one defendant, even though partially responsible for the plaintiff's injury, can be required to pay the full judgment awarded by the jury. Awards tend to fall in greater amounts on defendants with the better insurance. This is the "deep pockets" concept: Whoever has the most pays the greater percentage of the award.

APPEALS

An appellate court reviews a case on the basis of the trial record as well as written briefs and, if requested, concise oral arguments by the attorneys. A brief summarizes the facts of a case, testimony of the witnesses, laws affecting the case, and arguments of counsel. The party making the appeal is the appellant. The party answering the appeal is the appellee. After hearing the oral arguments, the court takes the case under advisement until such time as the judges consider it and agree on a decision. An opinion is then prepared explaining the reasons for a decision.

Grounds for appeal may result from one or more of the following: (1) the verdict was excessive or inadequate in the lower court, (2) evidence was rejected that should have been accepted, (3) inadmissible evidence was permitted, (4) testimony was excluded that should have been admissible, (5) the verdict was contrary to the weight of the evidence, or (6) the court improperly charged the jury. Notice of appeal must be filed with the trial court, the appellate court, and the adverse party. A "stay of execution" should also be filed by the party wishing to prevent execution of an adverse judgment until such time as the case has been heard and decided by an appellate court.

The appellate court may modify, affirm, or reverse the judgment or reorder a new trial on an appeal. The majority ruling of the judges in the appellate court is binding on the parties of a lawsuit. If the appellate court's decision is not unanimous, the minority may render a dissenting opinion. Further appeal may be made, as set by statute, to the highest court of appeals. If an appeal involves a constitutional question, it may eventually be appealed to the United States Supreme Court.

When a case is decided by the highest appellate court in a state, a final judgment results, and the matter is ended. The instances when one may appeal the ruling of a state court to the Supreme Court of the United States are rare. A federal question must be involved, and even then the Supreme Court must decide whether it will hear the case. A federal question is one involving the Constitution of the United States or a statute enacted by Congress, so it is unlikely that a negligence case arising in a state court would be reviewed and decided by the Supreme Court.

EXECUTION OF JUDGMENTS

Once the amount of damages has been established and all the appeals have been heard, the defendant must comply with the judgment. If he fails to do so, a court order may be executed requiring the sheriff or other judicial officer to sell as much of the defendant's property as necessary, within statutory limitations, to satisfy the plaintiff's judgment.

NOTES

1. Kern v. Gulf Coast Nursing Home of Moss Point, Inc., 502 So. 2d 1198 (Miss. 1987) at 1202.
2. Pierce v. Ortho Pharmaceutical Corp., 417 A.2d 505, 509 (N.J. 1980).
3. Roberts v. Ray, 45 Tenn. App. 280, 322 S.W.2d 435 (1958).
4. Spirito v. Temple Corp., 466 N.E.2d 491 (Ind. Ct. App. 1984).
5. S. EMANUEL, STEVEN, TORTS 184, 185 (1988).
6. *Kentucky: Malpractice Limit Struck*, 13 NATIONAL LAW JOURNAL, November 5, 1990, at 6.
7. 57A AM. JUR. 2D §342 (1989).

Chapter 5

Introduction to Long-Term Care

> Far from being a disease, normal human aging may simply be nature's way of telling a person to slow down and smell the roses, appreciate the wonder of life, and bequeath to younger generations a legacy of maturity. Old age is also a time for new fulfillments, particularly involving the use and sharing of knowledge and experience that has accumulated over a lifetime.[1]

THE AGING POPULATION

The first official census of the United States was not taken until 1790, shortly after George Washington became President. Inferences about the earlier part of this period are somewhat fragmentary.[2] The federal government has conducted a comprehensive enumeration of the U.S. population every ten years since 1790.

> As specified in Article 1, Section 2, of the Constitution, the purpose of these decennial censuses is to ensure fair apportionment of congressional representatives among the various states. Although apportionment remains the primary reason for conducting the census, the findings from the census serve many additional purposes today. In addition to enumerating the population, the census since 1790, has collected data on the number and characteristics of all housing units in the U.S. Such detailed population and housing data give government officials a basis for allocating funds and evaluating needs for public services . . . .[3]

The America of 1990 bears little resemblance to the America of 1790, or to the America of 1890. In 1790, if all went well, a person could travel from New York to Washington in eight days by horseback or coach. That's how long it took George Washington to get from his home outside what is now Washington, D.C. to New York City for his inauguration as President in 1789.

The nation's population in 1790 was nearly 4 million; 63 million in 1890; and 250 million in 1990 (see Figure 5-1). The proportion of the aging population is increasing rapidly. "At the beginning of the century, about 7.1 million persons, less than 10 percent of the total U.S. population were age 55 and over. In 1982 over one-fifth of the American population was 55 years old or over, an estimated 48.9 million persons."[4] "The older population—persons 65 years or older—numbered 31.0 million in 1989. They represented 12.5% of the U.S. population, about one in every eight Americans. The number of older Americans increased by 5.3 million or 21% since 1980, compared to an increase of 8% for the under-65 population."[5]

The nation's largest city, New York, had a population of 33,131 in 1790. The capital, Philadelphia, was second with a population of 28,522 (Washington, D.C. became the capital in 1800). Boston came in third with a population of 18,320. Only six cities contained more than 8,000 people. Just over 5 percent of the total population lived in urban areas, using the current definition of 2,500 or more residents.

The median age was estimated to be 17.8 years in 1840; 22.0 in 1890; 29 in 1940; and 33.0 years in 1990 (see Figure 5-2). As the baby boomers move into the "Gray Zone," there will be more concern and emphasis on the quality and costs of long-term care.[6] Persons reaching age 65 can look forward to a greater number of years of life. In 1978 life expectancy at age 65 was 16.3 years. By 1987 life expectancy at age 65 had increased to 16.9 years, for a total of 81.9 years. In other words, people who attained age 65 in 1987 could expect to live, on average, about another 17 years.[7] According to a Newsday interview with Dr. Arthur Feinberg, the lifespan of Americans is possibly 110 years.

> The population is aging and the fact that we are pretty good at controlling some of the diseases means that more and more people are going to be alive longer. As far as we know, lifespan is maybe 110 years. This country is nowhere near prepared for that—financially, in terms of the support systems, in terms of the institutions, in terms of the trained physi-

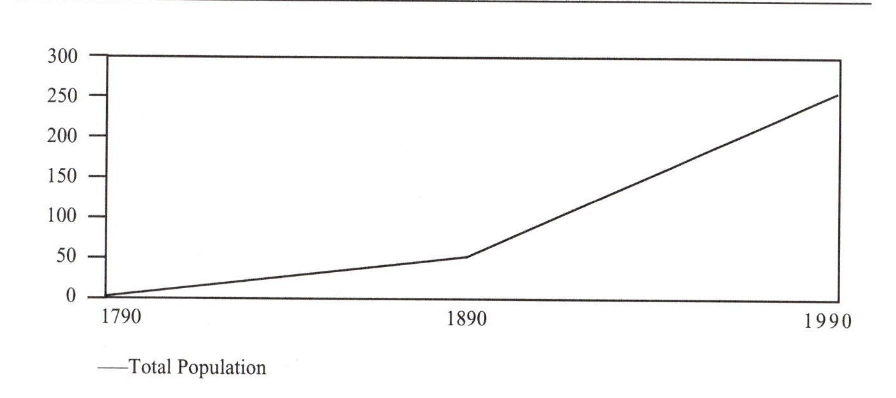

Figure 5-1 U.S. Population Growth (in millions)

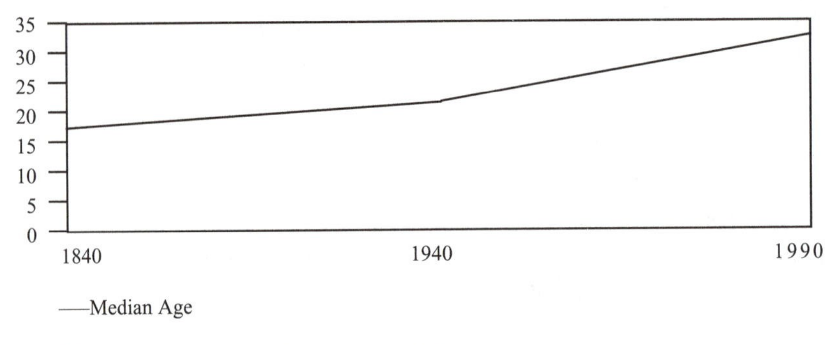

Figure 5-2 U.S. Median Age for 1840, 1940, and 1990

> cians and nurses. We're at the early Model T Ford stage in our approaches to dealing with elderly people.[8]

The first baby boomer will turn 50 in 1996.[9] By the year 2010, because of the maturation of the baby boom group, the proportion of older to younger Americans will rise dramatically—one-fourth of the total U.S. population (74.1 million) is projected to be at least 55 years old.[10] A child born in 1988 could expect to live 74.9 years, about 28 years longer than a child born in 1900. By the year 2000, persons over 65 are expected to represent 13 percent of the population, and this percentage may climb to 21.8 percent by the year 2030.[11]

LONG-TERM CARE SERVICES

Approximately 21 percent of America's elderly (those over the age of 65) experience a functional disability or disabilities requiring long-term care services to help them cope with the rudimentary activities of daily living.[12] A variety of long-term care facilities provide various levels of care for the elderly. The more common of these are discussed below.

Home Health Care

Home health care is an alternative for those who fear leaving the secure environment of their home. Such care is available through home health agencies. These agencies provide a variety of services for the elderly living at home. Such services include part-time or intermittent nursing care; physical, occupational, and speech therapy; medical social services, home health aide services, and nutritional guidance; medical supplies, other than drugs and biologicals prescribed by a physician; and the use of medical appliances. Depending on individual needs, these services are available on a daily, weekly, or even monthly basis.

Adult Day Care Centers

Adult day care centers are facilities where the elderly receive care one to five days a week in a structured setting. The care is generally provided on a full or half day basis. Adult day care programs generally involve such services as meals, transportation, social activities, leisure-time activities, self-care training, rest, nutritional services, and a variety of therapies (e.g., art and music). Some centers provide speech and physical therapy services. Services provided by adult day care centers, according to responses from some 1,400 hospitals surveyed, are presented in Table 5-1 below.

Financial Difficulties

Adult day care centers are experiencing severe financial difficulties. "More than 50 percent of about 1,400 adult day care centers surveyed said that they were operating at a deficit, according to Rick Zawadski, Ph.D., principal investigator for the 1989 national adult day center census, which was conducted by the University of California, San Francisco. Zawadski says the census identified 2100 adult day centers nationally."[13]

Assisted Living Facilities

Assisted living facilities provide custodial care for those who have minimal assistance needs. Custodial care in a communal residence includes the activities of daily living (e.g., bathing, dressing, and eating) and, if not prohibited by statute, some medication assistance. Assisted living facilities, as with most other facilities,

Table 5-1 Services Provided by Adult Day Care Centers

Service	Percent
Meals	98%
Recreational Therapy	98
Social Services	90
Family Counseling	83
Transportation	81
Personal Care	80
Nursing	77
Physical or Occupational Therapy	60
Medical Assessment	56

Based on responses from 1,400 hospital programs

Source: University of California, San Francisco, Institute for Health and Aging, 1989.

may be either non-profit (e.g., religious facilities) or proprietary. Such care is covered only minimally by Medicaid and private long-term care insurance. As indicated in Table 5-9 below, the cost for care in an assisted living facility ranges between $1,000 and $2,000 monthly.

Continuing Care Retirement Communities/Life Care Communities

Continuing care retirement communities, also referred to as life care communities, have been developed for the elderly, combining residential living with the availability of medical and nursing services in specialized premises on the facilities. The life care community is a financially self-sufficient residential community. A life care community consists of a major apartment complex. It has dining and recreational facilities. Health care is available on a skilled level, on an intermediate level, and in some on a home assistance living unit level.

Skilled Nursing Services in Hospitals/Transitional Care Units

Acute care hospitals are offering a wider range of programs for the elderly by opening transitional care units. Such units offer continuity of care for residents who do not need placement on an acute care unit but do require rehabilitative as well as recuperative care. Skilled nursing care provided in hospitals tends to be more intensive, requiring higher staffing ratios. In addition, bed turnover tends to be much higher than that experienced by free-standing skilled nursing facilities. According to a survey conducted by the AHA's Section for Aging and Long-Term Care Services, "the primary discharge destination for hospital-based SNF patients was to their homes or to a community residence (42.3 percent). And, while only 15.3 percent of hospital-based SNFs' discharges were to a hospital, 33.5 percent of the discharges from freestanding SNFs were to a hospital."[14]

Nursing Facilities

Skilled Nursing Facility

A skilled nursing facility (SNF) is a nursing home that provides 24-hour-a-day skilled nursing care for residents who have serious health needs but do not require the more intense level of care provided in a hospital. Skilled nursing facilities participating in the federal Medicare and/or Medicaid programs must meet both federal and state nursing home licensing standards.

Intermediate Care Facility

An intermediate care facility (ICF) provides a lower level of care than that provided by SNFs. ICFs serve residents whose physical or mental condition require limited medical attention. ICFs provide care for people unable to live independently but who are largely ambulatory (either on foot or in a wheelchair) and are able to handle their basic personal needs, such as grooming and dressing.

Nursing Facility

The Omnibus Budget Reconciliation Act of 1987 (OBRA 87) removed the distinction between SNFs and ICFs for Medicaid recipients, effective October 1, 1990. SNFs and ICFs are now classified as "nursing facilities" (NFs).

> (4) Section 1919 (a)–(d) of the Act creates a new term, 'nursing facility' in the Medicaid program, which replaces the terms skilled nursing and intermediate care facility effective October 1, 1990.
>
> (b) Scope. The provisions of this part contain the requirements that an institution must meet in order to qualify to participate as a SNF in the Medicare program, and before October 1, 1990, as a SNF or ICF in the Medicaid program and, effective October 1, 1990, as a nursing facility in the Medicaid program. They serve as a basis for survey activities for the purpose of determining whether a facility meets the requirements for participation in Medicare and Medicaid.[15]

Population Characteristics

As presented in Table 5-2 below, the most rapidly growing age group of nursing home residents for all races is 85 years of age and over. The number of nurs-

Table 5-2 Number and Rate per 1,000 Population of Nursing Home Residents in United States, 1973–74, 1977, and 1985

Total Residents All Ages	*1973–74*	*1977*	*1985*
Under 65 Years	114,300	177,100	173,100
65 Years and Over	961,500	1,126,000	1,318,300
65–74 Years	163,100	211,400	212,100
75–84 Years	384,900	464,700	509,000
85 Years and Over	413,600	449,900	597,300

Source: The National Nursing Home Survey, 1985 Summary for the United States, U.S. Department of Health and Human Services, Hyattsville, MD, January 1989, at 23.

ing home residents for the population 85 years of age and over increased from 413,600 in 1973–74, to 449,900 in 1977, and to 597,300 in 1985. The total number of nursing home residents in this age group increased 33 percent from 413,600 in 1973–74 to 597,300 in 1985, reflecting the rapid growth of this age group in the U.S. population.

Growing Need for Nursing Homes

A study by investigators at the agency for Health Care Policy Research in Rockville, Maryland, projects that 900,000 or 43 percent of the 2.2 million United States residents over the age of 65 will become nursing home residents at some point in their lives. Statistics indicate that the longer an individual lives the greater the likelihood that he or she will spend some portion of his or her lifetime in a nursing facility.[16] Seventy-five percent of nursing homes are proprietary, 19.7 percent are voluntary nonprofit, and 5.3 percent government operated (see Figure 5-3). Proprietary facilities control 1,121,500 beds, 69.1 percent of all nursing home beds (see Table 5-3). Voluntary non-profits control 19.0 percent (370,700 beds) and government controls 8.1 percent (131,900 beds). Large multi-organizational systems control 41.3 percent (7,900) of the homes and 49.3 percent (800,000) of the beds. Independents control 52.6 percent (10,000) homes and 41.9 percent (680,700) beds. Government controlled operations account for 5.3% (1,000) homes and 8.1 percent (131,900) beds.

At the end of 1984 there were approximately 1.4 million residents being cared for in 23,000 nursing homes.[17] "Although the number of nursing home beds grew substantially between 1976 and 1986, the rate of growth did not keep pace with that for the population 85 years and over. . . ."[18] Today, there are nearly 26,000 nursing homes dedicated to the care of the elderly.

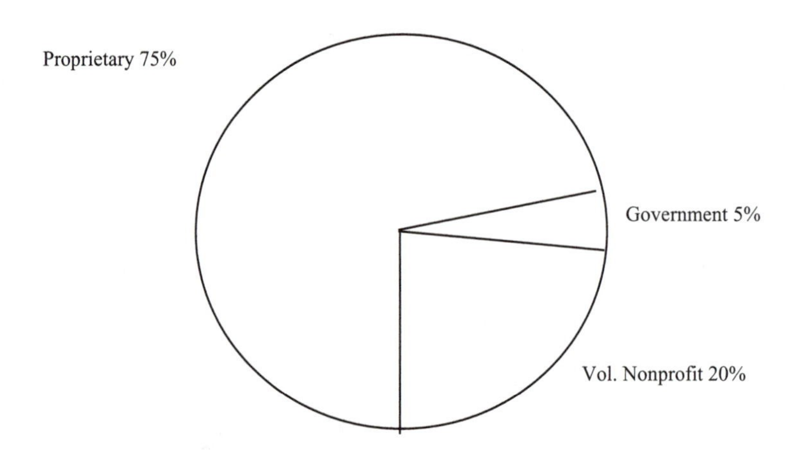

Figure 5-3 Nursing Home Distribution by Ownership

Table 5-3 Number and Percent Distribution of Nursing Homes and Beds

	Nursing Homes		*Beds*	
	Number	*Percent Distribution*	*Number*	*Percent Distribution*
All facilities	19,100	100.0	1,624,200	100.0
Ownership				
Proprietary	14,300	75.0	1,121,500	68.7
Voluntary Nonprofit	3,800	19.7	370,700	22.8
Government	1,000	5.3	131,900	8.1
Affiliation				
Chain	7,900	41.3	800,000	49.3
Independent	10,000	52.6	680,700	41.9
Government	1,000	5.3	131,900	8.4
Unknown	*	*	*	*

Source: The National Nursing Home Survey, 1985 Summary for the United States, U.S. Department of Health and Human Services, Hyattsville, MD, January 1989, at 7.

Reasons for Admission

Table 5-4 below presents the percent of nursing home discharges by reasons for admission and prior state of health as reported by the residents' next of kin. As one might expect, the incidence of hip fractures increases with age, 4.8 percent in the 65–74 age group, 7.9 percent in the 75–84 age group, and 8.5 percent in the 85+ age group.

The general reasons for admission are somewhat consistent in all age groups, see Table 5-5 below. The percentages do not total 100 percent because there are often multiple reasons for admission to a nursing facility (e.g., need for more care than household members can provide and not sufficient funds available for home care). According to a report released by the Department of Health and Human Services, "About 10 percent of hospitalized elderly patients were discharged to skilled-nursing or intermediate care facilities."[19]

The state of health of nursing home residents prior to admission is presented in Table 5-6 below. The gradual deteriorating condition of residents is the major reason for admission across all age groups, and increases from 31.6 for those under 65 to 49.5 percent for those 85 years of age and older.

Nursing Home Services

Table 5-7 illustrates selected services available in nursing homes to residents and nonresidents.

Table 5-4 Percent of Nursing Home Discharges by Medical Reasons for Admission by Age Group

Medical Reason for Admission	*Under 65*	*65–74*	*75–84*	*85+*
Hip Fracture		4.8	7.9	8.5
Other Fracture			2.7	2.1
Arthritis		2.9	2.0	2.3
Other Condition of Bones, Muscles or Joints		3.9	2.5	3.1
Stroke	9.9	14.9	14.8	12.5
Artherosclerosis			1.6	2.8
Other Heart or Circulatory Condition		9.5	8.6	10.3
Cancer, All Types	7.5	8.7	6.4	3.6
Alzheimer's Disease		5.5	5.2	2.8
Confused or Forgetful			1.6	2.6
Organic Brain Syndrome			2.1	3.3
Other Emotional, Mental, or Nervous Condition	17.5	8.2	3.8	4.8
Parkinson's Disease			2.2	
Central Nervous System, Diseases, or Injuries	13.4	4.2	1.9	
Dizziness, Fainting, or Falls				1.8
Loss of Vision or Hearing				1.5
Respiratory Condition	5.6	5.8	3.9	2.2
Diseases of the Digestive or Endocrine Systems	6.8	3.6	4.5	3.3
Genitourinary Diseases			3.4	1.5
No Main Medical Reason		3.1	2.9	3.2
General Debilitation			2.0	5.2
Other Medical Reasons or Unknown	18.5	13.6	17.3	21.1

Source: The National Nursing Home Survey, 1985 Summary for the United States, U.S. Department of Health and Human Services, Hyattsville, MD, January 1989, at 118.

Table 5-5 Percent of Nursing Home Discharges by General Reason for Admission by Age Group

General Reason for Admission	*Under 65*	*65–74*	*75–84*	*85+*
Recuperation from Surgery or Illness	47.9	53.7	51.3	41.3
No One at Home to Provide Care	46.6	53.3	56.5	58.3
Not Enough Money to Purchase Nursing Care at Home	42.0	41.9	36.3	33.4
Required More Care than Household Members Could Give	75.8	79.0	79.6	76.9
Problems in Doing Everyday Activities	71.4	79.6	77.9	74.6
Because Spouse Entered		3.2	2.6	2.7

Source: The National Nursing Home Survey, 1985 Summary for the United States, U.S. Department of Health and Human Services, Hyattsville, MD, January 1989, at 118.

Table 5-6 State of Health before Admission by Age Group

State of Health before Admission	*Under 65*	*65–74*	*75–84*	*85+*
Suddenly Ill or Injured	18.7	21.1	25.2	23.4
Gradually Worsening	31.6	44.6	46.5	49.5
In Poor Condition Most of Year	28.0	22.9	18.6	13.3
Other Health Status	13.9	7.8	7.3	11.4
Unknown	7.8	3.7	2.5	2.5

Source: The National Nursing Home Survey, 1985 Summary for the United States, U.S. Department of Health and Human Services, Hyattsville, MD, January 1989, at 118.

Table 5-7 Selected Services to Residents and Nonresidents

Total facilities	19,100
Services to Residents	
Personal Care	18,800
Prescribed or Nonprescribed Medicines	17,700
Equipment or Other Devices	17,000
Social Services	17,300
Transportation	16,600
Medical Services	16,500
Other Medical Services	16,200
Nursing Services	16,200
Nutrition Services	16,000
Mental Health Services	12,900
Physical Therapy	14,500
Speech Therapy	13,000
Occupational Therapy	10,600
Hospice Services	5,400
Sheltered Employment	2,400
Vocational Rehabilitation	2,700
Special Education	2,300
Other	6,300
Services to Nonresidents	
Day Care	900
Physical Therapy	1,200
Social Services	1,100
Other	1,700

Source: The National Nursing Home Survey, 1985 Summary for the United States, U.S. Department of Health and Human Services, Hyattsville, MD, January 1989, at 12.

National Staffing Characteristics of Nursing Homes

Table 5-8 presents full-time equivalent (FTE) staffing characteristics for nursing homes at a rate per 100 beds. Physician employment in nursing facilities is minimal, accounting for only 0.2 FTE per 100 beds. Under OBRA regulations, physician involvement in resident care is likely to increase.

Nursing Home Regulations

The United States Senate Special Committee on the Aging has concluded that more than 50 percent of nursing homes in the United States have

Table 5-8 Nursing Home Full-Time Equivalent Employees per 100 Beds

*Occupational Category**	*Total*
All Full-Time Equivalent Employees**	48.9
Administrative and Medical Staff	
Administrator or Assistant Administrator	1.6
Physician, Resident, Intern***	.2
Dietitian or Nutritionist	.4
Registered Medical Record Administrator	.2
Other Health Personnel****	1.1
Therapeutic Staff	
Registered Physical Therapist	.2
Activities Director	1.2
Social Worker	.6
Other Therapeutic Staff*****	.1
Nursing Staff	
Nurse's Aide and Orderly	30.8
Licensed Practical Nurse	7.4
Registered Nurse	5.1

* Includes only employees providing direct health-related services to residents.

** 35 hours of part-time employees' work is considered equivalent to 1 full-time employee. Part-time employees were converted to full-time equivalent employees by dividing the number of hours worked per week by 35.

*** Includes medical doctor and doctor of osteopathy.

****Includes dentist, pharmacist, psychologist, x-ray technician, and others.

*****Includes registered occupational therapist, radiological service personnel, speech pathologist and/or audiologist.

Source: The National Nursing Home Survey, 1985 Summary of the United States, U.S. Department of Health and Human Services, Hyattsville, MD, January 1989, at 14.

> substandard or life-threatening conditions, and that nursing home placements is a bitter confirmation of the fears of a lifetime, in that seniors fear change and uncertainty, poor care and abuses, loss of health and mobility, loss of liberty and human dignity, and exhaustion of savings and "going on welfare."[20]

The large number of elderly persons who will spend some portion of their lifetime in a nursing home, coupled with the need to improve nursing home conditions, has resulted in extensive federal, state, and municipal regulation (e.g., OBRA discussed below). State regulation generally involves some form of licensing and related requirements. 53 A.L.R. 4TH 689, at 702 (1987). Federal regulations provide that to obtain certification from the Secretary of Health and Human Services or a state survey agency as a qualified medicaid provider of nursing facility services, a nursing facility must meet state nursing home licensing standards. *Id.* at 702. Municipal ordinances generally include fire prevention regulations, ventilation and sanitation requirements, isolation procedures for persons suffering communicable diseases, board of health inspections, etc. "Municipal ordinances providing for the licensing and regulation of nursing homes have been held valid police regulations except when pre-empted by state law." *Id.* at 782.

> As life expectancy has continued to increase, so has the emphasis on improving the quality of life of persons who live to age 65 and well beyond. Major objectives are to make the remaining years of life as healthy, active, and enjoyable as possible and to reduce the prevalence of such chronic problems as diabetes, respiratory conditions, and injuries through diet, exercise, modifications in lifestyle and behaviors (for example, smoking and alcohol consumption), and the adoption and practice of safety measures, especially in and about the house.[21]

Nursing Home Licensure

Most types of nursing homes must be licensed. Nursing home regulations are standards promulgated by the state licensing agency, which must be satisfied by a facility in order for the facility to be licensed by the state. Such regulations deal with virtually every aspect of the operation of the facility, including qualifications of the administrator, which vary in their specifics from state to state.

Overview of Services for the Aging

There is a wide range of services available for the elderly. The various levels of care are illustrated in Table 5-9 below. As described in Table 5-9, there is a wide variety of alternatives for older people needing various levels of long-term care. The options range from home care and continuing-care retirement communities for the relatively healthy older person to nursing facilities that provide skilled nursing services. The costs, which continue to rise, can be staggering for those living on fixed incomes.

HEALTH PLANNING

The National Planning and Resource Development Act of 1974 (P.L. 93-641), with its emphasis on regional planning to reduce cost and improve quality and

Table 5-9 Overview of Services for the Aging

Category	*Description*	*Gov't/Private Costs*	*Coverage*
Home Care	Caregivers visit or live in the elderly person's home	Average/hr: personal-care worker or home health aide, $10–$20; physical therapist, $4–$60; LPN $15–$40; RN $25–$70; social worker, $50–$60	Limited coverage by Medicare, Medicaid, and long-term insurance policies
Adult Day Care	Elderly person visits care center one to five days weekly for half to full day of programs	$125–$175 per day; medical $100–$200 per day	Social models: coverage; medical models: limited coverage
Care Managers	Supervise and coordinate home care and other services	$20–$130 per hour	No coverage unless care includes direct services billable as home health care
Adult Homes	Apartments for independent living	Fees comparable to local rents plus costs of any services provided	No coverage
Assisted Living Facilities	Custodial care in a communal residence, includes: minimal assistance with activities of daily living; some medication supervision	$1,000–$2,000	Limited coverage by Medicaid and private long-term care insurance
Continuing-Care Retirement Communities	Complete range of housing and health-care services for well elderly through those nursing	Entry fees: $38–$100,000+; Monthly fees: $650–$2,300	No coverage. Many require that you purchase long-term insurance to cover possible need for care in their nursing home
Nursing Homes	Full range of nursing, medical rehabilitative, recreational, and social activities	$15–$50,000+ per year	Limited coverage by Medicare and Medigap and long-term care insurance; full coverage by Medicaid for the indigent

Source: Reprinted by permission of Consumers Digest Inc., from *Complete Guide to Quality Long Term Health Care* by Diana Benzaia, November/December 1990.

access to health services and facilities, represents a comprehensive approach toward remedying those problems that have been plaguing our health care delivery system.

The act itself has two parts. The first part, Title XV, creates health systems agencies (HSAs), state health planning and development agencies (SAs), and statewide health coordinating councils (SHCCs) that are responsible for health planning resource development. It also establishes within the Department of Health and Human Services (previously known as the Department of Health, Education and Welfare) a National Council for Health Planning that is responsible for developing national guidelines for health planning according to the national health priorities set forth in the act. The second part of the act, Title XVI, provides federal financial assistance for facility construction and modernization.

HOUSE SELECT COMMITTEE ON AGING

The champion of the rights and needs of the elderly was the late Claude Denson Pepper, a Congressman from the great state of Florida. Congressman Pepper served as Chairman of the "House Select Committee on Aging," which was to become one of the most powerful and influential committees of the House. With the passing of time, members of the House considered it to be an honor to serve as a member of the committee. Congressman Pepper considered it his duty to represent the nation's aging population in the United States Congress, and this he did well. The committee, with 35 members, became operational in June 1975. The number soon grew to 65 members.[22]

The committee held hearings and conducted research into the problems of older Americans. Accomplishments of the committee include increased home care benefits for the aging population, a package of reform bills targeted at reducing abuses against nursing home residents, bills reforming nursing home operations, and a bill establishing Alzheimer's research and care centers.[23] The following is a summary of the Pepper Commission's 1990 recommendations on long-term care to the Congress.

> The Pepper commission's proposal would provide coverage to all Americans for home and community-based long-term care services and protection against impoverishment in nursing homes.

1. Home and community-based care
   - Severely disabled persons of all ages are eligible for social insurance for home and community-based care.
2. Nursing home care
   - The plan establishes a Nursing Home Program (NHP) for nursing home care to provide an ample floor of financial protection, ensuring that no one faces impoverishment.

  - In addition, all nursing home users are entitled to social insurance for the first three months of nursing home care. This "front-end" insurance allows people who have short stays to return home with resources intact.
3. Financing and administration
   - The federal government finances the home and community-based care program and the three-month "front-end" nursing home care.
   - The federal and state governments share financial responsibility for the NHP.
   - All three components of the plan are administered by the states according to federal guidelines.
   - States are responsible for cost containment, quality assurance, and consumer protection within federal standards.
4. Private sector role
   - Private long-term care insurance fills gaps not covered by this plan, subject to government standards and oversight.
   - The federal government encourages the development of private long-term care insurance through clarification of the tax code.
5. Phase-in
   - For both administrative and fiscal reasons, the benefits will be phased in over time.[24]

Major components of the Pepper Commission recommendations were signed into law in 1990. The enactments include new standards for long-term care insurance and Medigap policy sales.[25] Both the federal and state governments share responsibility for standards and oversight of the long-term care market. The Pepper Commission recommendations provided that:

- The federal government establishes minimum standards that private long-term care policies must meet to be eligible for the tax clarification, and establishes methods of disseminating to consumers non-biased, professional information regarding private long-term care policies.
- States regulate private long-term care insurance, using federal or stricter standards. The federal government will encourage states to strengthen civil penalties for misrepresenting policy standards, knowingly selling duplicative insurance, or marketing unapproved policies by direct mail. In addition, states should train benefits specialists regarding private long-term care insurance and the availability of state information on that insurance.[26]

Another component of the Pepper Commission report signed into law in 1990 was the creation of a new state option under Medicaid for establishing home and community care for the disabled elderly.[27] The Pepper Commission recommendations for social insurance for home and community-based care provided that

- Severely disabled individuals of all ages are eligible for this program. This includes individuals who need hands-on or supervisory assistance with three out of five ADLs (Activities of Daily Living—eating, transferring, toileting, dressing, bathing), or who are severely cognitively impaired.
- Eligibility is determined by a state or local government or a federally funded non-profit assessment agency using standardized assessment criteria. This agency conducts annual audits of case managers (described below) and monitors the quality of care.
- Case managers determine the number of hours of care and mix of services the beneficiary receives.
  —The case manager develops an individual care plan tailored to the needs of the beneficiary. The availability of informal supports is included in the decision to allocate resources.[28]
  —The case manager operates within a budget set by the federal government, and conducts periodic assessments of the beneficiary with special consideration to be given to cost containment. The case manager budget, in conjunction with other available services, will be sufficient to provide all services needed by the patient.
- The benefits include:
  —Home health care
  —Physical, occupational, speech, and other appropriate therapy services
  —Personal care services (feeding, transferring, personal hygiene)
  —Homemaker chore services (meal preparation, laundry, housework)
  —Grocery shopping and transportation
  —Medication management
  —Adult day health and social day care
  —Respite care for caregivers
  —Cost effective training of family members for delivery of home-based family care, and support counseling for family caregivers.

OMNIBUS BUDGET RECONCILIATION ACTS

OBRA 87 and OBRA 90 include federal laws that set mandatory minimum standards for nursing homes participating in the Medicare and Medicaid programs. OBRA addresses such areas as resident rights, quality of life, quality assurance, and facility practices. OBRA 87 and OBRA 90 were implemented as of October 1, 1990. They affect long-term care providers that participate in the Medicare and Medicaid programs, including about 1,200 hospitals with beds classified as skilled nursing facilities (SNFs).[29] OBRA regulations "serve as a basis for survey activities for the purpose of determining whether a facility meets the requirements for participation in Medicare and Medicaid."[30]

OBRA 87 is structured into four main sections: Resident Rights, Resident Behavior and Facility Practices, Quality of Care, and Quality of Life. Employees of nursing facilities, through in-service education, should be instructed as to their job responsibilities in implementing each section of the act.

Major Changes

The major changes affecting nursing facilities under the OBRA 87 nursing home reforms are described below.

Nurse Aide Training and Competency Evaluation Programs

The purpose of these programs is to ensure that nurse aides have the education, practical knowledge, and skills needed to care for residents of nursing facilities.[31]

The Secretary of Health and Human Services (HHS) may not refuse to enter into an agreement or cancel an existing agreement with a state to determine provider compliance on the basis that the state failed to meet OBRA requirements on competency evaluation through procedures other than passing a written examination before the effective date of regulations issued by the Secretary, if the state demonstrates to the satisfaction of the Secretary that it has made a good faith effort to meet such requirement before such effective date.[32]

Nurse Aide Registry

A nurse aide registry is required to be maintained by the various states. Information to be maintained by the registries includes a listing of all individuals who have satisfactorily completed a nurse aide training and competency evaluation program approved by the state. The registry must include specific documented findings of resident neglect or abuse or misappropriation of resident property. Individuals may file a brief statement disputing the findings. The proposed regulations provide that the registry would have 10 days to respond to a facility inquiry. A hiring decision would have to be delayed until the inquiry is completed.

Preadmission Screening and Annual Review (PASARR)

New documentation requirements have been mandated for preadmission screening and annual resident review. The Multiple Data Set (MDS) must be completed within 14 days after admission. The resident assessment involves a great deal of paper work. It includes obtaining a specific set of personal information for each resident, which has been identified as the "minimum data set." Preadmission screening requirements do not apply to nursing facility residents who are being readmitted to a facility after a hospital stay or to persons (1) who are admitted to a nursing facility directly from a hospital in which that individual has received acute inpatient care, (2) who require nursing facility services for the condition for which the individual received care in the hospital, and (3) who have been certified by an attending physician as likely to require less than 30 days of nursing facility services.[33]

Quality of Life Maintenance and Enhancement

Nursing facilities must maintain or enhance the quality of life of each resident.

Residents' Rights

Under OBRA 87, there is a comprehensive residents' bill of rights, including

- appeals of discharges and transfers
- access and visitation rights
- admissions policy guaranteeing equal access to quality care
- protection of residents' funds

The Health Care Financing Administration (HCFA) has expanded upon the statute in the regulatory requirements it has published for facility participation. The expanded requirements include

- posting of survey results
- standards regarding charges for services
- restrictions on the use of restraints and psychopharmacologic drugs

Economic Implications under OBRA

The financial implications of implementing OBRA are substantial for both the federal government and nursing facilities. For example, certification of facilities to conduct in-house training programs to satisfy state approval requirements can be very costly. Some nursing facility chains have estimated that nurse aide training cost them $100 per aide prior to OBRA. These same chains believe that, under OBRA's requirements, it could cost them as much as $1,000 per aide to provide the course and pay the aide's salary during the training period.[34] It is argued that the training requirements will create staffing shortages, inflate compliance costs, and be detrimental to resident care. Providers say that neither they nor the government have definitive answers for these concerns and that it might be years before they do.[35]

Long-term care administrators caution that these changes will only ensure high quality care for nursing facility residents if adequate reimbursement follows. Poor reimbursement will serve only to push long-term care providers into deeper fiscal difficulties.[36] The long-term care community closely watched *Wilder v. Virginia Hospital Association*, in which hospitals tested the providers' ability to sue the government for adequate reimbursement. The Supreme Court confirmed the right of a health care provider to sue holding that a provider could sue under 42 U.S.C.S. §1983 to challenge the adequacy of a state's reimbursement rates for medical services provided under the Medicaid program.[37] Although OBRA 87 instructs HCFA to ensure that states reimburse providers for the costs of implementing the law, the question of who will pay for the "which" and "how much" of the costs of implementation remains an unknown.

> The Congressional Budget Office has estimated that it will cost approximately $400 million to implement the nursing home provisions of the 1987 budget legislation. The federal portion is estimated to be approximately $240 million, which will be financed through the Medicare and Medicaid programs. The law requires that in computing rates of payment to nursing homes, HHS and state Medicaid agencies take into account the added costs of compliance.[38]

Although there are many unknowns about OBRA, physicians suspect it will hurt them economically. The new regulations will require more comprehensive medical evaluations of residents, and the perception that physician reimbursement is inadequate means that there will continue to be a shortage of physicians in long-term care.[39]

Survey Process

The survey process is the means used by the federal government to assess compliance with federal health, safety, and quality standards. The survey process centers on the "outcomes" of the care residents receive in addition to how the outcomes are achieved as the primary means to establish the compliance status of facilities. For example, if someone is attending an activity, what is the expected outcome of the activity for the resident? Further, it speaks to attitudes of personnel. How do we treat people? Do we knock when we come to their door? Do we treat them respectfully? OBRA also looks at our attitudes. Do we react or act? The idea is to act and predict concerns.

> [b](2) . . . Specifically surveyors will directly observe the actual provision of care and services to residents, and the effects of that care, to assess whether the care provided meets the needs of individual residents.
> (3) Surveyors are professionals who use their judgment, in concert with Federal forms and procedures, to determine compliance;
> (4) Federal procedures are used by all surveyors to ensure uniform and consistent application and interpretation of Federal requirements;
> (5) Federal forms are used by all surveyors to ensure proper recording of findings and to document the basis for the findings.
> (c) The State survey agency must use the survey methods, procedures, and forms that are prescribed by HCFA.[40]

The survey process reinforces and reminds employees that the resident is the focus of the facility's tasks. Jobs must be viewed as a mechanism for enacting each resident's ability to function at his or her highest potential. With OBRA, now more than ever, the facility within which a resident resides must be seen as the resident's home. The environment should be an integral part of our change in attitude. How a resident functions and interacts in a long-term care setting is an important aspect of OBRA, taking into consideration what the resident was like prior to admission. A resident is not merely a recipient of care, but will be the mechanism for monitoring the delivery of care to residents.

The purpose of the survey process is to assess whether the quality of care, as intended by the law and regulations, and as needed by the resident, is actually being provided. The goal of OBRA is to to assist residents in maintaining their independence and dignity by giving them control over the way they spend their days in the facility (e.g., providing choices) and by encouraging them to stay in touch with their outside world (e.g., family, friends, and outside interests). Although on-site review procedures have been changed, facilities must continue to meet all applicable conditions and standards in order to participate in Medicare/ Medicaid programs. The methods utilized to compile information regarding compliance with law and regulations are changed; the law and regulations themselves are not changed. Surveyors will confirm, through interviews with residents and staff, that resident needs are indeed met on a regular basis. In most reviews, surveyors will ascertain whether the facility is actually providing the required and needed care and services, rather than whether or not the facility is capable of providing the care and services.

Survey Elements

An SNF survey must include the following elements:

1. an entrance conference
2. a resident-centered tour of the facility
3. an in-depth review of a sample of residents, including observation, interview and record review
4. observation of the preparation and administration of drugs for a sample of residents
5. evaluation of a facility's meals, dining areas and eating assistance procedures
6. a description in the survey report of all deficiencies found during the survey
7. an exit conference
8. follow-up surveys, as appropriate.[41]

Resident Council

Each nursing facility must have a resident council. The surveyors may meet with the council to ascertain strengths and/or problems, if any, from the consumer's perspective. The meeting is conducted in a manner that allows for comments about any aspect of the facility. Staff members do not attend unless they are specifically invited by council members. A sampling of questions that surveyors might ask the council includes

- What is best about this home?
- What is worst?
- What would you like to change?

In order to get more detail, surveyors might use questions such as

- Can you be more specific?
- Can you give me an example?
- What can anyone else tell me about this?

If surveyors wish to obtain information about a topic not raised by the residents, they might use an approach such as

- Tell me what you think about the food/staff/cleanliness here.
- What would make it better?
- What don't you like?
- What do you like?[42]

A sampling of questions that surveyors might ask residents with regard to their medical condition and treatment include

- Has your doctor discussed your health with you? How is it, what's wrong, and what you can expect in the future?
- Have you had the opportunity to help plan what you need and how you are taken care of?
- Do you know that you can refuse treatment or medication?
- Have you ever refused medication or treatment? What happened when you did?[43]

Required Documents and Reports

The following is a sampling of documents and reports that must be available to surveyors at the time of the survey.

- resident medical records
- incident reports
- infection control records
- resident assessment and care plans
- disaster drill documentation
- departmental policy and procedure manuals, safety manuals, etc.

Facility Tour/Resident Needs

The surveyors will conduct a tour of the nursing facility in order to: (1) develop an overall picture of the types and patterns of care delivery present within the facility; (2) view the physical environment; and (3) ascertain whether randomly selected residents are communicative and willing to be interviewed. While touring a nursing facility, the surveyors will focus on the residents' needs (e.g., physical, emotional, psychosocial, and spiritual) and whether they are being met. Specific areas of observation will include

- personal hygiene, grooming and appropriate dress
- position
- assistive and other restorative devices
- rehabilitation issues
- functional limitations in activities of daily living (ADL)
- hydration and nutritional status
- resident rights
- activity for time of day (appropriate or inappropriate)
- emotional status
- level of orientation
- awareness of surroundings
- behaviors
- cleanliness of immediate environment (wheelchair, bed, bedside table, etc.)
- odors
- adequate clothing and care supplies, as well as maintenance and cleanliness of same.[44]

Environmental Assessment

Environmental assessment will include the monitoring of facility temperature, humidity, air circulation, and odors. Space requirements will be reviewed to determine adequacy of environment (e.g., dining and recreational facilities).

Disclosure of Survey Results

Survey and certification information is to be made available to the public within 14 calendar days after this information is made available to the facilities.

Correcting Deficiencies

Nursing facilities must closely monitor the survey process and be sure to correct any deficiencies or violations found. Repeated violations can result in stiff penalties, including the loss of licensure. Nursing facilities should

- challenge those violations with which they disagree[45]

- take prompt action to correct any and all citations[46]
- maintain clear and accurate records of all remedial actions taken to correct any deficiency that might affect a resident's health or safety
- accurately record all dates, times, and actions taken, by which individuals, to correct violations
- document any new incidents that might occur following correction of a previously cited deficiency
- carefully document any incidents that occur that result in harm or have the potential to result in harm to a resident

LONGEVITY AND QUALITY LIVING

The diseases that impair, disable, and handicap Americans today are not the same as they were 50 years ago. This is an age of transition, in which even people at 100 years of age and older can live longer, healthier, and happier lives with minds that are alert and continue to thirst for knowledge. Health impairment among adults in the United States is substantially attributable to risk factors, such as poor nutritional habits, use of cigarettes, drug and alcohol abuse, lack of exercise, failure to take control of stressful situations, and social deprivation. These risk factors are primarily attributable to learned, socially reinforced behavior, to lifestyles rather than "biology."

> Changes in lifestyle habits, not a massive infusion of federal dollars, is the surest way to improve the overall health status of Americans yet save money, according to one of Bush's top domestic policy advisors.
>
> "The greatest opportunities to become a healthier nation lie outside the health care system," said Roger B. Porter, assistant to the president for economic and domestic policy.[47]

A committee of the Institute of Medicine, in a report entitled "The Second Fifty Years: Promoting Health and Preventing Disability," has concluded that a great deal more could be done to promote health and prevent disease in the elderly.[48] Specific recommendations of the committee include the following:

- Medicare and other insurance should pay for blood pressure screening, and ways should be found for detection and treatment of high blood pressure in older people who have limited access to health care.
- Research on understanding sensory impairment, its effects, and the effectiveness of services or devices that help prevent disability due to sensory impairment should be priority.
- Physicians should periodically review all drugs taken by their older patients and older people themselves should be alert to dangers of multiple medication.

* * *

- Health care professionals should access the diet and nutritional status of elderly patients, and, since there are more of the very old living alone at home, there should be better services for delivering meals in a group setting.[49]

A twelve-year study was conducted of the elderly in Manitoba, Canada, assessing the determinants of successful aging. The study found that a significant group of the elderly do age successfully. Those who aged successfully were shown to have greater satisfaction with life and made fewer demands on the health care system than those who aged less well. Of the predictors for successful living, not having one's spouse die or enter a nursing home was shown to be an important factor to successful aging.[50] "Individuals at particular risk of not aging successfully include those with poor self-assessed health, whose spouse has died, whose mental status is somewhat compromised, who developed cancer, and those who are forced to retire or retire because of poor health."[51]

When it becomes necessary to admit an individual to a nursing facility, every effort should be made to provide an environment that is conducive to the well-being of the resident. In light of this study and others, improving the lifestyle for the aging population must be an ongoing process. Efforts to improve the quality of life in nursing facilities involve

- providing a common room in those instances where both spouses are residents of a nursing facility
- protecting vulnerable adults from improper limitations of medical treatments in institutions
- financial planning for nursing facility care
- finding alternatives to institutional care
- protecting residents from abusive persons
- implementing patient rights
- establishing and enforcing safety standards
- providing and implementing a long-term care ombudsman program
- controlling costs
- offering education and training
- supporting research
- improving the image of nursing facilities

The practical side of quality aging includes, when and where possible, implementation of the following improvements in each resident's lifestyle:

- placing greater importance on each resident's health and provide for continuity and regulation in

—diet
—work
—social activities, play, leisure
—physical exercise

- assisting the resident in developing realistic life goals, regardless of age
- improving the resident's self-confidence and self-image, to add quality years to his or her life
- reducing stress-causing activities and replacing them with the things the resident enjoys
- assisting the resident in arranging for "get away" time with family and/or friends
- providing opportunities for mixing with a variety of age groups
- encouraging and assisting the resident in pursuing childhood hobbies
- adopting a pet program
- helping the resident to get involved in
  —continuing education
  —theater
  —art
- helping the resident to keep in touch and get involved in community and national politics by
  —exercising the right to vote
  —attending political meetings and presenting his or her point of view (if resident can't go, have someone represent the resident)
  —attending, for example, a specially arranged town board meeting in the facility
  —having his or her voice heard (through, e.g., petitions, letter writing, and phone calls) on an issue in which the resident has a particular interest (e.g., environmental pollution)
- helping the resident develop a circle of friends
- helping the resident become a positive thinker
- providing the opportunity for the residents to worship and attend a religious service

CONCLUSION

The acute care needs of the nation's population must be properly balanced with the nation's long-term care needs. As the aging population increases, so must the efforts to improve the quality of life for the elderly.

Caregivers are also aging along with the general population and they too will be tomorrow's elderly citizens. The average staff nurse is already 40 and will be 45 in the year 2000.[52]

With all of the many advances in health care, much more emphasis must be placed on prevention.

> Until very recently, prevention efforts in the US were focused on the young. People older than 60 were excluded from most prevention trials . . . .
>
> * * *
>
> Delaying the onset of dependency and disability is essential for improving the older person's quality of life. It is also essential for the nation as a whole. Unless we reduce dependency among older people, there will be more people needing care and fewer individuals to provide it.[53]

The Robert Wood Johnson Foundation is right on target with its "New Goals" for the nineties which are to assure that Americans of all ages have access to basic health care, to improve the way services are organized and provided to people with chronic health conditions, and to promote health and prevent disease by reducing harm caused by substance abuse.[54]

NOTES

1. U.S. DEPARTMENT OF HEALTH AND HUMAN SERVICES, PUBLIC HEALTH SERVICE, NATIONAL INSTITUTES OF HEALTH, OLDER & WISER 43, September 1989.

2. D.J. BOGUEL,THE POPULATION OF THE UNITED STATES 18 (1985).

3. GUIDE TO 1980 U.S. DECENNIAL CENSUS PUBLICATIONS: ABSTRACTS V. (1986).

4. U.S. DEPARTMENT OF COMMERCE, BUREAU OF THE CENSUS, AMERICA IN TRANSITION: AN AGING SOCIETY 3 (1983).

5. AMERICAN ASSOCIATION OF RETIRED PERSONS, A PROFILE OF OLDER AMERICANS—1990, at 1 (1990).

6. U.S. DEPARTMENT OF COMMERCE, BUREAU OF THE CENSUS (1990).

7. NATIONAL CENTER FOR HEALTH STATISTICS, HEALTH, UNITED STATES 1989, 23 (1990).

8. R.C. Firstman, *Dr. Arthur Feinberg, Old and Sick Are His Concern*, THE NEWSDAY MAGAZINE 26, (January 13, 1991).

9. Baby boomers are the approximately 75 million Americans born between 1946 and 1964. *Health Care's Changing Face: The Demographics of the 21st Century*, 65, HOSPITALS, April 5, 1991, at 36.

10. AMERICA IN TRANSITION: AN AGING SOCIETY, *supra* note 4, at 3.

11. A PROFILE OF OLDER AMERICANS, *supra* note 5, at 1, 2.

12. P. Willging, *Policy Perspective, The Financing of Long Term Care*, 16, PROVIDER 10 (May 1990).

13. Reprinted from Hospitals, Vol. 64. No. 21, by permission, November 5, 1990, Copyright ©1990, American Hospital Publishing Inc., at 34.

14. *Skilled-Nursing Services in Hospitals vs. Freestanding Facilities: There's a Difference*, 27(21) AHA News, May 27, 1991, at 6.

15. 42 C.F.R. §483.1 (1990).

16. P. Kemper & C.M. Murtaugh, *Lifetime Use of Nursing Home Care,* 324, NEW ENGLAND J. MEDICINE, 595–600 (1991).

17. J.M. HAMME, *Case Law Update*, LONG TERM CARE AND THE LAW, TENTH ANNUAL SYMPOSIUM 3 (1986).

18. NATIONAL CENTER FOR HEALTH STATISTICS, *Health, supra* note 7.

19. *Health Care Utilization Among Elderly is High: HHS Study*, 27(23) AHA News, June 10, 1991, at 6.

20. 53 A.L.R. 4TH 689, at 782 (1987).

21. NATIONAL CENTER FOR HEALTH STATISTICS, *supra* note 7, at 24.

22. C.L. PEPPER & H. GOREY, EYEWITNESS TO A CENTURY, 261–262 (1987).

23. *Id.* at 262–265.

24. RECOMMENDATIONS TO THE CONGRESS BY THE U.S. BIPARTISAN COMMISSION ON COMPREHENSIVE CARE, ACCESS TO HEALTH CARE AND LONG-TERM CARE FOR ALL AMERICANS 3 (March 2, 1990) (hereinafter THE PEPPER COMMISSION).

25. M. BURKE, *Congressional Leaders Outline Their Health Agendas: Sen. Jay Rockefeller*, 65 HOSPITALS, January 5, 1991, at 26.

26. THE PEPPER COMMISSION, *supra* note 24, at 16.

27. Burke, *supra* note 25, at 26.

28. THE PEPPER COMMISSION, *supra* note 24, at 13.

29. *Effectiveness of 1990 Long-Term Care Reforms Questioned*, 26(50) AHA News, December 24, 1990, at 4.

30. 42 C.F.R. §483.1 (1990).

31. 55 Fed. Reg. 10,938 (1990).

32. Key Medicare and Medicaid Legislation: 1990, OBRA 1990, Special Member Briefing, Chicago: American Hospital Association, January 1991, at 19.

33. *Id.* at 159.

34. L. DUNCAN, *OBRA, Data Rules Force Chain to Switch Gears*, MODERN HEALTHCARE'S ELDERCARE BUSINESS, November 12, 1990, at 14.

35. *Implementing OBRA: LTC Providers Fear Poor Reimbursement*, HOSPITALS, August 20, 1990 at 54, 56.

36. *Id.* at 56.

37. *Wilder v. Virginia Hospital Association*, 110 L. Ed. 2d 455, 110 S. Ct. 2510 (1990).

38. H. G. Collier, *Legal Issues in Long Term Care*, 1989 HEALTH LAW HANDBOOK 60, (Ed. A.G. Gosfield) (1989).

39. S.J. D'Amico, *Don't Neglect Physician Relations Now*, MODERN HEALTHCARE'S ELDERCARE BUSINESS, November 12, 1990, at 16.

40. 42 C.F.R. §488.26 (1990).

41. 42 C.F.R. §488.26 (1990).

42. 42 CFR §488.110 (1990).

43. 42 CFR §488.115 (1989).

44. 42 CFR §488.110 (1990).

45. *Recertification Attained Through Aggressive Challenge*, 16(6) PROVIDER FOR LONG TERM CARE PROFESSIONALS, June 1990, at 28–29.

46. *Serving Cold Mashed Potatoes Could Lead to Indictments*, 15(10) PROVIDER FOR LONG TERM CARE PROFESSIONALS, October 1989, at 53–54.

47. *Lifestyle Habits Impede Health Care Progress: Policy Adviser to Bush*, 27(5) AHA News, February 4, 1991, at 2.

48. *Much More Health Promotion Could Be Done for Elderly: Report*, XXI(1) THE NATION'S HEALTH, January 1991, at 5.

49. *Id.*

50. N.P. Roos & B. Havens, *Predictors of Successful Aging: A Twelve Year Study of Manitoba Elderly*, 81 AMERICAN J. PUBLIC HEALTH 63–68 (1991).

51. *Id.* at 67.

52. *Health Care's Changing Face: The Demographics of the 21st Century, supra* note 9 at 36.

53. *Older Americans Present a Double Challenge: Preventing Disability and Providing Care*, 81 AMERICAN J. PUBLIC HEALTH, 287 (1991).

54. *Foundation Announces New Goals for Nineties*, IV(1) ADVANCES, THE ROBERT WOOD JOHNSON FOUNDATION, Spring 1991, at 1

Chapter 6

Liability of Long-Term Care Facilities

The typical nursing facility is incorporated under state law as a free-standing for-profit or not-for-profit corporation. The corporation has a governing body, which is generally referred to as a board of directors, or board of trustees. The governing body has ultimate responsibility for the operation and management of the facility with a necessary delegation of appropriate responsibility to administrative employees and the medical staff.

Under federal regulations, OBRA requires that nursing facilities have a governing board or designated persons functioning as a governing body that is legally responsible for establishing and implementing policies regarding the management and operation of the facility. The governing body is responsible for the appointment of an administrator who is licensed by the state. The administrator is responsible for the day-to-day management of the facility.[1]

Not-for-profit nursing facilities are usually exempt from federal taxation under Section 501(c)(3) of the Internal Revenue Code of 1986, as amended. Such federal exemption usually entitles the organization to an automatic exemption from state taxes as well. Such tax exemption not only relieves the nursing facility from the payment of income taxes, sales taxes, and the like, but also permits the nursing facility to receive contributions from donors who then may obtain charitable deductions on their personal tax returns.

Although long-term care facilities may operate as sole proprietorships or partnerships, most function as corporations. Thus, an important source of law applicable to governing boards and to the duties and responsibilities of their members is found in state corporation laws. An incorporated long-term care facility is a legal person with recognized rights, duties, powers, and responsibilities. Because the legal "person" is in reality a "fictitious person," there is a requirement that certain humans be designated to exercise the corporate powers and that they be held accountable for corporate decision-making. These natural persons comprise the governing board. In an unincorporated facility, the powers and duties are held by one or more natural persons. There is no recognized fictitious person. This chapter discusses some of the major responsibilities as well as legal risks of long-term care facilities and their boards.

AUTHORITY OF LONG-TERM CARE CORPORATIONS

The governing board is organized to oversee and control all the activities of the corporation. It is therefore essential that the governing board have an appropriate degree of authority. In this way there will be a rational and practical transition from formulating policy to implementing practice and procedure. Authority is conferred by corporation laws, regulations, and corporate charters.

Long-term care corporations—governmental, charitable, or proprietary—have certain powers expressly or implicitly granted to them by state statutes. Generally, the authority of a corporation is expressed in the law under which the corporation is chartered and in the corporation's articles of incorporation. The existence of this authority creates certain duties and liabilities for governing boards and their individual members. Members of the board of directors of a facility have both express and implied corporate authority.

OBRA requirements provide that the governing board is responsible for assuring that the facility has an overall plan that includes an annual operating budget and a capital expenditures plan that covers a three-year period. The plan must be submitted to the state and updated on an annual basis. The plan must be prepared under the direction of the governing body of the institution by a committee consisting of representatives of the governing body, the administration, and the medical staff.[2]

State nursing home codes generally provide that a nursing facility have a governing body that is legally responsible for establishing and implementing policies regarding the management and operation of the facility. The general responsibilities of a nursing facility include: (1) policy formation; (2) oversight of the management and operation of the facility; (3) assurance of the financial viability of the facility; (4) appointment of a qualified administrator; (5) provision of a safe physical plant equipped and staffed to maintain facility and services in accordance with any applicable local and state regulations that may apply to federal programs in which the facility participates; (6) adoption of written policies assuring the protection of residents' rights and resident grievance procedures; (7) determination of the frequency of meetings of the governing body and documentation of such meetings; and (8) adoption of a written policy concerning potential conflict of interest on the part of members of the governing body, the administration, the medical and nursing staff, and other employees who might influence corporate decisions.

Express Corporate Authority

Express corporate authority is the authority that is specifically delegated by statute. A long-term care corporation derives its authority to act from the laws of the state in which it is incorporated. The articles of incorporation set forth the purpose(s) of the corporation's existence and the powers the corporation is authorized to exercise in order to carry out its purposes.

Implied Corporate Authority

Implied corporate authority is the authority to perform any and all acts necessary to exercise a corporation's expressly conferred authority and to accomplish the purpose(s) for which it was created. Much of the litigation concerning excesses of corporate authority involve questions of whether a corporation has the implied authority, incidental to its express authority, to perform a questioned act.

Generally, implied corporate authority arises from situations where such authority is required or suggested as a result of a need for corporate powers not specifically granted in the articles of incorporation. A board of directors, at its own discretion, may establish new bylaws, rules, and regulations; purchase or mortgage property; borrow money; purchase equipment; select personnel; adopt corporate resolutions that delineate decision making responsibilities; etc. These powers can be enumerated in the articles of incorporation and, as such, would be categorized as express rather than implied corporate authority.

Ultra Vires Acts

A board can be held liable for acting beyond its scope of authority, which is either expressed (e.g., in its articles of incorporation) or implied in law. Acts of this nature are referred to as ultra vires acts. The governing body acts in and on behalf of the corporation. If any action is in violation of a statute or regulation, it is illegal. An example of an illegal act would be the employment of an unlicensed person in a position which by law requires a license. The state, through its attorney general, has the power to prevent the performance of an ultra vires act by injunction. Governing boards should have their corporate charters periodically reviewed by legal counsel to make certain that their express powers are consistent with the activities in which they presently engage or plan to undertake in the future.

Members of an institution's governing board, as well as its corporate officers, may in certain circumstances be individually responsible for ultra vires acts. This might be true, for example, if a member of a governing board or corporate officer exceeded the powers of the corporation for individual benefit.

DOCTRINE OF RESPONDEAT SUPERIOR

Respondeat superior ("let the master respond") is the legal doctrine holding employers liable, in certain cases, for the wrongful acts of their employees. This doctrine has also been referred to as vicarious liability whereby an employer is answerable for the torts committed by employees. In the health care setting, a nursing facility is liable for the negligent acts of its employees, even though there has been no wrongful conduct on the part of the facility. In order for liability to be imputed to the employer: (1) a master–servant relationship must exist between the employer and the employee and (2) the wrongful act of the employee must have occurred within the scope of his or her employment. The question of liability frequently rests on whether or not persons treating a resident are independent agents (responsible for their own acts) or employees of the facility. The answer to this depends on whether or not the facility can exercise control over the particular act that was the proximate cause of the injury.

The basic rationale for imposing liability upon an employer developed from the fact that the employer possesses the right to control the physical acts of its employees. It is not necessary that the employer actually exercise control, but only that it possesses the right, power, or authority to do so.

Generally, the plaintiff's attorney will file suit against both employer and employee. This is done out of practical considerations, since the employer is generally in a better financial condition and also very likely will have insurance to cover the judgment.

The employer is not without remedy if liability has been imposed against it under respondeat superior for an employee's negligent act. Since the law holds negligent persons responsible for their negligent acts, employees are not absolved from liability when a health care facility is held liable through the application of respondeat superior. Not only may the injured party sue the employee directly, but also the employer, if sued, may seek indemnification—that is, compensation for the financial loss occasioned by the employee's act—from the employee.

The plaintiff has the burden for establishing an employee–employer relationship. This can be difficult in long-term care facilities, especially in the case of independent physicians.

In the instance of wrongful conduct by an independent contractor, the doctrine of respondeat superior does not apply. An independent contractor relationship is established when the principal has no right of control over the manner in which the agent's work is to be performed. The independent contractor is generally responsible for his or her own negligent acts.

The doctrine of respondeat superior may impose liability on a health care facility for a nurse's acts or omissions that result in injury to the resident. Whether such liability attaches depends on whether the conduct of the nurse was wrongful and whether the nurse was subject to the control of the facility at the time the act in question was performed. Determination of whether the nurse's conduct was wrongful in a given situation depends on the standard of conduct to which the nurse is expected to adhere. In liability deliberations, the nurse who is subject to the control of the facility at the time of the negligent conduct is considered an employee and is not the borrowed servant of a staff physician or surgeon.

An officer or director of a corporation is not, merely as a result of his or her position, personally liable for the torts of corporate employees. To incur liability, the director or officer ordinarily must be shown to have in some way participated in or directed the tortious act.

DUTIES OF LONG-TERM CARE CORPORATIONS

Along with the corporate authority that is granted to the governing board, duties are attached to its individual members. These responsibilities we call duties because they are imposed by law and they can be enforced in legal proceedings. Membership on a governing board should not be considered merely a recognition of social or community standing or financial well-being. Governing board members are considered by law to have the highest measure of accountability. They have a fiduciary duty that requires acting primarily for the benefit of the corporation. The general duties of a governing board are both implied and express. Failure of a board to function may constitute mismanagement of such a degree that the appointment of a receiver to manage the affairs of the corporation may be warranted.

Administration

Federal regulations under OBRA specify that a facility must be administered in a manner that enables it to use its resources effectively and efficiently to attain or maintain the highest practicable physical, mental, and psychosocial well-being of each resident. The facility must be licensed in accordance with state law and provide services in compliance with all federal, state, and local laws, regulations, and codes.[3]

Duty To Comply with Statutes, Rules, and Regulations

The governing board in general and its agents (assigned representatives) in particular are responsible for compliance with federal, state, and local rules and regulations regarding the operation of the long-term care facility. Depending on the scope of the wrong committed and the intent of the board, failure to comply could subject the board members and/or their agents to civil liability and even, in rare instances, to criminal prosecution.

A board is required to comply with the statutes, rules, and regulations governing its facility's operations. The nursing facility in *Moon Lake Convalescent Center v. Margolis*, 535 N.E.2d 956 (Ill. App. Ct. 1989), was found to have violated the state's Minimum Standards, Rules and Regulations for the Licensure of Skilled Nursing Facilities and Intermediate Care Facilities (1980) Rule 03.01.01.00, by failing to provide an adequate means for employees to follow its policy of preventing accidents by ensuring that water temperatures did not exceed 100 degrees. The facility also violated Rule 03.01.01.00 by leaving a resident unattended in his bath in violation of written policy. The resident received severe burns over 40 percent of his body and expired of complications. The facility lost its license for violating state regulations, as well as its own policy and procedures.

Failure of nursing facilities to comply with applicable statutory regulations can be costly. This was the case in *People v. Casa Blanca Convalescent Homes, Inc.*, 206 Cal. Rptr. 164 (1984), where there was evidence of numerous and prolonged deficiencies in resident care. The nursing home's practice of providing insufficient personnel constituted not only illegal practice, but also unfair business practice in violation of Business and Professions Code Section 17200. The trial court was found to have properly assessed a fine of $2,500 for each of 67 violations, totaling $167,500, where the evidence showed that the operator of the nursing home had the financial ability to pay that amount.

Duties Specified by Corporate Law

A corporation has certain duties that are specified by the state's corporation laws. These include

- duty to hold meetings
- duty to establish policy
- financial duties
- provide adequate insurance
- duty to pay taxes

The general duty to use due care in the management of the property and assets of the facility and the specific duty to manage its financial aspects includes maintenance of the physical plant and appropriating funds for such purpose as necessary. The governing board has a duty to protect the facility from the risk of loss because of fire, other destruction or liability for the negligence of its employees. The governing board has a duty to pay all taxes that become due upon any property, so that no penalties are incurred.

Duty To Appoint an Administrator

Members of the governing board are responsible for appointing a licensed administrator to act as their agent in the management of the facility. The administrator is responsible for the day-to-day operations of the facility. Federal law requires that nursing facility administrators be appropriately licensed.

> *Section 431.702 State Plan Requirement*
>
> A state plan must provide that the state has a program for licensing administrators of nursing homes that meets the requirements of Section 431.703 through 431.713 of this subpart.

Section 431.703 Licensing Requirement

The state licensing program must provide that only nursing homes supervised by an administrator licensed in accordance with the requirement of this subpart may operate in the state.

Section 431.713 Continuing Study and Investigation

The agency or board must conduct a continuing study of nursing homes and administrators within the State to improve: (1) licensing standards; and (2) the procedures and methods for enforcing the standards.[4]

In order to comply with federal requirements, the various states have incorporated licensing requirements in their regulations. Administrators are licensed under the laws of their individual states. Minimum qualifications for administrators are contained in licensing statutes as well as in the rules and regulations promulgated under them. Statutes generally provide that the administrator of a facility be licensed in accordance with state law.

A $5,000 fine was imposed on a home for operating a nursing facility without a licensed administrator for 54 days in *Magnolias Nursing and Convalescent Center v. Department of Health and Rehabilitation Services*, 438 So. 2d 412 (Fla. Dist. Ct. App. 1983). The statute prohibiting operation of a nursing home without a licensed administrator was not considered vague or ambiguous, nor unconstitutional.

Where minimum qualifications exist, the governing board must at least satisfy these requirements in the appointment of an administrator. If the circumstances of a particular facility necessitate employing an administrator of a higher level of qualification and competency, the governing board, at its discretion, may select an administrator that meets that need.

The responsibilities and authority of the administrator should be expressed in an appropriate job description, as well as in any formal agreement or contract that the facility has with the administrator. State health codes and licensing boards describe the responsibilities of administrators in broad terms. They generally provide that the administrator shall be responsible for: (1) the overall management of the facility; (2) the enforcement of any applicable federal, state, and local regulations, as well as the facility's bylaws, policies, and procedures; (3) the appointment of, with the approval of the governing body, a qualified medical director; (4) liaison between the governing body and the medical and facility staff; and (5) the appointment of an administrative person to act during the administrator's absence from the facility.

States requiring administrators to be licensed provide penalties ranging from fine to imprisonment for those administrators functioning without a license. Reciprocity, the granting of a license to one previously licensed by another state in recognition that both states impose essentially the same requirements, is found in all nursing home administrator licensing laws.

The failure to remove an incompetent administrator or any other incapable agent of a long-term care facility is as much a breach of a board's duty as is its failure to appoint competent employees. Termination of an administrator due to incompetence must be in accordance with facility bylaws, which should set forth the administrator's due process rights. These rights should be included in an appropriately written contract for the administrator.

The general duty of a governing board is to exercise due care and diligence in supervising and managing the facility. This duty does not cease upon the selection of a competent administrator. A governing board can be liable if the level of resident care becomes inadequate because of the board's failure to properly supervise the administrator's management of a facility.

In some facilities, the administrator fills a dual role by serving as a member of the governing board in addition to his position as the facility's chief executive officer. When the administrator is a board member, he frequently serves in the capacity as secretary of the board. If the administrator is a non-voting member, his position on the board is for the most part honorary.

Duty To Supervise and Manage

The duty to supervise and manage is as applicable to the trustees of a facility as it is to the managers of any other business corporation. In both instances there is a duty to act as a reasonably prudent person would act under similar circumstances. The facility board must act prudently in administering the affairs of the facility and exercise its powers in good faith.

The basic management functions of the governing board include

- selection of corporate officers and agents
- general control over the compensation of such agents
- delegation of authority to the CEO/administrator and the administrator's subordinates for administrative actions
- selection and monitoring of the medical staff members and the delineation of clinical privileges
- establishment of institutional goals, policies, and procedures
- supervision and vigilance over the welfare and assets of the corporation

Specific management duties peculiar to nursing facilities include determining the policies of the facility in connection with community health needs, maintaining proper professional standards in the facility, assuming a general responsibility for adequate resident care throughout the facility, and providing adequate financing of resident care, and assuming businesslike control of expenditures.

Duty To Provide Propitious Treatment

Nursing facilities can be held liable for delays in treatment if a resident suffers injury because of the delay.

Duty To Avoid Self-Dealing/Conflict of Interest Situations

There should be full disclosure of each board member's dealings with the facility. Transactions between a board member and a facility must be just and reasonable. Board members must refrain from self-dealing and avoid conflict-of-interest situations. Membership on the board or its committees should not be used for private gain. Board members are expected to disclose potential conflict-of-interest situations and withdraw from the board room at the time of voting. Board members who suspect a conflict-of-interest situation have a right and a duty to raise pertinent questions regarding any potential conflict. Conflict of interest is presumed to exist when a board member or a firm with which he or she is associated may benefit or lose from the passage of a proposed action.

Membership on the board of a facility is deemed a public service. Neither the court nor the community expects or desires such public service to be turned to private profit. Thus, the standards imposed on board members regarding the investment of trust funds, self-dealing transactions, or personal compensation may be stricter than are those for directors of business corporations. The essential rules regarding self-dealing are clear. Generally, a contract between a facility and a trustee financially interested in the transaction is voidable by the facility in the event that the interested trustee spoke or voted in favor of the arrangement or did not fully disclose the material facts regarding his or her interest. This resolution of the self-dealing problem is based on the belief that if an interested board member does not participate in the board's action and does make full disclosure of his or her interest, the disinterested remaining members of the board are able to protect the facility's interests. If the fairness of the transaction is questioned, the burden of establishing fairness falls on the trustee involved.

Underlying the controversy of self-dealing is the knowledge that sometimes the most advantageous contract for the facility would be with one of its trustees or with a company in which the director is interested. These considerations are of great importance when dealings between a charitable corporation and a member of the board are involved. A rule denying this opportunity to the corporation would be too severe. However, statutory provisions in some states specifically forbid self-dealing transactions altogether, irrespective of disclosure or the fairness of the deal.

Under Sections 1877(b) and 1909(b) of the Social Security Act, it is considered a felony for anyone to knowingly and willfully offer, pay, solicit, or receive any payment in return for referring an individual to another for the furnishing, or the arranging for the furnishing, of any item or service that may be paid for by the Medicare or Medicaid programs. Persons convicted under these provisions are subject to fines of up to $25,000 and/or imprisonment of up to five years. The inspector general of the U.S. Department of Health and Human Services has identified the following arrangements as examples of potential violations of the Social Security Act:

- payment of a "finder's fee" to respiratory therapists, physical therapists, or other therapists working in a facility for referring patients to durable medical equipment suppliers who supply oxygen equipment, wheelchairs, or other equipment or supplies to patients
- payment to social workers or discharge planners by home health agencies for referring patients in need of home health services once they are discharged from a facility

Duty To Provide Adequate Facilities and Equipment

A nursing facility is under a duty to exercise reasonable care to furnish adequate equipment, appliances, and supplies for use in the diagnosis or treatment of residents. "The facility must be designed, constructed, equipped and maintained to protect the health and safety of residents, personnel and the public."[5] The general rule seems to be that the facility's equipment should be fit for the purposes and uses intended. The regulations state

> (h) Level B requirement: Environment.
>
> The facility must provide—
>
> (1) A safe, clean, comfortable and homelike environment, allowing the resident to use his or her personal belongings to the extent possible;
> (2) Housekeeping and maintenance services to maintain a sanitary, orderly and comfortable interior;
> (3) Clean bed and bath linens that are in good condition;
> (4) Private closet space in each resident room . . .;
> (5) Adequate and comfortable lighting levels in all areas;
> (6) Comfortable and safe temperature levels. Facilities initially certified after August 1, 1989, must maintain a temperature range of 71–81 (degree) F; and
> (7) For the maintenance of comfortable sound levels.[6]

Within its duty to provide adequate facilities and equipment, the board must exercise reasonable care and skill in supervising and managing facility property. This obligation includes protecting property from destruction and loss.

The nursing facility should be designed, constructed, equipped, and maintained to provide a safe, healthy, functional, sanitary, and comfortable environment for residents, personnel, and the public. Buildings and equipment should be maintained and operated so as to prevent fire and other hazards to personal safety. Fires should be promptly investigated and a written report of the investigation containing all pertinent information regarding the fire should be maintained on file.

Resident rooms should be designed and equipped for adequate nursing care, comfort, and privacy for residents. Mechanical, electrical, and resident care equipment should be maintained in a safe operating condition.

The nursing facility, Driftwood Convalescent Hospital, operated by Western Medical Enterprises, Inc., in *Beach v. Western Medical Enterprises, Inc.*, 171 Cal. Rptr. 846 (Cal. Ct. App. 1981), was fined $2,500 in civil penalties because of nonfunctioning hallway lights and the facility's failure to provide the required type and amount of decubitus preventive equipment necessary for resident care as required by Health and Safety Code regulations. The regulations require that equipment "necessary for care to patients, as ordered or indicated" be provided.

> Though no evidence was introduced to show that the decubitus equipment had been ordered by a physician, the phrase "as indicated" supports an inference that when a patient's condition requires certain equipment, the fact that no physician has ordered that equipment does not relieve the hospital (nursing facility) of the responsibility for providing equipment necessary for patient care.

Id. at 852.

Duty To Provide Adequate Insurance

One basic protection for tangible property is adequate insurance against fire and other risks. This duty extends to keeping the physical plant of the nursing facility in good repair and appropriating funds for such purpose when necessary.

The duty of a board is to purchase insurance against various risks. Nursing facilities face as much risk of losing their tangible and intangible assets through judgments for negligence as they do through fires or other disasters. Where this is true, the duty to insure against the risks of negligence is as great as the duty to insure against fire, and the amount of insurance must be adequate for the circumstances.

Duty To Provide Satisfactory Resident Care

The most important aspect of a governing board's duty to operate a nursing facility with due care and diligence is its responsibility to provide satisfactory resident care. It is only through the fulfillment of this duty that the basic purpose of the facility will be accomplished; this duty includes the maintenance of a satisfactory standard of medical care through supervision of the medical, nursing, and ancillary staffs. At the option of the state, the resident's health care can be provided under the supervision of a nurse practitioner, clinical nurse specialist, or physician's assistant who is not an employee of the facility, but who is working in collaboration with a physician. This provision is effective October 1, 1990, regardless of whether final regulations have been promulgated.[7]

Inadequate Care and Treatment

The estate of a nursing home resident, who had expired as the result of multiple infected bedsores, brought a malpractice action against the nursing home in *Montgomery Health Care Facility v. Ballard*, 565 So. 2d 221 (Ala. 1990). First American Health Care, Inc. is the parent corporation of the Montgomery Health Care Facility, a nursing home. The trial court entered a judgment on a jury verdict against the home, and an appeal was taken. The Alabama Supreme Court held that reports compiled by the Alabama Department of Public Health concerning deficiencies found in the nursing home were admissible as evidence. Evidence showed that the care given to the deceased was deficient in the same ways as noted in the survey and complaint reports, which indicated that deficiencies in the home included

> inadequate documentation of treatment given for decubitus ulcers; 23 patients found with decubitus ulcers, 10 of whom developed those ulcers in the facility; dressings on the sores were not changed as ordered; nursing progress note did not describe patients' ongoing conditions, particularly with respect to descriptions of decubitus ulcers; ineffective policies and procedures with respect to sterile dressing supplies; lack of nursing assessments; incomplete patient care plans; inadequate documentation of doctor's visits, orders or progress notes; a.m. care not consistently documented; inadequate documentation of turning of patients; incomplete "activities of daily living" sheets; "range of motion" exercises not documented; patients found wet and soiled with dried fecal matter; lack of bowel and bladder retraining programs; incomplete documentation of ordered force fluids . . . .

Id. at 223, 224.

From a corporate standpoint, the parent corporation of the nursing home could be held liable for the nursing home's negligence, where the parent company controlled or retained the right to control the day to day operations of the home. The defendants had argued that the punitive damage award of $2 million against the home was greater than what was necessary to meet society's goal of punishing them. The Supreme Court of Alabama, however, found the award not to be excessive. "The trial court also found that because of the large number of nursing home residents vulnerable to the type of neglect found in Mrs. Stovall's case the verdict would further the goal of discouraging others from similar conduct in the future." *Id.* at 226.

Duty To Provide Adequate Staff

A nursing facility must provide sufficient numbers of caregivers in accordance with statutory requirements and resident needs. The Secretary of HHS is required under OBRA 90 to conduct a study and report to Congress by January 1, 1992, on the appropriateness of establishing minimum caregiver-to-resident ratios and minimum supervisor-to-caregiver ratios for Medicare and Medicaid nursing facilities.[8]

Each resident in a facility must be under the care and supervision of a physician. Provision should be made by the facility to obtain the services of at least one physician to oversee the quality of medical care in the facility.

Nursing services are essential to the facility. It is not surprising, therefore, to find that various regulations are explicit with regard to the numbers, qualifications, and duties of the nursing staff. The federal rules relating to nursing services that must be provided by the home are found in OBRA and state public health regulations.

The states are more exacting than the Medicare regulations in expressing the number of nurses that must be present in nursing homes. Nursing staff regulations for nursing homes, requiring sufficient staff to meet the needs of the residents, were held valid by *Koelbl v. Whalen*, 406 N.Y.S.2d 621 (N.Y. App. Div. 1978). Regulations requiring the employment of sufficient personnel to provide for resident needs in nursing or convalescent homes have been found to be sufficiently clear to avoid their being held unconstitutionally vague. 53 A.L.R. 4TH 689, at 739 (1987). State regulations vary in the methods utilized to establish the minimum nursing staff. Some states regulate the number of nurses and nurse aides according to the number of residents in the facility in order to provide appropriate care of residents housed in the facility 24 hours per day. State regulations are often developed to ensure that the resident receives treatment, therapies, medications and nourishments as prescribed in the resident care plans; the resident is kept clean, comfortable and well groomed; and the resident is protected from accident, infection, etc.

In addition to nurses and physicians, a variety of other health care workers in nursing facilities support the care and services provided to residents. They include dietitians, physical therapists, social workers, activity directors, etc. The members of this group have specialized training and usually are licensed or certified by the state to practice their specialty. They differ from the medical or nursing staff in that they may not be involved with all residents, but rather limit their activities to residents needing their special skills.

Failure to comply with regulations relating to the professional staff can have serious consequences. Facilities that fail to meet federal standards could lose certification as a provider of health services. This could then lead to the denial of federal monies and possibly the loss of license.

Failure of health care facilities to provide adequate staffing has given rise to lawsuits. In *Montgomery Health Care Facility v. Ballard*, discussed above, three nurses testified that the facility was understaffed. "One nurse testified that she asked her supervisor for more help but that she did not get it." *Id.* 565 So. 2d at 224.

Duty To Require Competitive Bidding

Many states have developed regulations requiring competitive bidding for work or services commissioned by public institutions. The fundamental purpose of this requirement is to eliminate, or at least reduce, the possibility that such abuses as fraud, favoritism, improvidence, or extravagance will intrude into an institution's business practices. Contracts made in violation of a statute are considered illegal and could result in personal liability for board members, especially if the members become aware of a fraudulent activity and allow it to continue. It should be noted that the mere appearance of favoritism toward one contractor over another could give rise to an unlawful action. For example, a board member's pressing the administrator to favor one ambulance transporter over others because of his or her social acquaintance with the owner is suspect and would most likely ring a bad note in the ears of the courts. A facility board should avoid even the appearance of wrongdoing by requiring competitive bidding.

Duty To Provide a Safe Environment for Residents and Employees

Because nursing facilities are liable for injuries to both employees and residents, they must provide them with a safe environment. Failure to do so could result in revocation of a facility's operating certificate. The license of a nursing facility was revoked in *Slocum v. Berman*, 439 N.Y.S.2d 967 (N.Y. App. Div. 1981), for violations of nursing home regulations relating to construction and safety standards. The most critical issues related to the structure, which was neither "protected wood frame" or "fire resistive" as required by regulation, amounting to a violation that adversely affected the "health, safety and welfare of the occupants." *Id.* at 968. It was determined that the nursing home "could not be made reasonably safe or functionally adequate for nursing home occupancy." *Id.*

The license of a nursing facility operator was revoked in *Erie Care Center, Inc. v. Ackerman*, 449 N.E.2d 486 (Ohio Ct. App. 1982), on findings of uncleanliness, disrepair, inadequate record keeping, and nursing shortages. The court held that although violation of a single public health regulation may have been insufficient in and of itself to justify revocation of the nursing home's operating license, multiple violations, taken together, established the facility's practice and justified revocation.

In *Nichols v. Green Acres Rest Home*, 245 So. 2d 544, 545 (La. Ct. App. 1971), action was brought for the death of a resident of the defendant nursing home. On an appeal by the plaintiff from a lower court's decision, the appeals court held that evidence establishing that the plaintiff's decedent was seen in his room at approximately 2:55 P.M. and was discovered missing shortly after 3:00 P.M. by the attendant, who immediately reported the decedent missing, and that the decedent was found face down in a puddle of water 25 to 45 feet from a river, supported a finding that the nursing home was not negligent and that the decedent, who was 81 years of age, did not expire from drowning. Although nursing facilities have a duty to provide reasonable and prudent care for their residents, taking into consideration their mental and physical conditions, that duty does not include having an employee following each resident around at all times. Sometime following this incident, the nursing home constructed a fence along the river. The plaintiff attempted to bring this into evidence; however, the court found it inadmissible.

Employees should be warned of any unusual hazards related to their jobs. Although one cannot guard against the unforeseeable, a facility is liable for injuries resulting from dangers that it knowingly failed to guard against or those that it should have known about and failed to guard against.

A maintenance man's skin condition was found to be compensable in *Albertville Nursing Home v. Upton*, 383 So. 2d 544 (Ala. Civ. App. 1980). The maintenance man had developed a severe skin condition on his hands and feet as a result of daily exposure to various caustic cleaning solutions that he used while performing his duties in the nursing facility. The court held that the claimant was entitled to disability benefits for a period of 26 weeks.

The proper test to determine whether a claimant's job caused his injury is set out in the case of *Newman Brothers, Inc. v. McDowell*, 354 So. 2d 1138 (Ala. Civ. App. 1987). That test is:

> If in the performance of his job he has to exert or strain himself or is exposed to conditions of risk or hazard and he would not have strained or exerted himself or been exposed to such conditions had he not been performing his job and the exertion or strain or the exposure to the conditions was, in fact a contributing cause to his injury or death, the test whether the job caused the injury or death is satisfied. 354 So. 2d at 1140.

Id. at 546.

Duty To Establish Infection Control Program

Nursing facilities are required to establish and maintain an infection control program that is designed to provide a safe, sanitary, and comfortable environment in which residents reside and to help prevent the development and transmission of disease and infection. Under OBRA:

> (a) Level B requirement: Infection control program. The facility must establish an infection control program under which it—
> (1) Investigates, controls and prevents infections in the facility;
> (2) Decides what procedures, such as, isolation, should be applied to an individual resident; and
> (3) Maintains a record of incidents and corrective actions related to infections.

(b) Level B requirements: Preventing spread of infection.
  (1) When the infection control program determines that a resident needs isolation to prevent the spread of infection, the facility must isolate the resident.
  (2) The facility must prohibit employees with a communicable disease or infected skin lesions from direct contact with residents or their food, if direct contact will transmit the disease.
  (3) The facility must require staff to wash their hands after each direct resident contact for which handwashing is indicated by accepted professional practice.

(c) Level B requirement: Linens. Personnel must handle, store, process, and transport linens so as to prevent the spread of infection.[9]

Duty To Protect against Falls

Falls by residents usually involve mixed allegations of a failure to restrain, supervise, assist, or attend the resident. Some plaintiffs have argued that, although restraints were applied, they were inadequately applied. The plaintiff in *Smith v. Gravois Rest Haven, Inc.*, 662 S.W.2d 880 (Mo. Ct. App. 1983), brought a lawsuit arising out of a fall and subsequent injuries and damages suffered by his 78-year-old mother. The plaintiff's mother required use of a "posey" restraining device because of previous falls in the facility. There was sufficient evidence to establish that the restraints had been improperly applied. Evidence showed that the plaintiff was a frail, elderly woman who had a history of crippling arthritis, among other ailments, and who had been administered a sleeping pill one hour before her fall, making it highly unlikely that she could have untied properly installed restraints and walk out of bed.

Nursing facilities, when transferring residents to another facility, should be sure to provide instructions as to any special needs that the resident may require. It was decided in *Krestview Nursing Home, Inc. v. Synowiec*, 317 So. 2d 94 (Fla. Dist. Ct. App. 1975), that the nursing facility, which sent a senile resident to a hospital for treatment, should have notified the hospital of the resident's tendency to wander. The patient had wandered off from the hospital and was found dead several days later from lack of attention.

Beds

Falls from beds are frequent occurrences in nursing facilities. A nursing facility resident and her husband filed a suit for damages sustained to her hip because of a fall from her bed in *Knutson v. Life Care Communities, Inc.*, 493 So. 2d 1133 (Fla. Dist. Ct. App. 1986). The trial court entered a judgment against the plaintiffs and they appealed. The appellate court held that the resident, who had settled a suit for injuries she suffered in a traffic accident, was not barred from suing the nursing facility for a hip injury sustained while convalescing.

Floors

Floors are often a major source of lawsuits. In order to reduce liability due to falls, floors should be properly maintained. Specifically

- Floors should not contain a dangerous amount of wax.
- "Slippery Floor" signs should be utilized where appropriate.
- Floors should be properly cared for and maintained on rainy or snowy days.
- Broken floor tiles should be promptly repaired.
- Foreign matter should be quickly and completely wiped from the floor.
- Signs, ropes, and lights should be used where appropriate.
- Appropriate precautions should also be taken for outdoor walkways, to guard against dangers such as icy conditions and construction hazards.

Windows

Reasonable care and diligence should be exercised in safeguarding residents, with reasonableness to be measured by their capacity to provide for their own safety. The administrator of the decedent's estate in *Flint City Nursing Home, Inc. v. Depreast*, 406 So. 2d 356 (Ala. 1981), brought a suit against the nursing facility because of a resident's fall from a window wherein he suffered injuries causing his death. The trial court entered judgment for the plaintiff and the nursing facility appealed. The Supreme Court of Alabama held that the trial court erred in admitting evidence concerning the licensure status of the nursing facility and its administrator at the time of the accident. The state department of health had cited the nursing facility for various deficiencies. The deficiencies were not admissible because they were not deficiencies that proximately caused or proximately contributed to the resident's injuries and ultimate death. The court did, however, state that "Even though we reverse the case, we are compelled to point out that the record contains sufficient evidence from which the jury could have found that the defendant was negligent on the occasion complained of . . . . " *Id.* at 362. Because of the prejudicial nature of the evidence regarding the facility's licensure status and the potential for such evidence to affect the size of the jury's award, the case was remanded for a new trial.

Duty To Safeguard Resident Valuables

Appropriate procedures should be developed for handling the personal property of residents. A nursing facility can be held liable for the negligent handling of a resident's valuables.

The evidence presented in *People v. Lancaster*, 683 P.2d 1202 (Colo. 1984), was found to have provided a probable cause foundation for information charging felony theft of nursing home residents' money by the office manager. Evidence showed that on repeated occasions the residents' income checks were cashed or cash was otherwise received on behalf of residents; that the defendant, by virtue of her office, had sole responsibility for maintaining the residents' ledger accounts; and that cash receipts frequently were never posted to the residents' accounts.

Duty To Be Ethically and Financially Scrupulous

Nursing facilities searching for alternate sources of income must do so scrupulously and not find themselves in what could be construed as questionable corporate activities.

A triable claim of illegal fee splitting was stated in *Hauptman v. Grand Manor Health Related Facility, Inc.*, 502 N.Y.S.2d 1012 (App. Div. 1986), by the allegations of a psychiatrist that a nursing home had barred him from continuing to treat its residents unless he joined a professional corporation, the members of which included owners of the nursing home. Under the proposed agreement, the nursing home would retain 20 percent of the fees collected on his behalf. Although Section 6509-(a) of the New York State Education Law §6509-a does not prohibit members of a professional corporation from pooling fees, the statute did not apply to forced conscription into a corporation at the price of surrendering a portion of one's fees unwillingly. Likewise, 8 N.Y. COMP. CODES R. & REGS. §29.1 [b][4] expressly forbids a professional corporation from charging a fee for billing and office expenses based on a percentage of income from a practice. The psychiatrist's allegations also showed possible violation of Public Health Law §2801-b, which prohibited exclusion of a practitioner on grounds not related to reasonable objectives of the institution.

MEDICAL STAFF

The role of the board in setting policy and supervision of the medical staff is extremely important. The facility's board should ensure that the facility's medical staff bylaws provide for the following:

- application requirements for clinical privileges and admission to a facility's medical staff
- emergency procedures to be followed in medical emergencies
- procedures for arranging medical consultations
- procedures for the review and appraisal of the quality and appropriateness of medical care rendered by each physician to the facility's residents
- procedures and responsibility for maintaining adequate medical records
- procedures for dealing with disruptive physicians and substance abuse (e.g., alcohol and drugs)

- procedures for corrective action (Disciplinary actions can take the form of a letter of reprimand, suspension, or termination of privileges.)

CEO/ADMINISTRATOR'S ROLE AND RESPONSIBILITY

The administrator is responsible for the supervision of the administrative staff and department heads, who assist in the daily operations of the facility. The administrator derives authority from the owner or board. The administrator of a nursing facility owned and operated by a governmental agency may be an appointed public official.

Administrators, as is the case with board members, can be personally liable for their own acts of negligence that injure others. When an administrator exceeds the limits of his or her authority, the question of whether the institution will be responsible for the administrator 's acts may arise. Questions of this nature most often occur where the administrator purports to enter into agreements on behalf of the nursing home with third parties. If the actions of the governing board give rise to a third party's reasonable belief that the administrator acts with the authority of the facility, and such belief causes the third party to enter into an agreement with the administrator, expecting that the facility will be obligated under the contract, the facility is generally responsible under the concept of "apparent authority." However, if a third party deals with the administrator in the absence of indications of the administrator's authority created by the board, and thereby unreasonably assumes that the administrator possess the authority to bind the facility to a contract, such third party deals with the administrator in an individual capacity, and not as an agent of the home. The administrator, not the facility, will personally be responsible.

There are times when an administrator may clearly exceed the limitations of his or her authority, but the governing board may subsequently approve such actions and undertake to accept any resulting responsibility as though it had been previously authorized. This is known as "ratification" by the board of the administrator's actions.

The duties of the administrator include the correction of any deficiencies found during facility surveys. There was an attempt by the Board of Nursing Home Administrators in *Carroll v. Gaddy*, 368 S.E.2d 909 (S.C. 1988), to remove the license of a nursing home administrator for his alleged failure to correct nursing home deficiencies. The deficiencies were found during several inspections of the facility, from November 1984 through January 1986, by the South Carolina Department of Health and Environmental Control (DHEC). The DHEC recommended in January 1986 to the Health Care Financing Administration (HCFA), the federal Medicare/Medicaid certifying agency, that the facility be decertified. HCFA declined to revoke the facility's certification. Subsequently, the Board of Nursing Home Administrators sought to revoke the administrator's license. A hearing was conducted by the Board in July and October of 1986, following which the administrator's license was revoked. The trial court reversed the Board's decision, holding that the record did not contain "substantial evidence" to support the Board's decision to revoke the administrator's license.

> Substantial evidence under Section 1-23-380(g)(5), Code of Laws of South Carolina, 1976, is neither a mere scintilla of evidence nor evidence viewed blindly from one side of a case, but rather is evidence which, considering the record as a whole, would allow reasonable minds to reach the conclusion that the administrative agency reached.

Id. at 911. On appeal by the Board, the Supreme Court of South Carolina affirmed the trial court's decision, holding that there was not substantial evidence to support revocation of the administrator's license, despite findings of deficiencies at the facility. Evidence indicated that the administrator was fully cooperative with DHEC inspectors and that he promptly corrected deficiencies. Although the administrator was exonerated in this case, it illustrates the potential for the abuse of power by administrative agencies.

The administrator must implement the policies of the board, as well as interpret policies to the staff. Appropriate action must be taken where noncompliance with rules occurs. The administrator is responsible for making periodic reports to the board regarding policy implementation in facility operations.

There may be occasions when the administrator believes that following a direction of the board may create a danger to the residents or others. If the administrator knows or should have known, as a reasonably prudent facility administrator, of a danger or unreasonable risk or harm that will be created by certain directed activity, but nevertheless proceeds as directed, he or she could become personally liable for any resulting injury. The administrator must, therefore, take appropriate steps to notify the board of any danger in carrying out policies that create dangers or unreasonable risks. Good communications with board members and suggestions for resolving policy issues will go a long way toward maintaining harmony with the board.

In some facilities, the administrator fills a dual role by serving as a member of the governing board in addition to his or her position as the facility's chief executive officer. If the administrator is a non-voting member, his or her position on the board is for the most part honorary.

The administrator is generally responsible for all activities involving the care and treatment of residents. While the administrator cannot assume the functions of the professional staff, he or she must ensure that proper admission and discharge policies and procedures are formulated and carried out. He or she must cooperate with the professional staff in maintaining satisfactory standards of medical care. The administrator must keep abreast of regulatory changes that affect nursing home operations. Periodic meetings to inform the facility's staff of regulatory changes affecting their duties and responsibilities should be conducted. The administrator should designate a representative for administrative coverage during those hours he or she is absent from the facility. This individual should be capable of dealing with minor administrative matters and be able to contact the administrator when major problems arise.

Nursing facility administrators are subject to state laws and administrative regulations that control to some degree the scope of their activities. They have historically been subject to greater regulation than hospital administrators because of federal requirements that states enact licensing laws for nursing home administrators.

Today's nursing facility administrator must be familiar with the sociological and psychological impact of geriatric group dynamics, the effects of drugs, the relationships between families and residents, management–employee relationships, institutional management, staffing, finance, community relations, fund raising, medical staff relationships, legal issues, regulations, and a host of other topics. Licensure represents a high level of achievement and represents a significant step forward for administrators functioning in an increasingly complex field encompassing a wide range of duties and responsibilities.

Tort Liability of Administrator

The wrongful injury to another by the administrator in the performance of his or her duties makes the administrator liable to the one injured. Since the administrator is subject to the control of the nursing facility, it may also be liable for the torts of the administrator that occur within the scope of his or her employment. When performing the duties he or she was hired to do, the administrator is working for the benefit of the facility, and not as an individual. Since the facility gains from the work performed by its employees, the law renders the facility legally responsible for the acts of employees while performing the work of the institution.

Administrator's Liability for the Acts of Others

The administrator is not liable for the negligent acts of other employees, so long as he or she personally took no part in the commission of the negligent act, and was not negligent in selecting or directing the person committing the injury. Under the doctrine of respondeat superior, the nursing facility can be liable for the employee's negligent acts.

Contract Liability of Administrator

The administrator is not personally liable on contracts entered into by him on behalf of the facility. However, if the administrator exceeds his or her authority, the facility will not be bound by the contract. The administrator may be liable for damages occurring to the contracting party. The administrator generally possesses the authority to enter into a contract for a needed piece of equipment, such as medication cabinets. The contract of sale by the administrator as the agent of the home becomes the obligation of the facility. However, if the board had imposed a limitation upon purchases that could be made without specific prior approval of the board, the price of the medication cabinets would determine whether the board was bound under the contract. If the cabinets were $7,000 and the limitation on purchases without specific board approval was $5,000, the administrator would have no authority to bind the nursing home for the purchase of the cabinets. The administrator would generally be liable to the supplier of the medication cabinets. As previously discussed, the two legal concepts of "apparent authority" and "ratification" may operate to alter the personal liability of the administrator.

Case Overviews

A fair number of cases over the years have dealt with administrators and their management of nursing facilities. In general, an administrator employed for the duration of satisfactory performance has no property right in the position, as was pointed out in *Bleeker v. Dukakis*, 665 F.2d 401 (C.A. 1st. Cir. Mass. 1981). The administrator of the Woodland Nursing Home had been hired under an oral agreement under which his continued employment was contingent upon satisfactory work performance. "[T]he assistant commissioner determined that Woodland was being managed improperly and that appellant should be replaced." *Id.* at 402. The administrator's appointment was considered to be at the will of the employers even though the nursing facility's policies provided a procedure for warning and an opportunity to correct work performance deficiencies. *Id.* at 403.

Dealing with the legal system can be a harrowing experience, even in those instances where the administrator is eventually exonerated from either negligence or criminal activity. Presented below are a few agonizing moments in the lives of some boards and their administrators.

- An administrator's license was revoked for concealment of the identities of the facility's owners in *Loren v. Board of Examiners of Nursing Home Administrators*, 430 N.Y.S.2d 402 (N.Y. App. Div. 1980). The court found that the record contained substantial evidence to support the board's finding. The administrator had actively participated in a scheme to divert checks belonging to the nursing home to undisclosed partners of the home. The crime of knowingly filing false statements as to the facility's ownership with the intent of defrauding the United States Government and the state of New York involved moral turpitude and subjected the administrator to disciplinary action.
- An administrator's plea to misdemeanor counts for mismanagement was considered a proper basis for suspending his nursing home license for one year. *Feuereisen v. Axelrod*, 473 N.Y.S.2d 870 (N.Y. App. Div. 1984).
- A nursing home's exclusion from a Medicaid rate incentive program was considered rationally related to the encouragement of superior health care after the administrator was indicted for accepting excessive payments from the residents' relatives. *Cliff House Nursing Home, Inc. v. Department of Public Health*, 463 N.E.2d 578 (Mass. App. Ct. 1984).
- Although cases of alleged wrongdoing do not always end in a finding for the plaintiff, going through the ordeal is at best a miserable situation for the defendant. The court in *State v. Serebin*, 338 N.W.2d 855 (Wis. Ct. App. 1983), held that the evidence of inadequate staffing and diet was found to be insufficient to support homicide charges against the administrator where the resident left the facility and died of exposure.

CONCLUSION

There is a need for a new legal definition of the duties and responsibilities of nursing facility board members. A board meeting is not a social function, and board members must not delegate all decision making to the administrator or make decisions too slowly or hastily. *Smith v. Van Gorkum*, 488 A.2d 858 (Del. 1985), involved a board of directors that authorized the sale of its company through a cash-out merger for a tendered price per share that was nearly 50 percent over the market price. Although that might sound like a good deal, the board did not make any inquiry to determine whether it was the best deal available. In fact, it made no decision during a hastily arranged, brief meeting in which it relied solely on the CEO's report regarding the desirability of the move. The Supreme Court of Delaware held that the board's decision to approve a proposed cash-out merger was not a product of informed business judgment and that it acted in a grossly negligent manner in approving amendments to the merger proposal.

The traditional business judgment doctrine is too vague in light of the goals and missions of today's modern health care institutions. Attending a monthly meeting of the board and serving on several committees are not sufficient commitment in light of the complexities and difficulties in operating multi-million dollar health care systems. Perhaps it is time to compensate board members in light of the time commitment they are required to make and the legal risks to which they are exposed. "[B]y examining the functions of corporate boards and their members, it is possible to create a new, more practical legal standard based upon the flow of responsibility, rather than on any single decision or action."[10]

NOTES

1. 42 C.F.R. §483.75 (1989).
2. 42 C.F.R. §483.75 (1989).
3. 42 C.F.R. §483.75 (1989).
4. 42 C.F.R. §431.702, 431.703, and 431.713 (1989).
5. 42 C.F.R. §483.70 (1989).
6. 42 C.F.R. §483.15 (1989).
7. Key Medicare and Medicaid Legislation: 1990, OBRA 1990, Special Member Briefing, Chicago: American Hospital Association, January 1991, at 161.
8. *Id.* at 164.
9. 42 C.F.R. §483.65 (1989).
10. Manning, *The Director's Duty of Attention*, CORPORATE BOARD, Sept.–Oct. 1984, at 1(21).

Chapter 7

The Medical Staff

This chapter provides an overview of the responsibilities and the medical and legal risks of physicians who practice in a nursing facility. The individual states have enacted medical practice acts that regulate the practice of medicine. The practice of medicine includes three basic functions: diagnosis, treatment, and prescription. A physician's license demonstrates that the state, as the representative of the public, is satisfied that the physician has the basic training and ability to make diagnostic judgments and prescribe courses of treatment that will alleviate or cure a patient's ailment.

Because the general population is aging and is suffering more chronic diseases, the need is growing for more physician specialists trained in long-term care. Unfortunately, according to preliminary survey results of a study by the American Medical Directors Association, the nursing home industry is losing one-quarter more medical physicians than it is gaining.[1]

The wide range of authority in treating patients has brought with it a broad range of lawsuits. The single most sued group of professionals is physicians. Malpractice suits have become part of the practice of medicine. Unfortunately, it is rare for the best of physicians to say they have not been involved in some kind of litigation. Medical acts, which often transpire over a few minutes' time span, are closely examined by the court years after the occurrence. This chapter discusses many of those areas where physicians tend to be most vulnerable to lawsuits.

PHYSICIAN SERVICES

The role of the physician in a nursing facility is to integrate a comprehensive approach to patient care. This includes caring for acute illnesses and monitoring chronic diseases, as well as providing educational and psychological support to the family or caregiver. On the federal level, OBRA provides that each resident must be under the care of a physician. The OBRA regulations read, in part:

The facility must ensure that—

(1) The medical care of each resident is supervised by a physician; and
(2) Another physician supervises the medical care of residents when their attending physician is unavailable.
(b) Level B requirement: Physician visits.

The physician must—

(1) Review the resident's total program of care, including medications and treatments, at each visit required by paragraph (c) of this section;
(2) Write, sign and date progress notes at each visit; and
(3) Sign all orders.
(c) Level B requirement: Frequency of physician visits.

Physician visits must conform to the following schedule:

(1) For skilled nursing facilities, the resident must be seen by a physician at least once every 30 days for the first 90 days after admission, and at least once every 60 days thereafter.
(2) For nursing facilities . . . .

* * *

(3) A physician visit is considered timely if it occurs not later than 10 days after the date the visit was required.
(4) Except as presented in paragraph (c)(5) of this section, all required physician visits must be made by the physician personally.
(5) At the option of the physician, required visits after the initial visit may alternate between personal visits by the physician and visits by a physician assistant or nurse practitioner in accordance with paragraph (c) of this section.[2]

Physician services must be available to nursing facilities for emergency care. OBRA requirements provide that each facility must provide or arrange for the provision of such care for its residents on a 24 hour per day basis.[3]

State regulations often require that nursing facilities have an organized medical staff. Medical staff members are required to possess a license for the practice of medicine. Appointments to the medical staff should be made in writing and delineate a physician's duties and responsibilities. The medical staff should be required to adhere to the written bylaws governing the medical staff and care of facility residents. The bylaws should be approved by the medical director and the governing body. Each member of the facility's medical staff should be required to sign a statement attesting to the fact that the medical staff bylaws have been read and understood and that the physician agrees to abide by the bylaws and other policies and procedures that may be adopted from time to time by the facility.

The quality of care can be greatly improved and the incidence of malpractice suits kept to a minimum by following established guidelines for providing medical care. For example, the American Medical Directors Association very adequately described the role of an attending physician in the following guidelines.

An Attending Physician's Guide to the Medical Role in Nursing Home Care*

Prior to admission

- Personally approve a resident's admission to a facility, and the level of care
- advise the facility if you know that a mentally ill or retarded prospective NF admission has not been appropriately screened by a state mental health agent prior to admission

On admission

- assess the resident, and write admission orders
- indicate whether the individual has discharge potential
- place a medical assessment on the chart within 48 hours of admission, which includes a medical review of past history and current status and an evaluation of physical and psychological condition and functional status
- advise the staff about a resident's decision-making capacity
- help ensure that the resident is informed of his health status, including medical condition, in a comprehensible language
- certify when residents are incapable of self-administration of medication
- help other staff understand the relationship of the medical plan of care with those of other professional disciplines
- write admission orders that reflect an individual's physical and psychological needs and wishes, as much as possible
- designate an activity level consistent with condition and prognosis, and specify pertinent limitations to, or precautions for, such activities
- advise the facility about whether the resident should receive Pneumovax or flu vaccine

---

*_Source_: Courtesy of American Medical Directors Association, Columbia, MD.

Physician visits

- arrange, or provide for, alternative coverage in case you are unavailable
- at each visit, review the resident's total care plan, including medications and treatments, and write, sign, and date a progress note
- visit a resident at least once every 30 days for the first 90 days after admission, and at least once every 60 days thereafter
- make scheduled visits within 10 days of the scheduled date
- make the initial visits personally
- arrange, where desired, for alternate visits to be made by an appropriately supervised physician assistant or nurse practitioner

During the resident's stay, as needed

- perform or request an appropriate assessment of functional levels and rehabilitation potential, and request or approve specific rehabilitation services
- encourage the limited and judicious use of restraints, protective devices, and psychotropic medications, and document periodically the reason for their continuation
- consider and order, as indicated, specific treatments and services that may help the staff maintain or enhance a resident's quality of life and self-determination
- prescribe activity levels consistent with a resident's needs, condition, and interests
- order appropriate measures to try to prevent and manage declines in ADL function
- order appropriate treatment and assistive devices to try to maintain vision and hearing capabilities
- order appropriate measures to prevent or treat pressure sores
- order appropriate evaluation and management of urinary incontinence
- appropriately assess behavior and mental status changes, and consider the possibility of treatable medical illness or psychiatric dysfunction as a cause
- order evaluation and treatment to try to maximize movement and prevent contractures
- order appropriate intervention, testing, and treatment to try to improve or maintain psychosocial functioning
- order appropriate evaluation, diet, or treatment to maintain adequate nutritional and hydration status
- order tube feedings appropriately and judiciously
- order appropriate measures and assistive devices to try to reduce a resident's risk of accidents

- order appropriate therapeutic diets, as indicated
- strive to order medications judiciously, and observe for untoward side affects and complications—especially regarding psychotropic medications
- monitor for possible drug complications in specific residents
- periodically review and sign off on an interdisciplinary care plan
- provide relevant medical information to other caregivers
- periodically re-evaluate a resident's physical status and needs, psychiatric and behavioral status and needs, mobility, functional limitations, nutritional status, rehabilitation potential and needs, activity level, and oral status and needs
- request evaluations, consultations, or tests as needed to help clarify a resident's condition, prognosis, and potential to benefit from programs and services
- respond in a timely manner to notification of problems or changes in condition and status, and order appropriate monitoring, tests, treatments, and transfers
- consider the value of certain primary, secondary, and tertiary preventive measures that might improve function, reduce pain and discomfort, enhance autonomy, reduce morbidity and mortality, prevent the spread of communicable illness, reduce subsequent need for more costly and prolonged medical care, or permit a more comfortable dying process
- periodically review the resident's use of, and need for, PRN (as necessary) medications
- specify whether a resident will require medications during a short- or long-term leave of absence, and authorize appropriate supplies
- periodically review the resident's level of care, to ensure that the resident's needs are being met and the placement is appropriate for that level of care
- write necessary medical orders for pads, mattresses, or cushions; splints or orthotic devices; protective devices; supplemental oxygen; respiratory therapy equipment or suctioning
- write orders for appropriate special precautions, consistent with an individual's condition or illness

Moving the resident

- certify and document the medical necessity or appropriateness of admissions, transfers, and discharges
- provide an appropriate discharge summary, which includes information about diagnoses, post-discharge rehabilitation potential, clinical course, current medical orders, and other information pertinent to the individual's care
- as necessary, make or facilitate transfer arrangements
- provide a pertinent and timely discharge summary

General

- ensure that your orders comply with established policies and procedures, and are consistent with standards of appropriate geriatric care
- respond appropriately and in a timely fashion to questions or items raised by the pharmacist consultant
- provide appropriate orders for necessary laboratory and radiology testing, and follow up in a timely fashion on the results of these reports
- include pertinent assessments, medical care plans, and progress notes in the medical record
- review and cosign physician assistant or nurse practitioner notes and orders on subsequent visits, as required by law or regulations
- complete medical information on the death certificate, in accordance with legal requirements
- as needed, fill out and complete the medical portion of any appropriate incident reports or forms

Special situations

- assist the medical director and facility in prevention, management, and reporting of significant infections and outbreaks
- order appropriate precautions, preventive measures, vaccinations, or treatment of actual infections, consistent with accepted standards of geriatric medical practice
- assist the medical director in informing staff caring for residents with potentially serious or reportable communicable illnesses
- ensure that the admission of any AIDS patient is consistent with applicable regulations, facility policy, and the capacity of the staff to provide needed care
- assist the staff in dealing with difficult families, by providing adequate and timely information and support

Resident rights and ethical issues

- attempt to help other staff to respect and enhance certain resident rights, including the rights
    1. to know the identity of his primary attending physician
    2. to receive information from a physician about his condition and prognosis
    3. to know about procedures and who will do them
    4. to refuse to be a research subject
    5. to be free from restraints, except as specified by a physician for justifiable medical and psychiatric needs

6. to be transferred or discharged only for medical reasons or personal welfare
7. to be involved in care planning and decisions about care and treatment
8. to exercise free choice of medical care
9. to preserve personal privacy and confidentiality

- inform the medical director if the resident's wishes, needs, or condition limit or restrict your ability to provide adequate and appropriate care
- offer the resident or family member appropriate information about care and treatment, or any changes in that care or treatment
- help ensure that the resident (unless incompetent or incapacitated) participates in planning care and treatment
- discuss the use of feeding tubes with the resident, or with family or other substitute decision maker, as appropriate, before ordering them
- assist the facility's staff in managing the terminally ill resident, including understanding the condition, prognosis, and care plan
- upon admission, clarify the status of any resident with a known terminal illness or condition
- determine, or request a review of, the resident's decision-making capacity
- inform the facility staff if you are aware of the existence of any documents, such as durable power of attorney or living will, or other statements of the resident's or family's wishes
- encourage the resident and family or other substitute decision maker to complete appropriate forms and documents to provide ample written evidence of their wishes and intentions
- order any appropriate medications to help relieve pain or make the dying process more comfortable
- help provide the resident, family, and facility staff with pertinent information about condition, prognosis, treatment options, and possible or likely outcomes of treatment
- consider whether the individual has previously expressed any treatment preferences, or issued any specific instructions for care
- present the treatment options to the competent resident, or to the substitute decision maker for the incompetent resident
- as necessary, inform the administration of any need for the facility's assistance in obtaining an appropriate substitute decision maker consistent with state law
- periodically review a Do Not Resuscitate order after reassessing the resident's condition, to ensure that the order remains appropriate, and consistent with the resident's needs and wishes
- clarify any implications of the advance directives for specific treatments such as antibiotic usage or transfer to an acute care facility.

MEDICAL DIRECTOR

The appointment of a medical director is crucial to the provision of efficient and effective medical care in the nursing facility. On the federal level, OBRA requirements provide that a facility must designate a physician to serve as medical director responsible for the implementation of resident care policies and the coordination of medical care in the facility.[4]

State nursing home codes often provide for the designation of either a full-time or part-time physician to serve as a medical director. Paid medical directors should have clearly written agreements with the facility as to their duties, responsibilities, compensation arrangements, etc. A suit was brought by a medical director in *Cohen v. Daughters of Sarah Nursing Home Company, Inc.*, 435 N.Y.S.2d 190 (N.Y. App. Div. 1981), for breach of an employment contract. The contract dispute centered around the medical director's right to hire and fire members of the nursing staff. Resolution of the dispute focused on two clauses in the contract. One clause in the employment contract provided that the medical director was responsible for organizing, developing, directing, and supervising the medical and paramedical services. A second clause subordinated the medical director to the supervision of the facility's executive director. The two clauses were considered ambiguous as to the rights of the medical director to hire and fire nursing personnel, and therefore precluded each party's request for summary judgment.

The medical director is generally responsible for taking corrective action in those instances where facility physicians fail to provide residents with care and services that meet generally accepted standards of practice. The responsibilities of the medical director are generally to: (1) enforce the facility's bylaws governing medical care, (2) assure that quality medical care is provided in the facility, (3) serve as a liaison between the medical staff and the administration, (4) assure that each resident in the facility has an assigned personal physician, etc.

Artificial or "paper" compliance with federal and state regulations will not protect a medical director from lawsuits if he inadequately performs his duties and responsibilities. The position of medical director must not be viewed as a "figurehead" appointment. "When a Texas nursing home was indicted by a grand jury in 1981 for the deaths of several residents, the medical director was also indicted. His plea that he merely signed papers and attended meetings did not absolve him of the responsibility 'to ensure the adequacy and the appropriateness of medical services . . . .' "[5]

The American Medical Directors Association's descriptions of the qualifications and responsibilities of the medical director follow.*

Qualification for the Medical Director

A candidate for the position of medical director should

- exhibit an interest in geriatrics in long-term care facilities

---

Source: Courtesy of American Medical Directors Association, Columbia, MD.

- come from a specialty practice in family medicine or internal medicine, which is usually, but not necessarily, the best background and preparation for dealing with the problems of the aged
- have patients within the institution he or she serves and continue to act as attending physician to these patients
- be knowledgeable about the institution he or she will serve
- guarantee availability for routine, regular visits to patients in the facility
- be willing to commit time, as is necessary, for emergency calls, in addition to any regular, routine visits
- show an inquiring mind into the problems of the aged and a desire to keep current in the field, as evidenced by attendance at continuing education meetings and subscription to appropriate journals, or articles submitted to publications in the field
- demonstrate an ability to address problems within the institution with an open mind, a scientific approach, and the ability to document activities
- be known by and enjoy the professional respect of the local physician community and the established health and medical care communities within the facility's service area
- have a thorough knowledge of the federal, state, and local codes and regulations applicable to skilled nursing care facilities; the standards for extended care and skilled nursing care facilities of the Joint Commission on Accreditation of Hospitals; and the professional service and administration requirements and expectations of public and private reimbursement programs within the state and local areas
- have an understanding of and a desire to support a multi-disciplinary approach to patient care and its planning within the long-term care setting

Position Responsibilities for the Medical Director

The Medical Director is responsible for

- making routine onsite visits to meet with the nursing staff to discuss administrative, dietary, and housekeeping issues; specific patient care problems; and professional staff needs for education or consultants
- offering solutions to problems and identifying areas where policy should be developed
- developing, amending, recommending, and implementing appropriate policies
- developing an ongoing program of continuing medical education for the professional staff of the institution in cooperation with the Director of Nursing
- meeting formally and informally with health care team members to discuss patient care

- participating, with the collaboration of the other health professionals and administration of the institution, in the development of formal patient care policies for the facility and, further, ensuring that such patient care policies must:
  —be developed with the advice of (and at least annual review by) this group of professional personnel, which shall include at least one other physician and one registered nurse
  —be available to admitting physicians, sponsoring agencies, patients, and the public
  —provide for the total medical and psychosocial needs of the patient
  —include admission, transfer, and discharge planning; range of services available to patients; and frequency of physician visits by category of patients admitted to the facility
  —provide for patients' rights as identified in the federally mandated Patient Bill of Rights
  —show compliance in execution of these patient care policies as reflected and documented in minutes of the various organized committees of the staff and the total institution
  —reflect compliance with appropriate utilization review committee recommendations
  —include written designation of a registered nurse (with the guidance of the medical director as an advisory physician) as responsible for the day-to-day execution of these policies
- developing and implementing a surveillance mechanism that will ensure that each patient's medical regime is incorporated appropriately into the patient care plan
- conducting periodic formal meetings with heads of each of the respective sections of the facility and committees, such as ethics committees and utilization review committees, where they exist. In this capacity, the medical director should review, revise, and certify existing policies, and review any current or potential problems or changes
- acting as a spokesperson for the medical staff, analogous to the chief-of-staff within a hospital. In this capacity, the medical director is responsible for developing, with the cooperation of the institution's administration and the approval of the governing body, the institution's rules, regulations and policies, which individual attending physicians are expected to observe in admitting and caring for their patients in the institution
- monitoring the activities of the medical staff with the ability and responsibility to intervene appropriately on behalf of patients or the administration of the facility
- assuming temporary responsibility for the care of a patient, in an emergency situation, when the patient's own attending physician is not available

- acting as a resource on patient care, new treatment modalities, and the pathophysiology of illness that the professional staff deals with on a daily basis
- obtaining qualified individuals in specific areas of medical care to serve as consultants, for example, in the areas of dentistry, podiatry, dermatology, orthopedics, etc.
- representing his or her facility in discussions and meetings with other institutions
- preparing a report which summarizes his or her actions, concerns, and recommendations on a regular basis
- making an ongoing evaluation of the health of employees of the facility, both in establishing policy and procedure and in direct physical examination of the employees
- maintaining membership in the American Medical Directors Association and other organizations that will keep him or her abreast of changes in medical care of the aged, advances in nursing modalities, and changes in the regulatory and legislative arenas
- assisting the staff of the institution in arranging for procedures to be followed in medical emergencies and in developing procedures to utilize the resources of acute hospitals of the community and its practicing doctors of medicine
- developing and implementing a mechanism for continuing surveillance of the health status of employees, including freedom from significant infection, pre-employment physical examinations and re-examinations, compliance with local and state health regulations, and written documentation of compliance
- assisting the administrator in ensuring a safe and sanitary environment for patients and personnel, including reviewing of incidents and accidents, identifying hazards to health and safety, and advising the administrator about possible correction or improvement of the environment
- assisting management in its review and response to any official medical review of the various official surveys and inspections

MEDICAL STAFF PRIVILEGES

Appointment and granting of medical staff privileges should be made only after the appropriate committee(s) of a facility's medical staff have made an effective and thorough investigation of the applicant. The medical staff is responsible to the board of managers for the quality of care rendered by members of the medical staff. The delineation of privileges should be facility specific, based on appropriate predetermined criteria that adhere to a national standard.

Most state laws clearly state that the governing boards of health care facilities are ultimately responsible for the selection of medical staff members and the delineation of clinical privileges. Trustees have a duty and obligation to protect residents from physicians they know, or should know, are unqualified to practice medicine at their facilities.

The duty to select members of the medical staff is legally vested in the governing board as the body charged with managing the health care facility and maintaining a satisfactory standard of care. While cognizant of the importance of medical staff membership to physicians, the governing board must meet its obligation to maintain standards of good medical practice in dealing with matters of staff appointment, credentialing, and the disciplining of physicians for such things as disruptive behavior, incompetence, psychological problems, criminal actions, and abuse of alcohol or drugs.

A facility owes its residents a duty of care, and this duty includes the obligation to protect them from negligent and fraudulent acts of those physicians with a propensity to commit malpractice. The courts will not permit any organization or institution to hide behind the cloak of ignorance in this responsibility.

Physicians have attempted to use state and federal antitrust laws to challenge determinations denying or limiting medical staff privileges. Generally these actions claim that the facility conspired with other physicians to ensure that the complaining physician would not be granted privileges so that competition among the physicians would be reduced. To date, physicians have generally been unsuccessful in pursuing these antitrust claims.

Credentialing

Nursing facilities have a duty to supervise the competence of their physicians. If a nursing facility has reason to know or should know that a physician lacks the necessary skill to care for patients, the facility has a clear duty to restrict, suspend, or require supervision of a physician who has demonstrated an inability to handle a certain type of problem.

Boards have responded to lawsuits in this area by demonstrating that they have followed pre-established policies and procedures. The board may exercise its authority to fix these policies through the promulgation of rules and regulations for the conduct of the facility, or, like other responsibilities of the board, policy making may be delegated. This delegation may be broad or narrow as determined by the board. It may take the form of permission for the administrator, the administrator's subordinates, or committees to make policies or formulate rules and regulations, subject to the review of the board. Policies made in this way (which do not contravene statute, charter, or bylaws) bind the facility; they will be effective in determining the rights of beneficiaries of the facility, its employees, and its professional staff.

The governing board is under no obligation to delegate any of its management or its policy-making functions. Those that are delegated are subject to revocation by the governing board at any time. In other words, there is no obligation to delegate any part of a board's function, and there is no obligation to continue such delegation once it is made.

Physician Monitoring

Health care facilities are responsible for monitoring the quality of care rendered by physicians to residents cared for within their walls. The landmark decision in this area occurred in *Darling v. Charleston Community Memorial Hospital*, 33 Ill. 2d 326, 211 N.E.2d 253 (1965), *cert. denied*, 383 U.S. 946 (1966), where it was decided that the hospital governing board had a duty to establish mechanisms for the medical staff to evaluate, counsel, and, where necessary, take action against an unreasonable risk of harm to a patient arising from the patient's treatment by a personal physician. Because the hospital has a responsibility for the quality of medical care afforded the patient in the institution, appropriate mechanisms for evaluating the competency of candidates for staff appointments and the privileges given physicians must exist.

Physician monitoring is best accomplished through a system of peer review. It involves the periodic evaluation of the competence of physicians by other physicians. Most states provide statutory protection from liability for peer review activities when they are conducted in a reasonable manner and without malice.

Disruptive Physicians

Criteria other than academic credentials, for example, the applicant's ability to work with others, should be considered prior to granting medical staff privileges. That factor was considered by the court in *Ladenheim v. Union County Hospital District*, 76 Ill. App. 3d 90, 394 N.E.2d 770 (1979), which held that the physician's inability to work with other members of the staff was in itself sufficient grounds to deny him staff privileges. The physician's record was replete with evidence of his inability to work effectively with other members of the hospital staff. The ability to work smoothly with others is reasonably related to the object of ensuring patient welfare. The conclusion seems justified since health care professionals are frequently required to work together or in teams. A staff member who, because of personality characteristics or other problems, is incapable of getting along with others could severely hinder the effective treatment of patients.

The court in *Pick v. Santa Ana-Tustin Community Hospital*, 130 Cal. App. 3d 970 (1982), held that the petitioner's demonstrated lack of ability to work with others in the hospital setting was sufficient to support the denial of his application for admission to the medical staff. There was evidence that the petitioner presented a real and substantial danger to patients treated by him and that they might receive other than a high quality of medical care.

Summary Suspension and Termination of Privileges

A physician whose privileges are either suspended or terminated must exhaust all remedies provided in a facility's bylaws, rules, and regulations prior to commencing a court action. A facility that denies a physician due process as provided in its medical staff bylaws could find itself involved in a lawsuit. The court in *Northeast Georgia Radiological Associates v. Tidwell*, 670 F.2d 507 (5th Cir. 1982), held that a contract with the hospital's radiologists, which incorporated the medical staff bylaws, sustained the plaintiffs' claim to a protected property interest entitling them to a hearing before the medical staff and the hospital authority.

Interference with Physician–Patient Relationship

Although a nursing facility is responsible for monitoring the care rendered to its residents, inappropriate interference with physician–patient relationships can be costly to the facility. The physician in *Boyer v. Grandview Manor Care Center, Inc.*, 759 S.W.2d 230 (Mo. Ct. App. 1988), brought an action against the nursing facility and Vada Mae Eder, an individual defendant from Grandview, for interference with his physician–patient relationship with a facility resident. Dr. Boyer had been hired as a house physician when the facility first opened in 1979. As a house physician, he was referred patients whose own physicians did not wish to continue to follow them once they entered the nursing facility. After several years of employment, some of Dr. Boyer's patients began to terminate their relationship with him. Twenty-five of his patients terminated their relationship with him between November 1982 and August 1983. In April of 1983, he was terminated by eleven patients. As a result of his continuing loss of patients, he decided to write a letter expressing his concern over the loss of his patients and tendered his resignation. He indicated, however, that he would continue to care for his remaining patients. After sending his letter, he began to receive notes from his remaining patients or parties responsible for their care that he was being discharged. The patients or responsible parties had been informed of Dr. Boyer's retirement.

> Eder testified that she began contacting the responsible parties for the patients of Dr. Boyer after she received the letter and told them that, "Doctor had resigned as the house physician, he was planning on retiring, we had three new doctors that had offices in town, they were accepting patients, what would they like to do." Her testimony differed markedly from an earlier affidavit in which she indicated that she had been receiving complaints about Dr. Boyer and beginning in November, 1982, she contacted each of the responsible parties for the residents under Dr. Boyer's care and explained that Dr. Boyer would no longer be serving as house physician and giving them a choice of continuing with Dr. Boyer or changing to a new physician.

Id. at 232.

Although Dr. Boyer alleged interference with 26 of his patients, the case was submitted to the jury on the basis of one physician–patient relationship. In this case, one of the facility's residents was in need of an antibiotic and a nurse indicated to Ms. Eder that she was going to notify Dr. Boyer of the change in the patient's status. At trial the nurse stated that Ms. Eder had told her to call the resident's family and that she, Ms. Eder, would speak to them. The nurse called the family and Ms. Eder spoke to them, claiming that Dr. Boyer refused to order antibiotics that the patient needed.

The trial court, after setting aside a jury verdict for the physician, ordered a new trial. On appeal by Dr. Boyer, the appeals court found that the trial court had abused its discretion in ordering a new trial. Actual damages of $340 and punitive damages of $300,000 against the home and $30,000 against the home's administrator were not considered excessive.

THE OBRA SURVEY

The Health Care Financing Administration's survey process for determining eligibility for participation in the federal Medicare and Medicaid programs includes a review of a nursing facility's physician services to residents. During an actual survey, surveyors will determine whether: (1) residents are under the care and supervision of qualified physicians; (2) physicians have prescribed a planned regimen of care based on a medical evaluation of each resident's immediate and long-term care needs; (3) a physician is available to provide care in the absence of any resident's attending physician; (4) medical evaluation is done within 48 hours of admission unless it is done within five days prior to admission; (5) each resident is seen once every 30 days for the first 90 days after admission; (6) each resident's total program of care, including medications and treatments, is reviewed during a visit by the attending physician at least once every 30 days for the first 90 days and revised as necessary; and (7) emergency services from a physician are available and provided to each resident who requires emergency care. During the survey process, surveyors will focus on interviewing residents and staff, and reviewing facility records.

Resident Interview

In interviewing residents, the following questions might be used.

- How often does the physician visit?
- Has physician discussed the plan of care and medical treatment?
- Does the resident feel treatment and/or plan of care meets his or her needs?
- What kinds of questions does the resident ask the physician about his or her health problems? (Cite examples).[6]

Staff Interview

In interviewing the staff, the following questions could be asked.

- How often does the physician visit, and is it often enough to meet the resident's needs?
- Does the physician participate in evaluation and re-evaluation of the resident's plan of care?
- Does the plan of care meet the resident's needs?
- Is the physician available in an emergency?
- Is the physician available to discuss the resident's treatment and care?[7]

In addition to staff interviews, the administrator may be asked to produce the facility's policies on physician visits and physician coverage for a resident when his or her regular attending physician is unavailable.

Record Review

Surveyors will conduct an in-depth review of selected medical records. Items to be reviewed include:

- a current plan of care that is based upon the physician's orders and the resident's needs
- evidence that the plan is reviewed and revised as needed
- evidence through the physician's progress notes, nurses' notes, and physician's orders that the physician participates in the resident's overall plan of care
- evidence that rehabilitation potential is addressed
- long range plans that include an estimate of the length of time for skilled nursing care and a discharge plan
- physician's orders for medications and treatments on admission and during stay
- a medical evaluation completed within 48 hours of admission unless done within 5 days prior to admission that includes attention to needs, such as diet, vision, hearing, speech, level of activity, and emotional adjustment
- a few closed records to determine whether residents were appropriately discharged by an order written by the attending physician, and discharge plans to assure that they were adequate and implemented
- verbal medication orders countersigned by a physician
- all medications orders reviewed by a physician every quarter
- records documenting an accident or a medical emergency to determine whether the patient was seen by a physician or the physician was notified promptly of the emergency

- physician's orders to see whether specific medications or treatments were ordered to treat emergency situation if applicable
- physician's progress notes to see whether emergency situation was addressed[8]

Survey Evaluation Factors

Factors to be used in evaluating the survey results include:

- Medical records should provide evidence that the residents are under the supervision of a physician by the coordination of the physician's orders and progress notes with the resident's plan of care and observations of residents needs. There should be evidence that the physician reviews and revises the plan of care as needed. There should be evidence that physician services are available to the residents when the residents need such services. An alternate schedule for physician visits may be established if the attending physician determines that the resident need not be seen every 30 days. Justification for the decision should be placed in the resident's medical record and be reviewed by the Utilization Review committee and state medical review team. Where there is a change in the resident's condition and the physician has failed to document his findings or evaluation of the condition, the physician has failed to provide evidence of his evaluation of resident needs and supervised care.
- A physician should be available to respond within a reasonable time when a resident needs medical attention.
- Surveyor should verify that there are readily available written procedures for securing a physician in case of an emergency.
- Names and telephone numbers should be posted on rolodex.[9]

PHYSICIAN LIABILITY

Because of the absence of high risk medical procedures in nursing facilities and the limited involvement of physicians in the day to day care of residents, the incidence of malpractice suits against physicians who treat residents is negligible. The following cases illustrate some of the areas in which physicians have been involved in medical malpractice lawsuits. They are by no means exhaustive and are merely representative of the wide range of potential legal pitfalls in which physicians might find themselves.

Abandonment

Although physicians are required to make periodic visits to residents, the amount of time actually spent with residents is miniscule. Physicians are generally called as determined necessary by the nursing staff. The response time of physicians to phone calls is often slow and at times nonexistent. There is also a tendency for physicians to prescribe over the phone when a visit to the facility would be more appropriate.

The professional relationship that exists between physician and patient continues, for the most part, until it is terminated with the consent of both parties. However, a relationship can be discontinued through dismissal of the physician by the patient, or through physician withdrawal from the case, or at such time when the physician's services are no longer required. Failing to follow up after the acute stage of illness has subsided or neglecting to provide a patient with necessary instructions could involve the physician in serious legal difficulties. Premature termination of treatment is quite often the subject of a legal action for abandonment, defined as the unilateral termination of a physician–patient relationship by the physician without notice to the patient. Closely related to this type of problem is one that occurs when the physician, though not intending to end the relationship with the patient, fails to ensure the patient's understanding that further treatment of the complaint is necessary.

All of the following elements must be established in order for a patient to recover damages for abandonment.

- Medical care was unreasonably discontinued.
- The discontinuance of medical care was against the patient's will. (Termination of the physician–patient relationship must have been brought about by a unilateral act of the physician. There can be no abandonment if the relationship is terminated by mutual consent or by dismissal of the physician by the patient.)
- The physician failed to arrange for care by another physician. (Refusal by a physician to enter into a physician–patient relationship by failing to respond to a call or render treatment is not considered a case of abandonment. A plaintiff will not recover for damages unless he or she can prove that a physician–patient relationship had been established.)
- Foresight indicated that discontinuance might result in physical harm to the patient.
- Actual harm was suffered by the patient.

The relationship between a physician and a patient, once established, continues until it is ended by the mutual consent of the parties, the patient's dismissal of the physician, the physician's withdrawal from the case, or the fact that the physician's services are no longer needed. A physician who decides to withdraw his or her services must provide the patient with reasonable notice so that the services of another physician can be obtained.

Wrongful Death

Death resulting from a negligent injury by a defendant gives rise to an action for wrongful death by the survivors. Most states have enacted wrongful death statutes allowing recovery by a defined group of persons for damages suffered through the loss of the decedent.

Alternative Procedures

The potential for liability affects the choice of treatment a physician will follow in treating his or her patient. Use of unprecedented procedures that create an untoward result may cause a physician to be found negligent even though due care was followed. However, if a physician can show that the treatment used was approved by a respectable minority of medical opinion, recovery will be denied unless the plaintiff can prove that the treatment was applied in a negligent manner. A physician's efforts do not constitute negligence simply because they were unsuccessful in a particular case.

Delay in Treatment

A patient afflicted with lung cancer was awarded damages in *Blackmon v. Langley*, 737 S.W.2d 455 (Ark. 1987), because of the failure of the examining physician to inform the patient in a timely manner that a chest x-ray showed a lesion in his lung. The lesion was eventually diagnosed as cancerous. The physician contended that because the evidence showed the patient had less than a 50 percent chance of survival at the time of the alleged negligence, his actions could not be the proximate cause of injury. The Arkansas Supreme Court found that the jury was properly entitled to determine that the patient suffered and lost more than would have been the case had he been promptly notified of the lesion.

Failure To Follow Up

The Tennessee Supreme Court in *Truan v. Smith*, 578 S.W.2d 73 (Tenn. 1979) entered judgment in favor of plaintiffs who brought action against a treating physician for damages alleged to have been the result of malpractice by the physician in the examination, diagnosis, and treatment of breast cancer. The court held that the evidence was sufficient to support a finding that the defendant was guilty of malpractice in failing to inform his patient that cancer was a possible cause of her complaints and in failing to make any effort to see his patient at the expiration of the observation period instituted by him.

Failure To Disclose/Informed Consent

A physician may be held liable for malpractice if, in rendering treatment to a patient, he or she does not make a proper disclosure to the patient of the risks involved in a procedure. See Chapter 10, Consent.

Failure To Order Diagnostic Tests

As medical technology becomes more advanced, it is likely that patients will claim that physicians should have ordered certain diagnostic procedures as opposed to the ones actually ordered by the physician. So long as the physician can demonstrate that the diagnostic procedure selected was consistent with the medical practice in the community, these claims will be difficult to sustain.

Judicial Notice and X-rays

The use of x-rays as a diagnostic aid in cases of fracture can be considered a matter of common knowledge of which a court, in the absence of expert testimony, could take judicial notice (the act by which a court, in conducting a trial or forming a decision, will of its own motion and without evidence recognize the existence and truth of certain facts bearing on the controversy at bar). Should a resident have a serious fall and a fracture is indicated, under the foregoing rule it is a matter of common knowledge that the ordinary physician in good standing, in the exercise of ordinary care and diligence, would have ordered x-rays.

Diagnostic Testing—An Acceptable Standard

Physicians must conform to accepted standards. A plaintiff who claims that a physician has failed to order proper tests must show the following:

- It is a standard practice to employ a certain diagnostic test under the circumstances of the case.
- The physician failed to utilize the test and therefore failed to diagnose the resident's illness.
- The resident suffered injury as a result.

No damages can be awarded unless it can be shown that an incorrect therapeutic act or omission either caused injury to the resident or deprived the resident of a substantial chance for a cure.

Failure To Seek Consultation

A physician has a duty to consult and/or refer a resident whom he or she knows or should have known needs referral to a physician familiar with and clinically capable to treat the resident's particular ailments. Whether or not the failure to refer constitutes negligence depends on whether referral is demanded by accepted standards of practice. In order to recover damages, the resident must show that the physician deviated from the standard of care and that the failure to refer resulted in injury.

The medical ethics statement of the American Medical Association indicates that physicians should seek consultations upon a patient's request, when the physician is in doubt, in difficult cases, or when it appears that the quality of medical service may be thereby enhanced.[10] Violation or failure to abide by medical ethics does not in and of itself constitute malpractice.

Not every treatment of a patient that falls short of complete success is malpractice because the attending physician has failed to consult a specialist. Before malpractice may be imputed to physicians, it must be shown that they knew or should have known that a condition to be treated was beyond their ability, knowledge, or capacity to treat.

A California Court of Appeals found that expert testimony is not necessary where good medical practice would require a general physician to suggest a specialist's consultation. The court ruled that since specialists were called in after the patient's condition grew worse, it is reasonable to assume that they could have been called in sooner. The jury was instructed by the court that a general practitioner has a duty to suggest calling in a specialist if a reasonably prudent general practitioner would do under similar circumstances. *Valentine v. Kaiser Foundation Hospitals*, 194 Cal. App. 2d 282, 15 Cal. Rptr. 26 (1961) (dictum).

A physician is in a position of trust, and it is his or her duty to act in good faith. If a resident is in need of medical attention by a specialty different from that of the attending physician, it is his or her duty to advise the resident. Failure to do so could constitute a breach of duty. Today, with the rapid methods of transportation and easy means of communication, the duty of a physician is not fulfilled merely by utilizing the means at hand in a particular area of practice.

The convalescent home resident in *Stogsdill v. Manor Convalescent Home, Inc. and Hiatt, M.D.*, 343 N.E.2d 589 (Ill. 1976), brought an action against the physician, the home, and a co-owner of the home for damages suffered when her leg was amputated as a proximate result of allegedly deficient medical and convalescent care. The resident had developed a decubitus ulcer on her left ankle and gangrene developed sometime before November 7, 1972. There was testimony by one of the nurses at the nursing facility that she had noticed gangrene in August or September. The treating physician, Dr. Hiatt, prescribed certain medications but did not prescribe any antibiotics until November 6, 1972, at which time he prescribed terramycin. Wet soaks, lab workup, and vascular studies also were not ordered. The treating physician did not request hospitalization or seek "consultation" from another physician. *Id.* at 592. On November 7, 1972, the resident's son called another physician to see his mother. He diagnosed the resident's condition as a wet gangrene involving the entire outer surface of the ankle. The resident was taken to the hospital the same day. At the hospital, an orthopedic surgeon recommended amputation. After building the patient up for surgery with the use of intravenous fluids and feedings, her leg was amputated on November 10, 1972. Dr. Loutfy, a specialist in internal medicine, in response to a hypothetical question, ". . . was of the opinion, based on a reasonable degree of medical and surgical certainty, that with proper care and treatment the leg could have been saved." *Id.* at 599. The defendant presented no witnesses at trial. The trial court directed a verdict for the home and co-owner and assessed damages against the physician in the amount of $40,000 for general damages and $80,000 for punitive damages. The defendant appealed. The appellate court affirmed the directed verdict for the home and co-owner. Testimony was found sufficient to establish that the loss of the leg was proximately caused by Dr. Hiatt's negligence.

Physicians cannot assume that instructions are adequate just because a reasonably prudent person would understand them. They must make orders clear for each resident, given his or her experience, education, and general knowledge and the nature of the disease. If a resident is incompetent, instructions must be given to an appropriate member of the family or other responsible person (e.g., a guardian).

If a consulting physician has suggested a diagnosis with which the treating physician does not agree, it would be prudent to consider obtaining the opinion of a second consultant who could either confirm or disprove the first consultant's theory. Failure to diagnose and properly treat a suspected illness is an open door to liability.

Lack of Documentation

The importance of maintaining records of care rendered to a resident must not be underestimated. It may be many years after a resident has been treated before litigation is initiated; therefore, it is imperative that records of treatment in the physician's office, as well as in the nursing facility, be maintained. A jury may consider lack of documentation as sufficient evidence for finding a physician guilty of negligence.

Misdiagnosis

Misdiagnosis is the most frequently cited injury event in malpractice suits against physicians. Although diagnosis is a medical art and not an exact science, early detection can be critical to a resident's recovery and well-being. Misdiagnosis may involve the diagnosis and treatment of a disease different from that which the resident actually suffers or the diagnosis and treatment of a disease which the resident in fact does not have. Misdiagnosis in and of itself will not necessarily impose liability upon a physician, unless deviation from the accepted standard of care and injury can be established.

Once a physician concludes that a particular test is indicated, it should be performed and evaluated as soon as practicable. Delay may constitute negligence. The law imposes on a physician the same degree of responsibility in making a diagnosis as it does in prescribing and administering treatment.

Psychiatry

Nursing facility residents may suffer a variety of behavioral disorders that often are the result of relocation and the numerous social losses experienced on admission to a facility. Residents many times receive minimal help or simply go untreated because of the lack of services and/or physicians who specialize in geriatric psychiatry. Because of the numerous physical problems suffered by residents, psycho-social problems often take the back seat to the resident's psychiatric and social needs. There is no question regarding the tremendous need for more physician involvement in the psycho-social treatment of nursing facility residents. Training and treatment programs should be encouraged through the facility's medical and nursing directors.

Medications

Physicians should encourage the limited and judicious use of psychotropic medications, and document periodically the reason for their continuation. Physicians should periodically review all drugs taken by residents and be alert to the dangers of multiple medication. OBRA regulations are extensive regarding the use of medications. Residents have a right to refuse medications and may even be asked during a survey if they ever refused medications and what happened when they did.[11]

Lawsuits due to medication errors are a risk for both physicians and nurses. Expert testimony in *Leal v. Simon*, 542 N.Y.S.2d 328 (N.Y. App. Div. 1989), a medical malpractice action, supported the jury's determination that the physician had been negligent when he reduced the dosage of a resident's psychotropic medication, Haldol. The resident, a 36-year-old retarded individual who had been institutionalized his entire life, was a resident in an intermediate care facility. The drug had been utilized for controlling the resident's self-abusive behavior. Expert medical testimony showed that the physician failed to familiarize himself with the resident's history. He failed to secure the resident's complete medical records and he failed to slowly wean the resident off the medication.

Medication violations led to the revocation of license of a personal care home in *Miller Home v. Department of Public Welfare*, 556 A.2d 1 (Pa. Commw. Ct. 1989), for repeated failures of the operator to correct violations of administrative regulations concerning medications, among others. During an inspection of the facility on July 12, 1985, medication violations were found and cited. The same violations were again cited during an unannounced visit on March 5, 1986, at which time the facility's regular license was revoked and a provisional license granted. The facility was inspected again on June 17, 1986 and October 28, 1986, at which time continuing violations were found. "Thus substantial evidence exists to support the Department's conclusion that Miller has repeatedly failed to comply with the plan of correction and to correct noncompliance items in violation of 55 Pa. Code Section 20.71(a)(4)." *Id.* at 3.

Treatment Outside Field of Competence

A physician should practice discretion when treating a patient outside his or her field of expertise or competence. The standard of care required in a malpractice case will be that of the specialty in which a physician is treating, whether or not he or she has appropriate credentials in that specialty.

CONCLUSION

The need for continuing education and training in the treatment of the elderly must be a major and ongoing priority of the medical profession.

> . . . there is ample evidence of a severe shortage of medical and nursing expertise relevant to the complex problems presented by many elderly patients. Disease and disability among the elderly are frequently misdiagnosed, mistreated, or simply written off as concomitants of normal aging. A condition that is aggressively treated in younger people may be mistakenly regarded as irreversible—or it may be perceived as a blessing.
>
> * * *
>
> Because of geriatrics' late entry in academia there is considerable need for continuing education programs in geriatrics. Such programs are the only way to reach the majority of health professionals whose formal education predated opportunities in geriatrics.[12]

NOTES

1. *Long-Term Care,* 65(2) HOSPITALS, January 20, 1991, at 20.
2. 42 C.F.R. §483.40 (1989).
3. *Id.*
4. 42 C.F.R. §483.75 (1989).
5. J.J. Patee, *Update on the Medical Director*, 28(6), FAMILY PHYSICIAN, December 1983, at 130.
6. 42 C.F.R. §488.115 (1989).
7. *Id.*
8. *Id.*
9. *Id.*
10. AMERICAN MEDICAL ASSOCIATION, OPINIONS AND REPORTS OF THE JUDICIAL COUNCIL (1966).
11. 42 CFR §488.115 (1989).
12. U.S. CONGRESS, OFFICE OF TECHNOLOGY ASSESSMENT, LIFE-SUSTAINING TECHNOLOGIES AND THE ELDERLY 363, PUB. NO. OTA-BA-306 (1987).

Chapter 8

Nursing and the Law

Under federal law, effective October 1, 1990, nursing facilities must have sufficient nursing staff to provide nursing and related services adequate to attain and maintain the highest practicable physical, mental, and psychosocial well-being of each resident, as determined by resident assessments and individual plans of care. Nursing facilities must provide 24 hour nursing services that are sufficient to meet the total nursing needs in accordance with patient care plans.[1] Unfortunately, there is a severe national shortage of nurses specializing in gerontology.[2] As nursing facilities are increasingly filled with older, disabled residents with ever-increasing complex care needs, the demands for highly educated and trained nursing personnel continues to grow.[3] The nursing profession itself acknowledged this situation in a position statement on long-term care prepared by the New York State Nurse's Association, which states that "long term care is becoming increasingly complex and requires attention and direction from the nursing profession."[4]

The need for trained nurses in nursing facilities further strains the limited supply of nurses already afflicting the health care industry. Health officials reported to the House Select Committee on Aging that the nation's shortage has hit long-term care providers hardest. Inadequate career ladders and wage scales lower than those found in acute care hospitals make it difficult for long-term care facilities to attract nurses. The House Aging Committee is considering legislation to remedy these inequities.[5] Although there is a serious nursing shortage, enrollment in nursing schools was up 14 percent in 1990, according to preliminary findings of a study conducted by the National League for Nursing.[6] However, since it will take several years before any gains in nursing personnel are realized from this increased enrollment, the crisis is far from over.

A wide variety of acts and omissions may constitute negligence on the part of a nurse. Some are quite generalized and others more specific to the long-term care setting. As with physicians, the exposure of nurses to negligence suits in a nursing facility is somewhat more narrow in scope than for those working in an acute care facility. This chapter describes many of the legal risks that nurses have encountered in a variety of settings, all of which apply to nurses, regardless of whether they work in a long-term care or acute care facility.

HISTORICAL PERSPECTIVE

Health care facilities of the 19th century were filled with discharging wounds. The atmosphere was so offensive that the use of perfume was often required to temper the odors. Nurses of that period are said to have used snuff in order to make working conditions tolerable. Physicians would wear their coats for months without washing them. The same bed linen served several patients. Pain, hemorrhage, gangrene, and infection were rife on the wards. Mortality from operations was as high as 90 percent.

Florence Nightingale's service in caring for the sick and injured was faithfully industrious. In order to appreciate her work, it must be remembered that for more than a century prior to her organization of nursing service health care facilities resembled the worst type of prisons. The ill were at the mercy of attendants who were both heartless and unsympathetic. By 1854, during the Crimean War, her opportunity came. The English government, disturbed by reports of conditions among the sick and wounded soldiers, selected Florence Nightingale as the one person capable of improving the nursing service. Upon her arrival at the military hospital in Crimea, she found that the sick were lying on canvas sheets in the midst of dirt and vermin. There was neither laundry nor clothing and beds were made of straw. With boundless energy and a small band of nurses she had assembled, she proceeded to establish order and cleanliness. She organized diet kitchens, a laundry service, and departments of supplies, often utilizing her own funds to finance her projects. Ten days after her arrival, the newly established kitchens were feeding 1,000 soldiers. Within three months, 10,000 were receiving clothing, food, and medicine. It is said that as a result of her work, the death rate was reduced from 40 percent to 2 percent.[7] Ms. Nightingale has been credited with writing, "A good nursing staff will perform their duties more or less satisfactorily under every disadvantage. But while doing so, their head will always try to improve their surroundings, in such a way as to liberate them from subsidiary work, and enable them to devote their time more exclusively to the care of the sick."[8]

As a result of her tremendous organizational skills, Florence Nightingale is considered by many to be the first true health care administrator. The culmination of her work came in 1860, after her return to England. There she founded the Nightingale School of Nursing at the St. Thomas Hospital. From this school a group of 15 nurses graduated in 1863. They later became the pioneer heads of training schools throughout the world.

In 1886 the Royal British Nurse's Association (RBNA) was formed. The RBNA worked towards the establishment of a standard of technical excellence in nursing. A charter granted to the RBNA in 1893 denied nurses a register, although it did agree to the maintenance of a list of persons who could apply to have their name entered thereon as nurses.[9]

A unique opportunity presented itself to the nurse leaders of the 1890's. Mrs. Bedford Fenwick, a nurse leader in the English nurse registration movement, came to Chicago in 1893 to arrange the English nursing exhibit to be displayed in the Women's building at the Worlds Fair. As part of the Congress on Hospitals and Dispensaries, a nursing section included papers on establishing standards in hospital training schools, the establishment of a nurses' association, and nurse registration.

* * *

The development of the hospital economics course at Teachers College, Columbia University, ushered in a new era in preparation of nurse leaders in America. This one-year certificate course was extended to a two-year postbasic training program in 1905. The commitment of key nursing leaders to advancing educational preparation for nurse faculty fostered the subsequent development of baccalaureate education in nursing during the first quarter of the 20th century.

* * *

Despite the opposition, the movement for legislation to protect the public from the untrained nurse spread across the country. Although New York nurses began to organize for passage of legislation in 1901, the first state to pass a nurse practice bill was North Carolina in 1903.[10]

Nursing today is significantly different than it was in the days of Florence Nightingale. It requires a wider variety of skills and specialized knowledge. As advances in medicine continue to develop, the duties and responsibilities of the nurse continue to expand as well. As nursing tasks become more complex, the element of risk to the patient increases, as well as the nurse's potential exposure to malpractice. This chapter provides an overview of some of the more common risks encountered by nurses.

THE PRACTICE OF NURSING

Each state has its own Nurse Practice Act that defines the practice of nursing. Although most states have similar definitions of nursing, differences generally revolve around the scope of practice permitted. New York defines the practice of nursing as follows:

> . . . registered professional nurse is defined as diagnosing and treating human responses to actual or potential health problems through such services as casefinding, health teaching, health counseling, and provi-

> sion of care supportive to or restorative of life and well-being, and executing medical regimens prescribed by a licensed physician, dentist or other licensed health care provider legally authorized under this title and in accordance with the commissioner's regulations. A nursing regimen shall be consistent with and shall not vary any existing medical regimen.
>
> . . . a licensed practical nurse is defined as performing tasks and responsibilities within the framework of casefinding, health teaching, health counseling, and provision of supportive and restorative care under the direction of a registered professional nurse or a licensed physician, dentist, or other care provider legally authorized under this title and in accordance with the commissioner's regulations.
>
> The practice of registered professional nursing by a nurse practitioner . . . may include the diagnosis of illness and physical conditions and the performance of therapeutic and corrective measures within a specialty area of practice, in collaboration with a licensed physician qualified to collaborate in the specialty involved, provided such services are performed in accordance with a written practice agreement and written practice protocols. The written practice agreement shall include explicit provisions for the resolution of any disagreement between the collaborating physician and the nurse practitioner regarding a matter of diagnosis or treatment that is within the scope of practice of both. To the extent the practice agreement does not so provide, then the collaborating physician's diagnosis or treatment shall prevail.[11]

"Professional nursing . . . is in a period of rapid and progressive change in response to the growth of biomedical knowledge, changes in patterns of demand for health services, and the evolution of professional relationships among nurses, physicians and other health professions."[12] Although the actual authority of nurses to act varies considerably from state to state, the expanding scope of nursing functions and licensure are clearly illustrated in the following examples:

- 1903—North Carolina enacted the first nurse registration act.[13]
- 1938—New York enacted the first exclusive practice act. This act required mandatory licensure of everyone who performed nursing functions as a matter of employment.
- 1957—The California Nurses Association met with representatives of medical and hospital associations to draw up a statement supporting nurses in performing venipunctures.
- 1966—The Michigan Heart Association favored the use of defibrillators by coronary care nurses.

- 1968—The Hawaii nursing, medical, and hospital associations approved nurses performing cardiopulmonary resuscitation.
- 1971—Idaho revised its nurse practice act by allowing diagnosis and treatment if such is jointly promulgated by the Idaho State Board of Medicine and the Idaho Board of Nursing.
- 1972—New York expanded its nurse practice act and adopted a broad definition of nursing.
- 1973—The first American Nurses Association Guidelines for nurse practitioners were written for geriatric nurse practitioners. These were later modified and adapted to apply to other practitioners.[14]
- 1975—Missouri Revised Statutes Section 335.016(8) (as revised in 1975) authorized a nurse to make an assessment of persons who are ill and to render a "nursing diagnosis." "The 1975 Act not only describes a much broader spectrum of nursing functions, it qualifies this description with the phrase 'including, but not limited to.' We believe this phrase evidences an intent to avoid statutory constraints on the evolution of new functions for nurses delivering health services." *Sermchief v. Gonzales*, 660 S.W.2d 683, 689 (Mo. 1983).
- 1985—New York revised its definition of nursing by providing that a registered professional nurse who has the appropriate training and experience may provide primary healthcare services as defined under the statutory authority of the Public Health Law and as approved by the hospital's governing authority. The term primary healthcare services means

  —taking histories and performing physical examinations,

  —selecting clinical laboratory tests and diagnostic radiology procedures, and

  —choosing regimens of treatment.

  A physician's responsibility for the medical care of his or her patient is not altered by these provisions. New York Public Health Law, Ch. 5, A, Art. 1, Part 400.10 (1985).
- 1989—New York allowed nurse practitioners to diagnose, treat, and write prescriptions within their area of specialty with minimum physician supervision.

The role of the nurse continues to expand due to a shortage of nurses as well as primary physicians in certain rural and inner city areas, ever-increasing specialization, improved technology, public demand, and expectations within the profession itself. A matter of concern to professional nurses is whether certain patient care activities infringe on an area of practice reserved by state licensing legislation for physicians. The question can arise in almost any patient care setting, although it would appear to be an issue raised more frequently in emergency rooms and on special care units. A nurse who engages in activities beyond the legally recognized scope of practice runs the risk of violating a state's medical practice act, and the nursing facility that employs the nurse could also be held responsible under criminal law for aiding and abetting the illegal practice of medicine.

The shortage of nursing staff and the resulting expansion of nurses' scope of responsibility can lead to over-extension and ultimately result in increased exposure to malpractice suits. The law in some states would allow a jury to infer that a nurse was negligent if the nurse performed functions restricted by law to physicians and if harm was suffered by a patient. The burden then shifts to the nurse who must establish that his or her performance was not of a negligent character. Even where such an inference is not recognized, a plaintiff's attorney has the opportunity to put a nurse's performance in an unfavorable light if the facts suggest an intrusion into medical practice. Nurses, however, have not generally encountered lawsuits for exceeding their scope of practice unless negligence is an issue.

A nurse who exceeds her scope of practice as defined by state nurse practice acts can be found to have violated licensure provisions or to have performed tasks that are reserved by statute for another health professional. Because of increasingly complex nursing and medical procedures, it is sometimes difficult to distinguish the tasks that are clearly reserved for the physician from those that may be performed by the professional nurse.

> The broadening of the field of practice of the nursing profession . . . carries with it the profession's responsibility for continuing high educational standards and the individual nurse's responsibility to conduct herself or himself in a professional manner. The hallmark of the professional is knowing the limits of one's professional knowledge. The nurse, either upon reaching the limit of her or his knowledge or upon reaching the limits prescribed for the nurse by the physician's standing orders and protocols, should refer the patient to the physician.

Sermchief v. Gonzales, 660 S.W.2d at 690.

NURSE LICENSURE

The common organizational pattern of nurse licensing authority in each state is to establish a separate board, organized and operated within the guidelines of specific legislation, to license all professional and practical nurses. Each board is in turn responsible for the determination of eligibility for initial licensing and relicensing; for the enforcement of licensing statutes, including suspension, revocation, and restoration of licenses; and for the approval and supervision of training institutions.

According to the Supreme Court of Idaho, a licensing board has the authority to suspend a license; however, it must do so within existing rules and regulations. In *Tuma v. Board of Nursing*, 593 P.2d 711 (Idaho 1979), a statute allowing the suspension of a professional nursing license for unprofessional conduct could not be invoked to suspend the license of a nurse who allegedly interfered with the physician–patient relationship by discussing alternative treatment with the patient without some board of nursing rules or regulations to adequately warn her that such actions were prohibited.

Requirements for Licensure

Formal professional training is necessary for nurse licensure in all states. The course requirements vary, but all courses must be completed at board-approved schools or institutions.

Each state requires that an applicant pass a written examination, which is generally administered twice annually. The examinations may be drafted by the licensing board, or they may be prepared by professional examination services or national examining boards. Some states waive their written examination for applicants who present a certificate from a national nursing examination board. Graduate nurses are generally able to practice nursing under supervision while waiting for the results of their exam.

There are four basic methods by which boards license out-of-state nurses: reciprocity, endorsement, examination, or waiver. Reciprocity may be a formal or informal agreement between states whereby a nurse licensing board in one state recognizes licensees of another state if the board of that state extends reciprocal recognition to licensees from the first state. To have reciprocity, the initial licensing requirements of the two states must be essentially equivalent.

While some nurse licensing boards use the term endorsement interchangeably with reciprocity, the two words actually have different meanings. In licensing by endorsement, boards determine whether the out-of-state nurse's qualifications were equivalent to their own state requirements at the time of initial licensure. Many states make it a condition for endorsement that the qualifying examination taken in the other state be comparable to their own. As with reciprocity, endorsement becomes much easier where uniform qualification standards are applied by the different states.

Licensing out-of-state nurses can also be accomplished by waiver and examination. Where applicants do not meet all the requirements for licensure, but have equivalent qualifications, the specific prerequisite of education, experience, or examination may be waived. Some states will not recognize out-of-state licensed nurses and make it mandatory that all applicants pass the regular examination.

A majority of the states grant temporary licenses for nurses. These licenses may be given pending a decision by the board on permanent licensure or may be issued to out-of-state nurses who intend to be in a jurisdiction for only a limited time.

Nurse licensing boards are cautious in licensing persons educated in foreign countries. Graduates of schools in other countries are required to meet the same qualifications as are nurses trained in the United States. Many state boards have established special training, citizenship, and experience requirements for students educated abroad, and others insist on additional training in the United States.

Nurses who have completed their studies in a foreign country are required to pass an English proficiency examination and/or a licensing examination administered in English. A few states have reciprocity or endorsement agreements with some foreign countries.

Suspension and Revocation

All nurse licensing boards have the authority to suspend or revoke the license of a nurse who is found to have violated specified norms of conduct. Such violations may include procurement of a license by fraud; unprofessional, dishonorable, immoral, or illegal conduct; performance of specific actions prohibited by statute; and malpractice.

Suspension and revocation procedures are most commonly contained in the licensing act; in some jurisdictions, however, the procedure is left to the discretion of the board or is contained in the general administrative procedure acts. For the most part, suspension and revocation proceedings are administrative, rather than judicial, and do not carry criminal sanctions.

Liability for Practicing without a License

Insofar as a nursing facility's liability is concerned, the general considerations of the doctrine of respondeat superior apply. The mere fact that an unlicensed practitioner was hired and utilized by a facility would not impose additional liability unless a resident suffered harm as a result of an unlicensed nurse's negligence.

AMERICAN NURSES ASSOCIATION

The American Nurses Association (ANA) is the national professional organization of graduate registered nurses in the United States and its territories. ANA membership is available to all graduate nurses who are licensed in any jurisdiction of the United States. The purpose of the ANA is to

> foster high standards of nursing practice and to promote the professional and educational advancement of nurses and the welfare of nurses to the end that all people may have better nursing care. The association helps provide health protection for the American people, aides nurses to become more effective members of their profession, and promotes better health care for the people of the world.[15]

The standards of practice as developed by the ANA are as follows:

*Standard I**

The collection of data about the health status of client/patients is systematic and continuous, the data are accessible, communicated, and recorded.

Standard II

Nursing diagnoses are derived from health status data.

Standard III

The plan of nursing care includes goals derived from the nursing diagnoses.

Standard IV

The plan of nursing care includes priorities and the prescribed nursing approaches or measures to achieve the goals derived from the nursing diagnoses.

Standard V

Nursing actions provide for client/patient participation in health promotion, maintenance and restoration.

Standard VI

Nursing actions assist the client/patient to maximize his health capabilities.

Standard VII

The client's/patient's progress or lack of progress toward goal achievement is determined by the client/patient and the nurse.

Standard VIII

The client's/patient's progress or lack of progress toward goal achievement directs reassessment, recording of priorities, new goal setting and revision of the plan of nursing care.[16]

**Source*: Reprinted with permission from *Standards of Nursing Practice* by American Nurses Association, © 1973.

NATIONAL LEAGUE FOR NURSING

The National League for Nursing (NLN) is a membership organization of individuals and agencies organized for the purpose of fostering development and improvement of hospital, public health, and other organized nursing service and nursing education through the coordinated action of nurses, allied professional groups, citizens, agencies, and schools so that the nursing needs of the people will be met.[17] The philosophy of the NLN is to bring together professional and para-professional health care workers and consumers to work together toward improving nursing services and nursing education. The NLN is involved in nursing research, recruitment of students, testing services, workshops, conferences, seminars, consultation services, accreditation of nursing schools, fellowship aid, publications, and films. The NLN is funded through membership dues and grantors, such as the American Hospital Association, the W.K. Kellogg Foundation and the Rockefeller Fund.[18]

DIRECTOR OF NURSES AND NURSING SUPERVISORS

Federal OBRA regulations describe the requirements for the director of nursing services as follows:

> (a) Level A Requirement: Director of Nursing Services.
>
> The director of nursing services is a qualified registered nurse employed full-time who has, in writing, administrative authority, responsibility, and accountability for the function, activities, and training of the nursing services staff, and serves only one facility in this capacity. If the director of nursing services has other institutional responsibilities, a qualified registered nurse serves as her assistant so that there is the equivalent of a full-time director of nursing services responsible for the development and maintenance of nursing service objectives, standards of nursing practice, nursing policy and procedure manuals, written job descriptions for each level of nursing personnel, scheduling of daily rounds to see all patients, methods for coordination of nursing services with other patient services, for recommending the number and levels of nursing personnel to be employed, and nursing staff development . . . .[19]

The health codes of many states describe the minimum qualifications and responsibilities for the Director of Nurses. Although the duties of the director of nurses vary from state to state, they are generally responsible for the supervision, provision, and quality of nursing care in the facility; the coordination and integration of nursing services with other resident care services; development of job descriptions for nurses and nurse's aides; development of nursing service procedures; selection of nursing staff members; and development of orientation and training programs.

Although a nursing supervisor is liable for his or her own negligent acts, the nursing facility is liable for the negligent acts of all employees, which include supervisors (e.g., directors of nursing, assistant directors of nursing, and head nurses). Supervisors are not liable under the doctrine of respondeat superior for the negligent acts of those being supervised. Nursing supervisors have the right to direct the nurses who are being supervised. The nursing facility is the employer, and the supervisor's powers are derived directly from the facility's right of control.

A supervisor who knowingly fails to supervise an employee's performance or assigns a task to an individual he or she knows, or should have known, is not competent to perform can be held personally liable if injury occurs. The health care facility will be liable under the doctrine of respondeat superior as the employer of both the supervisor and the individual who performed the task in a negligent manner. The supervisor is not relieved of personal liability even though the nursing facility is liable under respondeat superior.

In determining whether a nurse with supervisory responsibilities has been negligent, the nurse is measured against the standard of care of a competent and prudent nurse in the performance of supervisory duties. Those duties include the setting of policies and procedures for the prevention of accidents in the care of a facility's residents. The director of nursing in *Moon Lake Convalescent Center v. Margolis*, 535 N.E.2d 956, 966–967 (Ill. App. Ct. 1989), was found to have violated her duty to maintain standards of nursing practice by not following the center's own bath policy and in failing to develop standards to prevent accidents from excessive temperatures. The nursing facility was fined $618 because the director of nurses failed to maintain the nursing standards of the facility, a type B violation of Rules 06.02.02.00 and 06.02.02.06 of the Illinois Rules and Regulations for the Licensure of Skilled Nursing Facilities and Intermediate Care Facilities.

A supervisor may ordinarily rely on the fact that a subordinate is licensed or certified as an indication of the subordinate's capabilities in performing tasks within the ambit of the license or certificate. Nonetheless, where the individual's past actions have led the supervisor to believe that the person is likely to perform a task in an unsatisfactory manner, assigning the task to that person can lead to liability for negligence on the part of the supervisor because the risk of harm to the resident is knowingly increased. If charting a resident's fluid intake was assigned to a nurse's aide not instructed in performing this task, and if such an assignment was not normally made until the supervisor personally ascertained the aide's ability to chart fluids satisfactorily, the departure from the standard of care that causes a resident harm would justify imposing liability for negligence.

NURSE PRACTITIONER

An exciting and challenging role for nurses is that of the nurse practitioner. The nurse practitioner is a registered nurse who has completed the necessary education to engage in primary health care decision making.

> The American Nurses' Association offers . . . a certificate for geriatric nurse practitioners. The geriatric nurse practitioner certificate is offered to licensed nurse practitioners who have a masters degree in nursing and who have completed at least 9 months or 1 academic year of clinical and didactic training in a program that meets American Nurses' Association guidelines.[20]

The nurse practitioner is trained in the delivery of primary health care and the assessment of psychosocial and physical health problems such as the performance of routine examinations and the ordering of routine diagnostic tests. Unfortunately,

> For registered nurses who complete advanced training in geriatrics or gerontology, Federal reimbursement policy may actually restrict employment opportunities. The services of geriatric nurse practitioners are directly reimbursable by Medicare, but only when the geriatric nurse practitioner is supervised onsite by a licensed physician. In hospitals this requirement is easily met. In most nursing homes, however, this requirement makes reimbursement difficult to obtain. As a result, highly trained geriatric nurse practitioners are too expensive for most nursing homes to hire. Similarly, Medicaid's restricted payments for skilled nursing personnel appear to leave most nursing homes with a choice of paying high salaries to a few highly trained nurses or paying low salaries to a large number of unskilled aides.[21]

A study by Kane and his colleagues in 1976 reported

> . . . an innovative effort to use geriatric nurse practitioners as sources of primary care for nursing home residents. This care proved cost effective. Not only was improvement in functional status and resident satisfaction documented, but the savings due to fewer hospitalizations and other associated costs more than offset the cost directly attributable to the new service.[22]

A Veterans Administration hospital introduced a program for delivering health services for nursing home patients that included geriatric nurse practitioners as primary resources in its associated nursing home unit. Results of the study revealed fewer transfers to acute care hospitals and significant improvements in functional status, patients satisfaction, and morale.[23]

Federal regulations under OBRA provide that a physician may delegate certain tasks to a nurse practitioner. A physician may not delegate a task when regulations specify that the physician must perform it personally, or when the delegation is prohibited under state law or by the facility's own policies.[24]

The potential risks of liability for the nurse practitioner are as real as the risks for any other nurse are. In the long-term care setting, the nurse practitioner should work under the direction of a physician.

The standard of care required is generally set by statute. If not, the courts will determine the standard based on the reasonable person doctrine—that is, what would a reasonably prudent nurse practitioner do under the given circumstances? The standard would be established through the use of expert testimony of other nurse practitioners in the field. Although case law in this area is practically nonexistent, nurse practitioners are required to meet the standards recognized in the field as reflecting the current status of the art. According to the American Nurses' Association, as of October 1989 there were 12,117 certified nurse practitioners, of which 1,149 were GNPs.[25]

CLINICAL NURSE SPECIALIST

A clinical nurse specialist is a professional nurse with an advanced academic degree and a major in a specific clinical specialty such as pediatrics or psychiatry. The geriatric nurse specialist concentrates her practice of nursing in one specialized clinical setting by applying advanced nursing procedures and techniques. The standard of care expected of the clinical nurse specialist is determined in a manner similar to that of the nurse practitioner.

SPECIAL DUTY NURSE

A nursing facility is generally not liable for the negligence of a special duty nurse —a nurse hired by the resident or the resident's family to perform nursing services. Generally, the master–servant relationship does not exist between the facility and the special duty nurse.

Like a staff physician, a special duty nurse may be required to observe certain rules and regulations as a precondition to working in the facility. The observance of nursing facility rules is insufficient, however, to raise a master–servant relationship between the facility and the nurse. Under ordinary circumstances a special duty nurse is employed by the resident, and the facility has no authority to hire or fire the nurse. The facility does have the responsibility, however, to protect the resident from incompetent or unqualified special duty nurses.

Even though a special duty nurse is employed by a resident, a nursing facility can be liable for damages resulting from a nurse's negligent conduct. A nursing facility can also be liable for damages awarded in a malpractice action if a nurse and his or her registry have inadequate insurance to cover a jury award. In such instances, a nursing facility would then have a right to seek recovery from the nurse and the registry. If a master–servant relationship exists between the facility and the special duty nurse, the doctrine of respondeat superior may be applied to impose liability on the facility for the nurse's negligent conduct. Even though the resident pays a special duty nurse, the existence of an employer–employee relationship, which determines the applicability of respondeat superior, is a matter to be determined by the jury.

A special duty nurse should carry malpractice insurance. This is especially important if the nurse is providing a service in a patient's home. If a nursing registry has inadequate insurance coverage, there is always a possibility that recovery will be sought against a nurse's estate.

NURSING ASSISTANTS

A nursing assistant is an aide who has been certified and trained to assist licensed and/or registered nursing personnel in the care of residents. OBRA requirements provide that a facility must not use any individual working in the facility as a nurse aide for more than four months unless

(i) That individual is competent to provide nursing and nursing related services; and
(ii) That individual has completed a training and competency evaluation program approved by the State as meeting the requirements of Secs. 483.151–483.154 of this part; or
(iii) That individual has been deemed competent as provided in Sec. 83.150(a) and (b).[26]

Requirements for minimum hours of initial training must specify at least 75 hours in the case of initial training.[27] Various functions of nursing assistants include assisting with the personal needs (e.g., feeding, grooming, toileting, bathing, and skin care) of residents, assisting residents with limited mobility, interacting with residents in a caring and courteous manner, assisting residents in adjustment to the nursing facility, communicating relevant information regarding residents' needs in an effective and timely manner to appropriate members of the health care team, reporting abuse or neglect of residents, following appropriate nursing procedures (e.g., monitoring residents' temperatures, tracking fluid input and output, infection control, and safety precautions), following administrative procedures (e.g., evacuation and fire drills), recognizing life-threatening situations and taking appropriate action, and helping residents and family members to cope with death and dying situations.

States are required to specify those training and competency evaluation programs that satisfy the requirements for state approval under OBRA's mandate. The law specifically required this provision to become effective even in the absence of regulations established by the Secretary of Health and Human Services. The implementing regulations must define the areas to be covered by the training and competency evaluation, including at least basic nursing skills; personal care skills, cognitive, behavioral, and social care; basic restorative services; and residents' rights. Until issuance of the final regulations, the states have broad discretion in approving programs, including in-house programs that may not be eligible for approval under the final regulations. Nursing facilities must consult "any other" state nurse aide registry that the facility believes will include information about an aide being considered for employment.[28]

Several cases involving nursing assistants are presented below.

Failure To Follow Procedures

A resident died in *Moon Lake Convalescent Center v. Margolis*, 535 N.E.2d 956 (Ill. App. Ct. 1989), after immersion in a hot tub. Following an administrative hearing, the director of the Department of Public Health affirmed a hearing officer's decision to impose penalties and revoke Moon Lake's license. On administrative review, the trial court reversed the director's decision and the department appealed. On November 13, 1983, a nursing assistant prepared a tub bath for one of the center's residents, Benjamin Ovitz, a 73-year-old male who had suffered a stroke. He had paralysis of his left side and could only articulate the words yes and no. The nursing assistant checked the water with his hand and bathed the resident. Later in the day, a nurse noticed that the resident's leg was bleeding and his skin was sloughing off. The paramedics were contacted and they transferred the resident to the Evanston Hospital after determining that the patient had suffered a third degree burn. Dr. Drueck, ". . . the surgeon in charge at Evanston Hospital, observed that Ovitz had suffered third degree burns over 40% of his body, primarily on his back, buttocks, both sides, genitals and lower legs. Ovitz's knees were not burned, nor were there splatter burns. The burns were consistent with immersion in a discrete body of water." *Id.* at 959. Mr. Ovitz developed pneumonia during his hospitalization and died on January 15, 1984. There was testimony from Dr. Drueck that the cause of death was due to complications following the burns.

> Moon Lake's bathing policy, 'Prevent accidents—do not make water too hot (95 degrees to 100 degrees F.),' indicates it recognized the importance of safe water temperatures with elderly residents who are susceptible to burns. Moon Lake's daily temperature logs for November 1983 also indicate that it knew that the water temperature in the system at times fluctuated above its bathing policy, at times exceeding 110 degrees. Yet, Moon Lake failed to take adequate measures to protect elderly residents from accidents from excessive water temperatures.

Id. at 966.
Written procedure was not followed when the nursing assistant left the resident unattended in his bath. This was a violation of written policy. *Id.* at 967. The appellate court held that revocation of the facility's license was warranted in this case.

Resident Fall

A nursing assistant in *Kern v. Gulf Coast Nursing Home of Moss Point, Inc.*, 502 So. 2d 1198 (Miss. 1987), was attempting to give a nursing facility resident a whirlpool bath. The resident had been placed in a special rolling seat and was being lifted by a hydraulic lifting device that was used to place residents in the whirlpool. In the process of lifting the resident, the seat, which had been connected to the lift, became disconnected. The resident fell to the floor, hitting her head and breaking her hip. The seat had apparently been improperly connected to the lift. The trial court entered a verdict in the amount of $20,000 for the the plaintiff and the plaintiff appealed, stating that the award was "inadequate." The Supreme Court of Mississippi held that the "verdict was not so low as to shock the conscience of the court." *Id.* at 1198.

STUDENT NURSES

Student nurses are entrusted with the responsibility of providing nursing care to patients. When liability is being assessed, a student nurse serving at a nursing facility is considered an agent of the facility. This is true even if the student is at the facility on an affiliation basis. Student nurses are personally liable for their own negligent acts, and the facility is liable for their acts on the basis of respondeat superior. Students must be supervised by a registered professional nurse who is either the direct agent of the student's nursing school or one who has been designated by the school to serve in that capacity.

A student nurse is held to the standard of a competent professional nurse when performing nursing duties. The courts, in several decisions, have taken the position that anyone who performs duties customarily performed by professional nurses is held to the standards of professional nurses. Each and every patient has the right to expect competent nursing services even if the care is provided by students as part of their clinical training. It would be unfair to deprive the patient of compensation for an injury merely because a student was responsible for the negligent act. Until it is clearly demonstrated that student nurses are competent to render nursing services without increasing the risks of injury to patients, they must be more closely supervised than graduate nurses are.

ADEQUATE NURSING SERVICES

Nursing facilities participating in the Medicare and Medicaid programs are required to provide nursing services sufficient to meet the nursing needs of all residents at all hours of the day or night.[29] The Health Care Financing Administration's survey process for determining eligibility for participation in the federal Medicare and Medicaid programs includes a review of a facility's nursing services. Surveyors will determine compliance by interviewing nurses and residents and by reviewing medical records.

Nurse Interview

Staff interviews could include the following questions.

- What is your plan for alternating injection sites? Show me.
- What is the medication for and what are the potential adverse reactions?
- Is there nonspecific pain at the injection site or shooting pains down a limb?
- Is there skin irritation or lumps under the skin?
- If adverse reactions occur, how soon are they reported?
- Could this be given by any other route?[30]

Resident Interview

Resident interviews might include the following questions.

- What kind of medicine do you receive by injection/shot? Why do you need that medicine?
- Do you have pain or numbness at or around your injection site?
- Who gives the injection?
- Do you receive your injection according to a schedule?[31]

Record Review

The surveyors will conduct a review of selected medical records. Items to be reviewed include

- physician order sheet
- nursing notes for:
  —resident response to medication if appropriate
  —any problems noted at injection site
  —any other adverse reactions
  —site of injection
- plan of care
  —rotation of injection site
  —care for any special problems related to the injection
- infection control: reports for any infections connected with injections[32]

Survey Evaluation Factors

The following questions will also be addressed in the survey:

- Is the medication administered according to the physician order?
- Is proper technique used in preparation and administration, including site rotation?
- Does the nurse administering the medication know the expected reaction of the drug?
- Do infection control reports show infections at injection sites?
- Is the resident's response to the medication noted in the progress notes?[33]

Because the administration of medications is a major risk area for negligence, surveyors will make observations of the following:

- the preparation of injection—i.e., maintenance of sterility, correct dilution, handwashing before preparation, etc.
- the injection site for
  —redness
  —discoloration
  —swelling
  —lesions
- proper techniques when injection is given
  —correct site
  —correct needle size
  —correct volume of drug
  —maintenance of sterility
- any adverse resident reactions
- the disposal method for used needles or syringes[34]

Case Review

The nursing facility in *Our Lady of the Woods v. Commonwealth of Kentucky Health Facilities*, 655 S.W.2d 14 (Ky. Ct. App. 1982), was closed because of deficiencies found during an inspection of the facility, the most serious of which was the lack of continuous nursing care on all shifts. The court held that evidence that the nursing facility lacked continuous services required by regulation was sufficient to sustain an order to close the facility. The appellants in this case had been notified of the deficiencies and were ordered to correct them. Many witnesses testified concerning the deficiencies and even the administrator admitted to the most serious violation—lack of continuous nursing services. The hearing officer, while noting that the quality of care provided to the facility's residents was satisfactory, concluded

> The facts clearly reveal that the respondent has long violated one of the "Essential Functions of a Nursing Home" by not providing continuous graduate nursing supervision. To contend that such supervision can be provided from afar (by an "on-call" nurse) is to contend that a resident will never be confronted with a medical problem of such immediacy that his health or even his life would not be endangered while awaiting the arrival of the "on-call" professional. Such contention is unacceptable; the facility violated on a protracted basis one of its most substantative mandates. Absent proof that an adequate nursing staff could not be obtained (there is no such proof herein) it must be concluded that there is no justification for this violation.

Id. at 16. The court held that "deference is given to the trier of the fact and agency determinations are to be upheld if the decision is supported by substantial, reliable and probative evidence in the record as a whole." *Id.* at 17.

ADMINISTRATION OF DRUGS

Nurses are required to handle and administer a vast variety of drugs prescribed by physicians. Medications may range from aspirin to esoteric drugs that are administered via intravenous (IV) solutions. Nurses are exempted from the various pharmacy statutes when administering a medication upon the oral or written order of a physician. The improper administration of medications can lead to malpractice suits. The more common complaints involve administering (1) the wrong drug (2) in the wrong dose (3) to the wrong resident (4) in the wrong manner or (5) at the wrong time.

The Wrong Medication

The injection of the wrong medication into a resident can lead to a malpractice suit. In *Abercrombie v. Roof*, 28 N.E.2d 772 (Ohio 1940), a solution was prepared by an employee and injected into the patient by a physician. The physician made no examination of the fluid and the patient suffered permanent injuries as a result of the injection. An action was brought against the physician for malpractice. The patient claimed that the fluid injected was alcohol and that the physician should have recognized its distinctive odor. The court in finding for the physician stated that he was not responsible for the misuse of drugs prepared by an employee, unless the ordinarily prudent use of his faculties would have prevented injury to the patient.

The Wrong Dosage

A nurse is responsible for making an inquiry if there is uncertainty about the accuracy of a physician's order. In the Louisiana case of *Norton v. Argonaut Insurance Co.*, 144 So. 2d 249 (La. Ct. App. 1962), the court focused attention on the responsibility of a nurse to obtain clarification of an apparently erroneous order from the physician. The medication order of the attending physician, as entered in the chart, was incomplete and subject to misinterpretation. The nurse did not contact the attending physician, but instead administered the misinterpreted dosage of medication. As a result, the patient died from a fatal overdose of the medication.

The court upheld the jury's finding that the nurse had been negligent in failing to get in contact with the attending physician before administering the medication. The nurse was held liable, as was the physician who wrote the ambiguous order that led to the fatal dose. In discussing the standard of care expected of a nurse who encounters an apparently erroneous order, the court stated that not only was the nurse unfamiliar with the medication in question, but she also violated the rule generally followed by the members of the nursing profession in the community, which requires that the prescribing physician be called when there is doubt about an order for medication. The court noted that it is the duty of a nurse, in such instances, to make absolutely certain what the doctor intended, regarding both dosage and route. The evidence leaves no doubt that a prescribing physician should be consulted about doubtful orders for medication. This clarification was not sought from the physician who wrote the order, and the departure from the standard of competent nursing practice provided the basis for holding the nurse liable for negligence.

Negligent Injection

In *Bernardi v. Community Hospital Association*, 166 Colo. 280, 443 P.2d 708 (1968), the attending physician had left written orders that the patient was to be given an injection of tetracycline every 12 hours. During the evening of the first day, the nurse injected the prescribed dosage of tetracycline in the patient's right gluteal region. It was claimed that the nurse negligently injected the tetracycline into or adjacent to the sciatic nerve, causing the patient to permanently lose the normal use of the right foot. The court concluded that if the plaintiff could prove the nurse's negligence, the hospital would be responsible for the nurse's act under the doctrine of respondeat superior. The physician did not know which nurse administered the injection since he was not present when the injection was given, and he had no opportunity to control its administration. The hospital was found liable under the doctrine of respondeat superior. The appellate court said: "The hospital was the employer of the nurse. Only it had the right to hire and fire her. Only it could assign the nurse to certain hours, designated areas and specific patients."

Unsterile Needle

The blood donor in *Brown v. Shannon West Texas Memorial Hospital*, 222 S.W.2d 248 (Tex. 1949), sought to recover from a serious injury allegedly caused by the use of an unsterile needle. The court held that the burden of proof was on the plaintiff to show, by competent evidence, that the needle was contaminated when used and that it was the proximate cause of the alleged injury. The mere proof, said the court, that infection followed the use of the needle or that the infection could possibly be attributed to the use of an unsterile needle was insufficient.

The Wrong Route

The nurse in *Fleming v. Baptist General Convention of Oklahoma*, 742 P.2d 1087 (Okla. 1987), negligently injected the patient with a solution of Talwin and Atarax subcutaneously, rather than intramuscularly. The patient suffered tissue necrosis as a result of the improper injection. The suit against the hospital was successful. On appeal, the court held that the jury's verdict for the plaintiff found adequate support in the testimony of the plaintiff's expert witness on the issues of negligence and causation.

Failure To Note an Order Change

Failure to review a resident's record before administering a medication to ascertain whether an order has been modified may render a nurse liable for negligence. The case of *Larrimore v. Homeopathic Hospital Association*, 54 Del. 449, 181 A.2d 573 (1962), concerned a female patient who had been receiving a drug by injection over a period of time. There came a time when the physician wrote an instruction on the patient's order sheet changing the method of administration from injection to oral medication. When a nurse on the patient unit who had been off duty for several days was preparing to medicate the patient by injection, the patient objected and referred the nurse to the physician's new order. The nurse, however, told the patient she was mistaken and gave the medication by injection. Perhaps the nurse had not reviewed the order sheet after being told by the patient that the medication was to be given orally; perhaps the nurse did not notice the physician's entry. Either way, the nurse's conduct was held to be negligent. The court went on to say that the jury could find the nurse negligent by applying ordinary common sense to establish the applicable standard of care.

Failure To Administer Medication

In *Kallenberg v. Beth Israel Hospital*, 45 A.D.2d 177, 357 N.Y.S.2d 508 (N.Y. App. Div. 1974), a patient died after her third cerebral hemorrhage due to the failure of the physicians and staff to administer necessary medications. When the patient was admitted to the hospital, her physician determined that she should be given a specific drug to reduce her blood pressure and make her condition operable. For an unexplained reason the drug was not administered. The patient's blood pressure rose, and after the final hemorrhage she died. The jury found the hospital and physicians negligent in failing to administer the drug and ruled that the negligence had caused the patient's death. The appellate court found that the jury had sufficient evidence to decide that the negligent treatment had been the cause of the patient's death.

Failure To Discontinue Medication

A nursing facility will be held liable if a nurse continues to inject a solution after noticing its ill effects. In the Florida case of *Parrish v. Clark*, 107 Fla. 598, 145 So. 848 (1933), the court held that a nurse's continued injection of saline solution into an unconscious patient's breast after the nurse noticed ill effects constituted negligence. Thus, once something was observed to be wrong with the administration of the solution, the nurse had the duty to discontinue its use.

Administration without Prescription

A nursing facility, director of nursing and a charge nurse were charged with second degree assault and individual defendants were charged with conspiracy to commit second degree assault in *People v. Nygren*, 696 P.2d 270 (Colo. 1985). Evidence was considered sufficient to establish probable cause for charging the nurses with second degree assault and conspiracy charges in the administration of unprescribed doses of Thorazine to a resident at a time when he was incapable of providing consent. The trial court was found to have erred in dismissing the information before the prosecution's first witness had completed his testimony. There was probable cause to believe that the defendants had committed the offense charged and that it would have been established if the prosecution had been permitted to present its witnesses, two of which would have testified that the nurses administered the unprescribed doses of the drug. The case was reversed and remanded for trial. It is interesting that the treating physician had told the special investigator from the Attorney General's office that Thorazine had never been prescribed for the resident while he was in the nursing facility. The resident was mentally retarded and incapable of consenting to administration of the drug. Medical evidence of the amount of Thorazine in the resident's blood was consistent with stupor and that it impaired physical and mental functions.

DUTIES OF THE NURSING STAFF

Duty To Follow Established Nursing Procedures

Failure of the nursing staff to follow proper nursing procedures can lead to malpractice suits. A practical nurse's license was revoked in *Homes v. Department of*

Professional Regulation Board of Nursing, 504 So. 2d 1338 (Fla. Dist. Ct. App. 1987), because of the nurse's failure to utilize proper aseptic techniques in inserting a catheter in a female patient who was observed to be in distress. The nurse had failed to properly assess and report a broken area on the patient's coccyx. The nurse's conduct constituted unprofessional conduct in violation of Florida statutes and was considered justification for revocation of her license. The revocation order by the Board of Nursing stated that the nurse was prohibited permanently from petitioning the board for reinstatement of her license. This was held to be improper because it conflicted with Florida statutes and with the rules of the Department of Professional Regulation.

Infection Control

OBRA 87 has removed the federal requirements for a separate infection control committee, allowing instead for its functions to be carried out by the quality assurance committee in an effort to reduce the number of committees in nursing facilities. The functions of such committees are still required. Nursing facilities must also comply with state laws that often provide minimum standards for infection control. Membership on infection control committees often includes representation from administration, medical staff, nursing, pharmacy, dietary, and housekeeping. Infection control committees are generally responsible for the development of policies and procedures for investigating, controlling, and preventing infections in the facility.

Failure to follow proper infection control procedures, such as proper hand washing techniques, can result in cross contamination between residents. Staff members who administer to residents, moving from one resident to another without washing their hands after changing dressings, giving back rubs, and carrying out routine procedures, can open up a nursing facility to major lawsuits.

In Staphylococcus infection cases, negligence of the defendant and injury resulting from that negligence must be demonstrated. The burden of proof is on the plaintiff to establish a causal relationship between the injury and a facility's deviation from the accepted standard of care. Negligence on the nurse's part can arise from failure to follow appropriate isolation procedures. Sterile technique must be followed even where a resident is suspected to have a Staphylococcus infection, though it has not been confirmed.

Staphylococcus infections can often be prevented by (1) requiring the staff to have periodic physicals, including cultures, (2) maintaining an active infections committee, (3) following predetermined isolation procedures (which should be maintained in writing), and (4) taking other reasonable precautions.

Decubitus Ulcers

The failure of nurses to follow adequate nursing procedures in treating decubitus ulcers was found to be a factor leading to the death of a nursing facility resident in *Montgomery Health Care v. Ballard*, 565 So. 2d 221 (Ala. 1990). "Two nurses testified that they did not know that decubitus ulcers could be life threatening. One nurse testified that she did not know that the patient's doctor should be called if there were symptoms of infection in the sore." *Id.* at 224. Such allegations would indicate that there was a lack of training and supervision of the nurses treating the patient. The seriousness of such failure was driven home when the court allowed $2 million in punitive damages.

Long-Term Care Survey/Skin Condition

Surveyors during a long-term care survey will evaluate the facility to determine if preventable pressure sores are occurring and how they are being treated. With the residents' permission, surveyor review will include the following:

- general condition of skin
  —redness
  —blanching
  —soft/dry/rough, etc.
  —rashes/irritation
  —bruises
  —scabs
  —freedom from above
- measures taken to prevent skin breakdown
- pressure sores
- pressure sores Rx
- factors contributing to prevention of pressure sores (overall cleanliness and maintenance of dry and aerated skin uncompromised by urine/feces/perspiration)
- padding for pressure points and bony prominences, including padding on bed and chair
- proper gentle massage to bony areas several times a day
- regular assistance for resident to turn or shift weight (e.g., bedrails, footboards, trapeze)
- bed linens, clothing, and underpads smooth and free from wrinkles
- elastic bandages or hose smooth and wrinkle free
- elastic bandages wrapped smooth with appropriate overlap
- dietary/nutritional support for skin integrity[35]

The staff of a nursing facility must be properly trained in the prevention and treatment of ulcers. An organized protocol and consistent plan of care should be implemented in order to help prevent ulcer formation and aid in the healing process.

Duty To Follow Physician Orders

A nursing facility can be held liable for the negligence of its nurses who fail to properly follow a physician's orders. Although this situation may more commonly arise in an acute care setting, it can also arise in a nursing facility, especially in those facilities where medical staff involvement in resident care is more intensive.

Duty To Report Physician Negligence

A nursing facility can be held liable for failure of its staff to take action when a resident's personal physician is clearly unwilling or unable to cope with a situation that threatens the life or health of a resident.

Duty To Report Changes in a Resident's Condition

Nurses have the responsibility to observe the conditions of those residents under their care and report those findings that may adversely affect their well-being to the attending physician. If the physician in charge fails to respond, there is a further duty to report the matter to the nursing supervisor or the appropriate departmental chairperson. Nursing facility policy and procedure should prescribe the guidelines for staff members to follow when confronted with a physician or other health professional whose action or inaction jeopardizes the well-being of a resident.

In *Goff v. Doctors General Hospital*, 166 Cal. App. 2d 314, 333 P.2d 29 (1958), the court held that nurses who knew that a woman they were attending was bleeding excessively were negligent in failing to report the circumstances so that prompt and adequate measures could be taken to safeguard her life.

Guidelines that are in place but not followed are of no value, as the following case illustrates. The plaintiff in *Utter v. United Hospital Center, Inc.*, 236 S.E.2d 213 (W. Va. 1977), suffered an amputation that the jury determined resulted from the failure of the nursing staff to properly report the patient's deteriorating condition. The nursing staff, according to written procedures in the nursing manual, was responsible for reporting such changes. It was determined that deviation from hospital policy constituted negligence.

As nursing procedures become more complicated, it is mandatory that the nursing staff promptly notify the resident's physician of significant changes in his or her condition. If a physician should fail to respond to a call for assistance and if such failure is likely to jeopardize a resident's health, the matter must be brought to the attention of the nursing supervisor, medical director, or administration. Failure to exercise that duty can lead to liability of the nurse as well as the nursing facility under the doctrine of respondeat superior.

Duty To Take Correct Telephone Orders

Failure to take correct telephone orders can be just as serious as failure to follow, understand, or interpret correctly a physician's orders. Telephone orders are necessary due to the nature of a physician's practice. Nurses must be alert in transcribing orders since there are periodic contradictions between what physicians claim they ordered and what nurses allege they ordered. Orders should be repeated, once transcribed, for verification purposes. Verification of an order by another nurse on a second phone is helpful, especially if an order is questionable. Any questionable orders must always be verified with the physician initiating the order. Nurses who disagree with a physician's order should not carry out an obviously erroneous order. In addition to confirming the order with the prescribing physician, they should report to the supervisor any difficulty in resolving a difference of opinion with a physician.

DUTY TO TAKE SAFETY PRECAUTIONS

Burns

Burns by hot water bottles, sitz baths, and heating pads can result in negligence suits.

The negligent use of a Bovie plate led to liability in *Monk v. Doctors Hospital*, 403 F.2d 580 (D.C. Cir. 1968), where a nurse had been instructed by the physician to set up a Bovie machine. The nurse placed the contact plate of the Bovie machine under the patient's right calf in a negligent manner and the patient suffered burns. The patient introduced instruction manuals, issued by the manufacturer, supporting a claim that the plate was improperly placed. These manuals had been available to the hospital. The trial court directed a verdict in favor of the hospital and the doctor. The appellate court found that there was sufficient evidence from which the jury could conclude that the Bovie plate was applied in a negligent manner. There was also sufficient evidence, including the manufacturer's manual and expert testimony, from which the jury could find that the physician was independently negligent. Appropriate safety precautions can prevent incidents such as this.

Resident Falls

Senior citizens are highly susceptible to falling and the consequences of falling are generally more serious with older age groups. Among senior citizens, falls represent the fifth leading cause of death and the mortality rate from falls increases significantly with age. For those age 75 and older, the mortality rate from falls is five times higher than for those in the 65 to 74 year age group, and the rate increases so that persons over 80 years old have eight times the chance of experiencing a fatal fall.[36]

The fall of a resident is not always attributable to negligence. The Court of Appeals of New York held that the evidence in *Stoker v. Tarentino*, 478 N.E.2d 184 (N.Y. 1985), did not support discipline of a nurse on a charge of having improperly left a wheelchair resident alone in the bathroom. The negligence charge against the petitioner was predicated upon a wheelchair resident having been left alone in the bathroom after the petitioner assisted another nurse in moving the resident from the bed to the wheelchair to the bathroom. All of the nurses who testified agreed that there was no order, written or verbal, requiring the nurse to remain with the resident while she was in the bathroom. Policies and procedures of the nursing facility and the health department contained no instructions concerning toilet procedures with respect to wheelchair residents. The court held that disciplinary action against the nurse should be annulled and expunged from the petitioner's personnel file.

CONCLUSION

The three major "Ls" when purchasing real estate are location, Location, and LOCATION. The three major "Es" for nurses in providing quality care to elder persons are education, Education, and EDUCATION. Although some gerontological content is included in most basic professional nurse training programs, there is a continuing need to offer full course programs in gerontological nursing.

NOTES

1. 42 C.F.R. §483.30 (1989).

2. U.S. CONGRESS, OFFICE OF TECHNOLOGY ASSESSMENT, LIFE-SUSTAINING TECHNOLOGIES AND THE ELDERLY 364, PUB. NO. OTA-BA-306 (1987).

3. *Educating and Licensing Nursing Home Administrators: Public Policy Issues*, 30 THE GERONTOLOGIST 582 (1990).

4. NEW YORK STATE NURSES ASSOCIATION, POSITION STATEMENT ON LONG TERM CARE 3 (1990).

5. *Committee on Aging Examines Dearth of LTC Nursing Personnel*, 27(10) AHA News, March 11, 1991, at 2.

6. *Enrollment in Nursing Schools Up 14% in 1990*, 27(1) AHA News, January 7, 1991, at 3.

7. M.T. MACEACHERN, HOSPITAL ORGANIZATION AND MANAGEMENT 17 (1962).

8. M.A. Byrnes, *Non-Nursing Functions: The Nurses State Their Case*, 82 AM J.. NURSING 1089 (1982).

9. *Registration: A Minor Victory*, 58(49) Nursing Times, Dec. 6, 1989, at 32.

10. D.J. MASON & S.W. TALBOTT, POLITICAL ACTION HANDBOOK FOR NURSES 11–12 (1985).

11. N.Y. NURSING LAWS §6902 (McKinney 1991).

12. DEPARTMENT OF HEALTH, EDUCATION AND WELFARE, EXTENDING THE SCOPE OF NURSING PRACTICE: A REPORT OF THE SECRETARY'S COMMITTEE TO STUDY EXTENDED ROLES FOR NURSES 8, PUB. NO. (HSM) 73-2037 (1971).

13. MASON & TALBOTT, *supra* note 10, at 11–12.

14. AMERICAN NURSES ASSOCIATION, GUIDELINES FOR SHORT TERM CONTINUING EDUCATION PROGRAMS PREPARING THE GERIATRIC NURSE PRACTITIONER (1974).

15. E. SPALDING, PROFESSIONAL NURSING: TRENDS/RESPONSIBILITIES/RELATIONSHIPS 351 (1959).

16. AMERICAN NURSES ASSOCIATION, STANDARDS OF NURSING PRACTICE 2–5 (1973).

17. SPALDING, *supra* note 15, at 363.

18. *Id.* at 371.

19. 42 C.F.R. §483.28 (1989).

20. U.S. Congress, Office of Technology Assessment, *supra* note 1, at 381.

21. *Id.* at 365.

22. R.A. Kane & R.L. Kane, Long-Term Care: Principles, Programs, and Policies 302 (1987).

23. D. Weiland, L. Rubenstein, J. Ouslander & S. Martin, Organizing an Academic Nursing Home, Impacts on Institutionalized Elderly, 255 J. Am. Med. A., 2622–2627 (1986).

24. 42 C.F.R. 483.40 (1989).

25. American Nurses Association, 1990 Certification Catalog (1990).

26. 55 Fed. Reg. 10, 948 (1990) (to be codified at 42 C.F.R. §483.75).

27. 55 Fed. Reg. 10, 938 (1990) (to be codified at 42 C.F.R. §483.152).

28. Key Medicare and Medicaid Legislation: 1990, OBRA 1990, Special Member Briefing, Chicago: American Hospital Association, January 1991, at 158.

29. 42 C.F.R. §488.115 (1989).

30. *Id.*

31. *Id.*

32. *Id.*

33. *Id.*

34. *Id.*

35. *Id.*

36. B. Hill & R. Johnson, *Reducing the Incidence of Falls in High Risk Patients*,18 J. Nursing Admin., 24 (1988).

Chapter 9

Nursing Facility Services

The needs of nursing facility residents cannot be met by nurses and physicians alone. There is a vast array of caregivers who provide a variety of health services to nursing facility residents. The combined services of physicians, nurses, social workers, physical therapists, physician assistants, nutritionists, activity therapists, etc., are all necessary and equally important in meeting the needs of residents.

> The growth of the elderly population, especially the population over age 85, and pressures for early hospital discharge have dramatically increased the need for beds in skilled nursing facilities (SNFs). . . . Obviously, more occupied nursing home beds create the need for more nursing home personnel.[1]

The National Advisory Committee on Rural Health has recognized the need for a variety of health care workers in rural areas and has recommended that the Department of Health and Human Services provide direct Medicare payments to physician assistants, nurse practitioners, and advanced practice nurses working in poor rural areas.[2]

> Information regarding geriatric specialization among allied health professionals is unavailable. In view of the limited opportunities for training, however, the numbers of allied health professionals with geriatric expertise are certainly inadequate.[3]

As with other professionals, allied health care workers are held to the standard of care expected of others practicing in the same profession.

> Health professionals caring for severely ill elderly patients must be knowledgeable about age-related physiological factors, and their interactions. To make correct diagnoses and treatment recommendations for

> elderly patients, caregivers must know that certain illnesses in elderly patients may be characterized by specific signs and symptoms that differ from the classic presentation of the same illness in younger adults, or frequently, by non-specific signs and symptoms that do not clearly indicate the affected organ system.[4]

Allied health care workers are liable for harm that results from their negligent acts. This chapter describes a variety of services provided in nursing facilities and reviews some of the legal risks of selected allied health care workers.

DENTAL SERVICES

Federal regulations require that a nursing facility must provide or obtain an outside resource to meet the dental needs of its residents. The services that must be provided are routine dental services (to the extent covered under the state plan) and emergency dental services.[5]

State regulations often require that oral hygiene care be provided to a nursing facility's residents. Nursing facilities should have arrangements with dentists to provide routine and emergency dental care. A facility's dentist is generally responsible for recommending oral hygiene policies and practices for the care of the residents and for developing oral hygiene programs for residents. Nursing facilities should maintain a list of dentists willing to treat residents who do not have their own private dentists.

As with all health professionals, a dentist is held to the prevailing standard of care required in his or her profession, which includes proper examination, diagnosis, treatment, and follow-up care. Nursing facility residents must be seen on a regular basis and proper procedures must be followed to assure that the dentists utilized by the facility are properly credentialed. High risk areas for dentists include extracting the wrong tooth and anesthesia complications.

DIETARY SERVICES

Nursing facilities provide dietary services that meet the nutritional needs of their residents. They must ensure that the special dietary needs of residents are met. Supervisory responsibilities for dietetic services should be assigned to a qualified dietitian, either on a full-time or consultation basis.[6] The potential for exposure to legal risks involve, for example, tray mix-ups that could be potentially harmful to an unsuspecting resident. The quality of nutritional support for residents is sometimes deficient because of a lack of information about their nutritional needs, appropriate nutritional support procedures, and properly trained staff.

Federal and state codes regulate dietary services for residents in nursing facilities. OBRA requirements provide

Level A Requirements: Dietary Services.

The facility must provide each resident with a nourishing palatable, well-balanced diet that meets the daily nutritional and special dietary needs of each resident.

(a) Level B Requirement: Staffing:

The facility must employ a qualified dietitian either full-time, part-time, or on a consultant basis.

(1) If a dietitian is not employed full-time, the facility must designate a person to serve as the director of food service.
(2) A qualified dietitian is one who is qualified based upon either registration by the Commission on Dietetic Registration of the American Dietetic Association, or on the basis of education, training, or experience in identification of dietary needs, planning and implementation of dietary programs.

(b) Level B requirement: Sufficient staff.

The facility must employ sufficient support personnel competent to carry out the functions of the dietary service.

(c) Level B requirement: Menus and nutritional adequacy. Menus must—

(1) Meet the nutritional needs of residents in accordance with the recommended dietary allowances of the Food and Nutrition Board of the National Research Council, National Academy of Sciences;
(2) Be prepared in advance; and
(3) Be followed.[7]

Nursing facilities must provide each resident with a nourishing, palatable well-balanced diet that meets the daily nutritional and special dietary needs of each resident. Failure to do so can lead to negligence suits. The daughter of a nursing facility resident in *Lambert v. Beverly Enterprises, Inc.*, 753 F. Supp. 267 (W.D. Ark. 1990), filed an action against the nursing facility claiming that the resident had been mistreated. The notice of intent to sue indicated that the deceased, Mr. Lee Brown, the plaintiff's father, "suffered various injuries and from malnutrition as a direct result of the acts or omissions of personnel of Meadowbrook Lodge" and that "Mr. Brown suffered actual damages which included substantial medical expenses and mental anguish due to the injuries he sustained." *Id.* at 268. The nursing facility sought to have the complaint dismissed. The motion to dismiss was denied.

LABORATORY SERVICES

OBRA requirements provide that a nursing facility must provide or obtain clinical laboratory services to meet the needs of its residents. The facility is responsible for the quality and timeliness of the services it provides. If the facility provides its own laboratory services, the services must meet the applicable conditions for coverage of the services furnished by independent laboratories. If the facility does not provide laboratory services on site, it must have an agreement to obtain such services from a laboratory that is approved for participation in the Medicare program as either a hospital or an independent laboratory.[8]

OCCUPATIONAL THERAPY

Occupational therapy is the art and science of evaluation and treatment of physical and psychological dysfunctions through the use of such activities as creative, manual, industrial, educational, recreational, social, and self-help activities to enable the resident to achieve his or her optimal level of self-care and productivity. Occupational therapy services, as well as a variety of other nursing facility services (e.g., physical therapy), are sometimes contracted to outside agencies. Contracts should be reviewed by a facility's attorney before any agreement is executed.

An occupational therapy consulting services contract was breached when the nursing facility failed to give a 180-day notice of termination as provided in the contract in *Zella Wahnon & Assoc. v. Bassman*, 398 N.E.2d 968 (Ill. App. Ct. 1979). The consulting service was entitled to recover the fees it would have earned during the 180-day period even though it provided no services to the facility. The owner of the nursing facility and not the corporation was personally responsible for the breach of contract where there was no reference in the contract to the corporation and it appeared from the circumstances surrounding the contract that the owner was acting individually in negotiating the contract. (There is a lesson to be learned here for nursing facility owners—be sure that all corporate contracts are in the corporation's name.)

PHARMACEUTICAL SERVICES

The practice of pharmacy essentially includes preparing, compounding, dispensing, and retailing medications. These activities may be carried out only by a pharmacist with a state license or by a person exempted from the provisions of a state's pharmacy statutes. The entire stock of drugs of a nursing facility is subject to strict government regulation and control. Pharmaceutical services in a nursing facility are provided under the supervision of a qualified pharmacist. The pharmacist is responsible for developing, coordinating, and supervising all pharmaceutical activities; reviewing the drug regimens of each resident on a regular basis; and reporting any irregularities to the medical director or administrator.[9]

Government Control of Drugs

All drugs stocked in a nursing facility are subject to government regulation at the federal, state, and local levels. It is important that the administrator, pharmacist, nursing and medical staffs, and other personnel authorized to handle drugs understand the manner in which they are controlled.

The power and authority to regulate drugs, their products, packaging, and distribution rests (as a general rule) with both the federal and state governments. Consequently there are often two sets of regulations and standards governing the same activity. In general, states have attempted to conform their laws to the federal laws. For example, the vast majority of states have adopted the Uniform Controlled Substances Act (UCSA). This uniform law is based upon and is in conformity with the federal Controlled Substances Act. A number of states have modified the UCSA in various ways, frequently setting more stringent standards than are already required under the federal law.

A nursing facility is often in a unique position with respect to drug handling. Unlike most hospitals, nursing facilities do not generally maintain in-house pharmacies. Drugs are generally purchased from off-site pharmacists and stored in in-house drug rooms. No dispensing has occurred when drugs are later removed from the drug room for administration to residents. Thus, many of the federal and state regulations governing dispensing do not apply to nursing facilities.

Federal Controls

Federal laws and regulations applicable to drugs include the OBRA regulations, the Controlled Substances Act, and the Federal Food, Drug and Cosmetic Act.

OBRA Regulations

OBRA requires that a facility must provide routine and emergency drugs and biologicals to its residents, or obtain them under agreement with a consulting pharmacy. Effective October 1, 1990, nursing facilities must provide pharmaceutical services (including procedures that assure the accurate acquiring, receiving, dispensing and administering of all drugs and biologicals) to meet the needs of each resident.[10]

> (d) Level B requirement: Service consultation. The facility must employ or obtain the services of a licensed pharmacist who—
>
> (1) Provides consultation on all aspects of the provision of pharmacy services in the facility;
> (2) Establishes a system of records of receipt and disposition of all controlled drugs in sufficient detail to enable an accurate reconciliation; and

(3) Determines that drug records are in order and that an account of all controlled drugs is maintained and periodically reconciled.
(e) Level B requirement: Drug regimen review.
(1) The drug regimen of each resident must be reviewed at least once a month by a licensed pharmacist.
(2) The pharmacist must report any irregularities to the attending physician or the director of nursing, and the nursing facility administrator, and these reports must be acted upon.
(f) Level B requirement: Labeling of drugs and biologicals. The facility must label drugs and biologicals in accordance with currently accepted professional principles, and include the appropriate accessory and cautionary instructions, and the expiration date.
(g) Level B requirement: Storage of drugs and biologicals.
(1) In accordance with State and Federal laws, the facility must store all drugs and biologicals in locked compartments under proper temperature controls, and permit only authorized personnel to have access to the keys.
(2) The facility must provide separately locked, permanently affixed compartments for storage of controlled drugs listed in Schedule II of the Comprehensive Drug Abuse Prevention and Control Act of 1970 and other drugs subject to abuse, except when the facility uses single unit package drug distribution systems in which the quantity stored is minimal and a nursing dose can be readily detected.[11]

Controlled Substances Act

The Comprehensive Drug Abuse Prevention and Control Act of 1970, commonly known as the Controlled Substances Act, was signed into law on October 27, 1970, as Public Law No. 91–513. Virtually all pre-existing federal laws dealing with narcotics, depressants, stimulants, and hallucinogenics were replaced by this law.

In certain states nursing facilities may register to operate a pharmacy while in others they may not. Where the law does not allow nursing facilities to register and operate a pharmacy, the facilities may maintain an emergency supply of controlled substances. The substances would be the property and responsibility of the prescribing physician, who must be registered with the Drug Enforcement Administration.

Federal Food, Drug and Cosmetic Act

The federal Food, Drug and Cosmetic Act (FDCA) applies to drugs and devices carried in interstate commerce and to goods produced and distributed in federal territory. The act's requirements apply to almost every drug that would be dispensed from a nursing facility's pharmacy, since almost all drugs and devices, or their components, are eventually carried in interstate commerce.

The FDCA provisions regarding labeling are of primary importance to a facility and its pharmacist. There are two major labeling provisions, consisting of a general rule and a section devoted to exceptions to that rule.

Section 502 of the act sets forth the information that must appear on the labels or the labeling of drugs and devices. The label must contain, among other special information: (1) the name and place of business of the manufacturer, packer, or distributor; (2) the quantity of contents; (3) the name and quantity of any ingredient found to be habit-forming, along with the statement "Warning—May be habit-forming"; (4) the established name of the drug or its ingredients; (5) adequate directions for use; (6) adequate warnings and cautions concerning conditions of use; and (7) special precautions for packaging.

The regulations (21 C.F.R. Section 1.106) implementing the labeling requirements of Section 502 exempt prescription drugs from the requirement that the label bear "adequate directions for use for laymen" if the drug is in the possession of a nursing facility pharmacy or under the custody of a practitioner licensed by law to administer or prescribe legend drugs. This particular exemption applies only to prescription drugs meeting the other requirements. Ordinary household remedies in the custody or possession of a practitioner or pharmacist would not fall under the labeling exemption.

If the drug container is too small to bear a label with all the required information, the label may contain only the quantity or proportion of each active ingredient and the lot or control number. The prescription legend may appear on the outer container of such drug units. The lot or control number may appear on the crimp of a dispensing tube, and the remainder of the required label information may appear on other labeling within the package.

In addition to the label itself, each legend drug must be accompanied by labeling, on or within the sealed package from which the drug is to be dispensed, bearing full prescribing information including indications; dosage; routes, methods, and frequency of administration; contraindications; side effects; precautions; and any other information concerning the intended use of the drug necessary for the prescriber to safely use the drug. This information is usually contained in what is known in the trade as the "package insert."

State Regulations

In addition to federal laws affecting the manufacture, use, and handling of drugs, the various states have controlling legislation. All states regulate the practice of pharmacy, as well as the operation of pharmacies. State regulations generally provide that: (1) each facility must assure the availability of pharmaceutical services to meet the needs of residents; (2) pharmaceutical services must be provided in accordance with all applicable federal and state laws and regulations; (3) pharmaceutical services must be provided under the supervision of a pharmacist; (4) space and equipment must be provided within the facility for the proper storage, safeguarding, preparation, dispensing, and administration of drugs; (5) each facility must develop and implement written policies and procedures regarding accountability, distribution, and assurance of quality of all drugs; and (6) each facility must develop and follow current written procedures for the safe prescribing and administering of drugs.

Most state laws require that pharmacies be licensed and that they be under the supervision of a person licensed to practice pharmacy. The pharmacist usually can be either an employee of the facility or a consultant pharmacist. The authority of a nursing facility to operate a pharmacy is conditioned upon compliance with licensing requirements affecting the pharmacy premises and its personnel. The statutes applying to pharmacies usually empower regulatory agencies, such as the state pharmacy board, to issue rules and regulations as necessary.

The nursing facility's administrator is responsible for overseeing the operation of the pharmacy to ensure that each pharmacist has a valid, current state license and that all personnel working within the facility who handle drugs comply with statutory requirements and regulations.

The nursing facility is subject to liability for the negligent acts of its professional and non-professional employees in the handling of drugs and medications within the facility. Both the pharmacist and the facility are subject to criminal liability, as well as civil liability, for the violation of statutory directives. Most states have regulations that dictate in detail the dispensation, distribution, administration, storage, control, and disposal of drugs within the facility.

Distributing, Dispensing, and Administration of Drugs

"Distributing" is the movement of a legend drug from a community pharmacy or institutional pharmacy to a nursing service area, while in the originally labeled manufacturer's container, labeled according to federal and state statutes and regulations.

The "dispensing" of medications is the processing of a drug for delivery or for administration to a resident pursuant to the order of a practitioner. It consists of checking the directions on the label with the directions on the prescription or order to determine accuracy; selecting the drug from stock to fill the order; counting, measuring, compounding, or preparing the drug; placing the drug in the proper container; and adding to a written prescription any required notations.

The "administration" of medications is an act in which a single dose of a prescribed drug is given to a resident by an authorized person in accordance with federal and state laws and regulations governing such act. The complete act of administration includes removing an individual dose from a previously dispensed, properly labeled container (including a unit dose container), verifying it with the physician's order, giving the individual dose to the proper resident, and recording the time and dose given.

Medications may be administered by licensed medical or nursing personnel in accordance with state regulations. Each dose of drug administered must be recorded on the resident's clinical records. A separate record of narcotic drugs must be maintained. The record must contain a separate sheet for each narcotic of different strength or type administered to the resident. The narcotic record must contain the following information: date and time administered, physician's name, signature of person administering the dose, and the balance of the narcotic drug on hand.

In the event that an emergency arises that requires the immediate administration of a particular drug, the resident's record should be properly documented, showing the necessity for administration of the drug on an emergency basis. Procedures should be in place for handling emergency situations. A list of on-call physicians should be maintained by the facility.

Storage of Drugs

Drugs must be stored in their original containers and must be properly labeled. The label should indicate the resident's full name, physician, prescription number, strength of the drug, expiration date of all time-dated drugs, and the address and telephone number of the pharmacy dispensing the drug. The medication containers must be stored in a locked cabinet at the nurse's station. Medications containing narcotics or other dangerous drugs must be stored under double lock (e.g., a locked box within the medicine cabinet). The keys to the medicine cabinet and narcotics box must be in the possession of authorized facility personnel. Medications for "external use only" must be clearly marked and kept separate from medications for internal use. Medications that are to be taken out of use must be disposed of according to federal and state laws and regulations.

Drug Substitution

Drug substitution may be defined as the dispensing of a different drug or brand in place of the drug or brand ordered. Several states prohibit this and penal sanctions, including loss of license, are imposed for violation of the law.

Some facilities may use a "formulary system," where physicians and pharmacists create a formulary, which is a list of drugs used in the institution. The formulary contains the brand names and generic names of drugs. Under the formulary system a physician agrees that his or her prescription, which calls for a brand name drug, may be filled with the generic equivalent of that drug, that is, a drug that contains the same active ingredients in the same proportions.

Authorization for using a generic equivalent should be given by the physician at the time he or she prescribes a formulary drug and should be evidenced by a written consent on the face of the prescription. When a formulary system is in use, the prescribing physician can require the use of a particular brand name drug, when he or she deems it necessary or desirable, by expressly prohibiting the use of the formulary system.

Case Reviews

The nursing facility and pharmacist are subject to liability for the mishandling or misuse of the items in the drug room. Failure of the facility to meet and maintain required standards in the handling of drugs could lead to criminal or civil liability and even to the revocation of its license. Violation of any drug statutes can lead to criminal liability as well as civil liability.

Medicaid Fraud

The court in *State of North Carolina v. Beatty*, 308 S.E.2d 65 (N.C. Ct. App. 1983), upheld a lower court's finding that the evidence submitted against the defendant pharmacist was sufficient to sustain a conviction for Medicaid fraud. The state was billed for medications that were never dispensed, was billed for more medications than some patients received, and in some instances was billed for the more expensive trade name drugs when cheaper generic drugs were dispensed.

The pharmacists in *People v. Kendzia*, 103 A.D.2d 999, 478 N.Y.S.2d 209 (1984), were convicted of mishandling drugs, and they appealed. The court held that the evidence supported a finding that the pharmacists sold generic drugs in vials with brand name labels and was sufficient to support a conviction. Investigators, working undercover, had been provided with Medicaid cards and fictitious prescriptions requiring brand name drugs to be dispensed as written. Between April and October 1979 the investigators had taken the prescriptions to the pharmacy where they were filled with generic substitutions in vials with the brand name labels.

Revocation of License

The court held in *Heller v. Ambach*, 78 A.D.2d 951, 433 N.Y.S.2d 281 (1980), that violation of statutes relating to the sale of controlled substances by a pharmacist amounted to unprofessional conduct and that the revocation of the defendant's license was justified for the protection of the public.[12]

Inaccurate Records

The operator of a pharmacy, in a disciplinary proceeding before the California Board of Pharmacy, was found negligent because of inaccurate record keeping in *Banks v. Board of Pharmacy*, 207 Cal. Rptr. 835 (Cal. Ct. App. 1984). The pharmacist had failed to keep accurate records of dangerous drugs, report thefts by employees, and report a burglary of pharmacy drugs. Such reporting was required by state statute.

PHYSICAL THERAPY

Physical therapy is the art and science of preventing and treating neuro-muscular or musculo-skeletal disabilities through the evaluation of an individual's disability and rehabilitation potential; the utilization of physical agents: heat, cold, electricity, water, and light; and neuromuscular procedures that, through their physiological effect, improve or maintain the patient's optimum functional level.

Because the aging process brings about a variety of physical disabilities, physical therapy is an extremely important component of a resident's total health care.

Common sense must prevail in the care of elderly residents. A lack of basic judgment is often the cause of problems for health professionals, as is illustrated in the following case.

A disciplinary proceeding was brought against a licensed physical therapist employed by a nursing facility for resident neglect. The therapist brought an Article 78 proceeding for judicial review. The proceeding was transferred to the Appellate Division by order of the Supreme Court, in *Zucker v. Axelrod*, 527 N.Y.S.2d 937 (N.Y. App. Div. 1988). The physical therapist in this case had been charged with resident neglect for refusing to allow an 82-year-old nursing facility resident to go to the bathroom before starting his therapy treatment session. Undisputed evidence at a hearing showed that the petitioner refused to allow the resident to be excused to the bathroom. The petitioner claimed that her refusal was based on the fact that she assumed that the resident had gone to the bathroom before going to therapy and that the resident was undergoing a bladder training program. The petitioner had not mentioned when she was interviewed following the incident or during her hearing testimony that she considered bladder training a basis for refusing to allow the resident to go to the bathroom. It is uncontroverted that the nursing facility had a policy of allowing residents to go to the bathroom whenever they wished to do so. The court held that the finding of resident neglect was sufficiently supported by the evidence.

PHYSICIAN'S ASSISTANT

Federal regulations under OBRA provide that a physician may delegate certain tasks to a physician's assistant. A physician may not delegate a task when regulations specify that the physician must perform it personally, or when the delegation is prohibited under state law or by the facility's own policies.[13] One of the solutions to the shortage of physicians in certain rural and inner-city areas has been to train allied health professionals such as a physician's assistant to perform the more routine and repetitive medical functions. The physician's assistant performs such tasks as suturing minor wounds, administering injections, and performing routine history and physical examinations. Physician's assistants are responsible for their own negligent acts. If the assistants are employees, employers can be held responsible on the basis of respondeat superior. A physician, as an employer of a physician's assistant, can also be held liable on the basis of respondeat superior.

Residents should be informed when a physician's assistant is assisting in their care; they must not be misled into thinking that they are being cared for by a physician.

In order to limit the potential risk of liability to a physician's assistant, the physician should closely monitor and supervise the assistant's work. Guidelines and procedures should also be established in order to provide a standard mechanism for reviewing an assistant's performance.

It is of interest that in *Washington State Nurses Association v. Board of Medical Examiners*, 605 P.2d 1269 (Wash. 1980), the nurses association brought an action challenging a regulation that authorized physician's assistants to issue prescriptions for medication and write medical orders for patient care. The trial court enjoined the board from effectuating the regulation, and the board appealed. The Washington Supreme Court held that the regulation did not exceed the statutory authority of the board, since statutes and regulations placed physician's assistants in the position of agent for their supervising physician, rather than of independent contractor, and thus nurses would not be exposed to statutory liability for executing prescriptions issued by physician's assistants.

RECREATION SERVICES

Recreation therapists plan and coordinate recreational activities for residents and supervise community volunteers. All facility volunteers should be trained as to policies and procedures applicable to them. Training should include a review of resident rights and the facility's health and safety policies.

RADIOLOGY SERVICES

OBRA requirements provide that a nursing facility must provide or obtain radiology and other diagnostic services to meet the needs of its residents. The facility is responsible for the quality and timeliness of the services. If the facility provides its own diagnostic services, the services must meet the applicable conditions of participation for hospitals. If the facility does not provide diagnostic services on site, it must have an agreement to obtain such services from a provider or supplier that is approved to provide such services under Medicare.[14]

REHABILITATIVE SERVICES

Nursing facilities should provide or obtain rehabilitative services, such as audiology, speech therapy, speech–language pathology, and occupational therapy, to every resident it admits. Services rendered should be in accordance with the resident's comprehensive plan to obtain or maintain the highest practicable physical well-being in accordance with generally accepted standards of rehabilitative care and services. Under OBRA:

> (a) Level B requirement: Provision of services.
>
> If specialized rehabilitative services are required in the resident's comprehensive plan of care, the facility must—

(1) Provide the required services; or
(2) Obtain the required services from an outside resource . . . .

(b) Level B requirement: Qualifications.

Specialized rehabilitative services must be provided under the written order of a physician by qualified personnel.[15]

RESPIRATORY THERAPY

The Health Care Financing Administration's survey process for determining eligibility for participation in the federal Medicare and Medicaid programs includes a review of a nursing facility's respiratory therapy services. The surveyors must determine that the facility is providing respiratory care by qualified persons with appropriate and safe equipment as ordered by the physician. During the survey process, surveyors will focus on the equipment, interview residents and staff, and review facility records.

Equipment

In order to determine that the necessary equipment is available, the surveyor will look for the following:

- Aerosol compressor or IPPB machine. Check that the machine is clean and operable.
- Tubing. (If tubing is not attached to the machine, ask to see it.) Check that it is stored dry and with consideration for cleanliness.
- Nebulizer cup. (If it is not attached to the tubing, ask to see it.) It should be filled with either the prescribed medicine or distilled water only if about to be used. It should not be stored wet.[16]

Resident Interview

Resident interviews could include the following questions:

- Do you ever feel short of breath?
- If yes, what is done when this occurs?
- Is the therapy helping you to feel better?
- Are there any problems with it?
- If so, how does the staff respond?

- Is the therapy consistently performed—both concerning time and method of providing it?[17]

Staff Interview

Staff interviews could include the following questions:

- What is the reason the resident is getting this therapy?
- What are the expected results?
- Can you demonstrate how you use the equipment?
- How often is the equipment cleaned?
- What are the infection control procedures in regard to use of respiratory equipment?
- Where is the emergency oxygen supply?[18]

Record Review

The surveyors will conduct a review of selected medical records. Items to be reviewed include

- whether respiratory/oxygen therapy is performed by appropriately trained staff
- whether there is a physician's order for therapy, that is specific as to rate of delivery, etc.
- if the physician's order is for PRN therapy, whether it specifies for what symptoms
- whether any information gained from resident or staff is verified in the record
- whether the assessment addresses both the need or reason for therapy and any problems or limitations which result from the need for therapy
- the kind, amount, frequency, and/or duration of therapy based on the physician's order
- specific goals to overcome to improve any identified problems and/or limitations[19]

Survey Evaluation Factors

Other factors to be evaluated by the surveyors include whether

- only qualified (trained) personnel should administer/assist with respiratory therapy

- therapy is provided as ordered
- the effectiveness of the therapy is periodically evaluated and therapy is revised as appropriate
- effective infection control measures are practiced
- needed safety precaution for the use of oxygen are practiced
- equipment is available and in working order[20]

Case Review

The court in *Poor Sisters of St. Francis v. Catron*, 435 N.E.2d 305 (Ind. Ct. App. 1982), held that the failure of nurses and an inhalation therapist to report to the supervisor that an endotracheal tube had been left in the plaintiff longer than the customary period of three or four days was sufficient to allow the jury to reach a finding of negligence. The patient experienced difficulty speaking and underwent several operations to remove scar tissue and open her voice box. At the time of trial, she could not speak above a whisper and breathed partially through a hole in her throat created by a tracheotomy. The hospital was found liable for the negligent acts of its employees and the resulting injuries to the plaintiff.

CERTIFICATION OF HEALTH CARE PROFESSIONALS

The certification of health care professionals is the recognition by a governmental or professional association that an individual's expertise meets the standards of that group. The standards established by professional associations generally exceed those required by government agencies. Some professional groups establish their own minimum standards for certification in those professions that are not licensed by a particular state. Certification by an association or group is a self-regulation credentialing process.

LICENSING OF HEALTH CARE PROFESSIONALS

Licensure can be defined as the process by which some competent authority grants permission to a qualified individual or entity to perform certain specified activities that would be illegal without a license. As it applies to health personnel, licensure refers to the process by which licensing boards, agencies, or departments of the several states grant to individuals who meet certain predetermined standards the legal right to practice in a health profession and to use a specified health practitioner's title.

The commonly stated objectives of licensing laws are to limit and control admission to the various health occupations and to protect the public from unqualified practitioners by promulgating and enforcing standards of practice within the professions.

The authority of states to license health care practitioners is found in their regulating power. Implicit in the power to license is the authority to collect license fees, establish standards of practice, require certain minimum qualifications and competency levels of applicants, and impose on applicants other requirements necessary to protect the general public welfare. This authority, which is vested in the legislature, may be delegated to political subdivisions or to state boards, agencies, and departments. In some instances, the scope of the delegated power is made quite specific in the legislation; in others, the licensing authority may have wide discretion in performing its functions. In either case, however, the authority granted by the legislature may not be exceeded.

CONCLUSION

As with physicians and nurses, the need for continuing education and training in the care of the elderly is an ever-present need for all allied health professionals. There is a

> . . . growing recognition that today's health professionals need to be prepared to deal with the ethical, legal, and economic constraints that modern medicine technologies bring to the fore. There is increased attention to the fact that decisionmaking about life-sustaining technologies demands caregivers who understand and are sensitive to ethical and humanitarian principles. These caregivers must not only know their profession and understand the patient population, they must show good judgment and caring, respect for patients' wishes, communication skills, ability to work as part of a health care team, and readiness to help even when healing is no longer possible.[21]

NOTES

1. U.S. Congress, Office of Technology Assessment, Life-Sustaining Technologies and the Elderly 377 Pub. No. OTA-BA-306 (1987).
2. *Direct Medicare Pay for Rural Mid-Level Providers Urged*, 27(1) AHA News, January 7, 1991, at 2.
3. U.S. Congress, Office of Technology Assessment, *supra* note 1, at 364.
4. *Id.* at 366.
5. 42 C.F.R. §483.55 (1990).
6. C.L. Johnson, L.A. Grant, The Nursing Home in American Society 128 (1985).
7. 42 C.F.R. §483.35 (1990).
8. 42 C.F.R. §483.75 (1990).
9. The Nursing Home in American Society, at 127.
10. 42 C.F.R. §483.60 (1990).
11. 42 C.F.R. §483.60 (1990).
12. *See also* Kupper v. Kentucky Board of Pharmacy, 666 S.W.2d 729 (Ky. 1984).

13. 42 C.F.R. §483.40 (1990).
14. 42 C.F.R. §483.75 (1990).
15. 42 C.F.R. §483.45 (1990).
16. 42 C.F.R. §488.115 (1989).
17. *Id.*
18. *Id.*
19. *Id.*
20. *Id.*
21. *Id.* at 357.

Chapter 10

Consent

Consent is the voluntary agreement by a person in the possession and exercise of sufficient mentality to make an intelligent choice to allow something proposed by another (e.g., administration of medication, performance of a procedure). Authorization for a touching is referred to as patient consent. Consent changes a touching that what would otherwise be nonconsensual to one that is consensual. It can be either express or implied.

Express consent can take the form of a verbal agreement to undergo a medical procedure or it can be accomplished through the execution of a signed consent form. In modern health care, written consent is the preferred method of obtaining consent.

Implied consent is consent that is manifested by some action or by the inaction of silence, which raises a presumption that consent has been authorized.

Consent must first be obtained from a patient, or from a person authorized to consent on a patient's behalf, before any medical procedure can be performed. Every individual has a right to refuse to authorize a touching. A touching of another without authorization to do so could be considered a battery. A competent patient's refusal must be adhered to, whether the refusal is grounded upon lack of confidence in the physician, fear of the procedure, doubt as to the value of a particular procedure or mere whim. If a patient asserts that a touching was unauthorized, it will be necessary to prove that a consent was obtained in order to avoid liability for the unwanted touching.

In the process of caring for residents in a nursing facility, it is inevitable that they will be touched and handled. Most touchings are generally routine and are performed by unskilled personnel. Typical touchings include bathing, dressing, or rendering assistance in and out of wheelchairs. Resident care may also include skilled care for such things as administering intravenous injections, irrigating wounds, inserting catheters, etc.

Not every touching results in a battery. When a person voluntarily enters a situation in which a reasonably prudent person would anticipate a touching (e.g., riding in an elevator or being transported as a resident), consent is implied. Consent is not required for the normal, everyday touching and bumping that occurs in life.

The law does require consent for the intentional touching that involves medical procedures to be performed, although exceptions do exist with respect to emergency situations. The question of liability for performing a procedure without consent is separate and distinct from any question of negligence or malpractice in performing a procedure. Liability may be imposed for a nonconsensual touching of a resident even if the procedure improved the patient's health. The eminent Justice Cardozo, in *Schloendorff v. Society of New York Hospital*, 211 N.Y. 125, 105 N.E. 92, (1914), stated

> Every human being of adult years and sound mind has a right to determine what shall be done with his own body and a surgeon who performs an operation without his patient's consent commits an assault, for which he is liable in damages, except in cases of emergency where the patient is unconscious and where it is necessary to operate before consent can be obtained.

211 N.Y. at 129, 105 N.E. at 93.

INFORMED CONSENT

An authorization from a resident, without an understanding of what he or she is consenting to, is not effective consent. Informed consent is a legal term that refers to a person consenting to a proposed medical intervention after being provided information deemed necessary to make that decision. Informed consent requires that a resident have a full understanding of that to which he or she has consented.

Some courts have recognized that the condition of the resident may be taken into account to determine whether the resident has received sufficient information. The person seeking consent, usually the attending physician, must weigh the importance of giving full disclosure to the resident against the likelihood that such disclosure will seriously and adversely affect the condition of the resident.

An elderly nursing facility resident suffering from hypertension could very well receive a modified disclosure if the attending physician has reason to believe that a full explanation of a contemplated treatment could aggravate the hypertension, which in turn could have a detrimental affect on the body systems already impaired by age or illness. A modified disclosure consistent with the resident's condition may be adequate if it can be shown that other physicians in the community would have also made a modified disclosure.

Residents must be given sufficient information to allow them to make intelligent choices from among the various alternative courses of available treatment for their specific ailments. They have a right to refuse a specific course of treatment even if the medical procedure is advisable. Residents have a right to be secure in their persons from any touching, and they are free to reject recommended treatment.

A physician should provide as much information about treatment options as is necessary based on a resident's personal understanding of the physician's explanation of the risks of treatment and the probable consequences of the treatment. The needs of each resident can vary depending on age, maturity, and mental status. A resident instituting a lawsuit would have to show that he or she was provided information insufficient for informed consent. Physicians are reminded that residents are concerned with the risks of death and bodily harm. Taking the time to sit at a resident's bedside and explain a resident treatment plan will produce a first-rate physician–resident relationship and most likely result in fewer lawsuits.

When questions do arise as to whether or not adequate consent has been given, some courts take into consideration the information that is ordinarily provided by other physicians. A plaintiff suing under the theory of informed consent must prove:

1. The defendant physician failed to adequately inform the plaintiff of a material risk before securing his or her consent to a proposed treatment.
2. If the plaintiff had been informed of the risk, he or she would not have consented to the treatment.
3. The adverse consequences that were not made known did in fact occur.
4. The plaintiff was injured as a result of submitting to treatment.

With regard to material risk, the court in *Scott v. Bradford*, 606 P.2d 554 (Okla. 1979), noted that "[t]here is no bright line separating the material from the immaterial, it is a question of fact. A risk is material if it would be likely to affect a patient's decision. When non-disclosure of a particular risk is open to debate, the issue is for the finder of the facts." *Id.* at 558. Since this decision imposed a new duty on physicians with respect to disclosure of the risk of treatment, the opinion was ordered to apply prospectively, affecting those causes of action arising after the date this opinion was promulgated.

PROOF OF CONSENT

Oral consent, if proved, is as binding as written consent for there is, in general, no legal requirement that a resident's consent be in writing. However, an oral consent is generally more difficult to corroborate. Written consent provides visible proof of a resident's wishes. A valid written consent must: (1) indicate the procedure or treatment consented to; (2) indicate that the patient understands the nature of any treatment, the alternatives, the risks involved, and the probable consequences of the proposed treatment; and (3) be dated, signed and witnessed.

The nurse, as well as other health professionals, has an important role in the realm of informed consent. He or she can be instrumental in averting major lawsuits by being observant as to doubts, changes of mind, confusion, or misunderstandings expressed by a resident regarding any proposed procedures he or she is about to undergo.

Since the function of a written consent form is to preserve evidence of informed consent, the nature of the treatment and the risks and consequences involved should be incorporated into the form. States have taken the view that consent, in order to be effective, must be an "informed consent."

General Consent

A general written consent form should be properly executed at the time of a resident's admission to a nursing facility. The general consent form records the resident's consent to routine services, general diagnostic procedures, medical treatment, and the everyday routine touchings of the resident. The admitting office should explain to the resident or his or her guardian the need for the consent form. The danger from its use arises from the potential of unwarranted reliance upon it for specific potentially high risk procedures or treatments.

Special Consent

A special consent form should be executed where a proposed treatment program may involve some unusual risk(s) to the resident, such as the use of restraints. (See Appendix B for an example of a restraint form.) A list of procedures and treatments requiring special written consent should be maintained and appropriate consent forms utilized by the nursing and medical staff. The special consent form should be signed, dated, and witnessed at the time the physician explains to the resident the procedure he plans to perform. An informed consent form should include the following elements:

- the nature of the resident's illness or injury
- the nature and purpose of the proposed treatment
- the risks of the proposed treatment
- the probability that the proposed treatment will be successful
- any alternative methods of treatment and their associated risks and benefits
- the risks and prognosis if no treatment is rendered
- the signatures of the patient, physician, and witnesses
- the date the consent is signed

Nursing facility personnel and physicians should be alert to any changes in a resident's decision or attitude to undergo a specified procedure or treatment after the consent is signed. In order for special consents to be effective, they should be signed within a reasonable period of time prior to a scheduled procedure or treatment.

Nonroutine Inoculations

A special form should be completed as part of a nursing facility program, such as an annual flu inoculation program. Inoculation should not be considered merely as a routine service of the facility and should be carried out under the supervision of a physician.

Experimental Procedures and Investigational Drugs

A written special consent form for the use of investigational drugs must be obtained from the resident. Federal regulations require that the nature of the drug and possible adverse consequences be explained.

Federal regulations control federal grants that apply to experiments involving new drugs, new medical devices, or new medical procedures. Generally, a combination of federal and state guidelines and regulations ensures proper supervision and control over research that involves human subjects. For example, federal regulations provide that a "resident has a right to refuse treatment, and to refuse to participate in experimental research."[1] Institutions conducting medical research on human subjects must fully disclose the inherent risks to the resident, make a proper determination that the resident is competent to consent, identify treatment alternatives, and obtain written consent from the resident.

Survey Process. The Health Care Financing Administration (HCFA) survey process includes a review of the rights of any residents participating in experimental research. Surveyor/s will review the records of residents identified as participating in a clinical research study. They will determine whether or not informed consent forms have been properly executed. The form itself will be reviewed to determine if all known risks have been identified. Appropriate questions may be directed to both the staff and residents or the residents' guardians. Questions may be directed to both residents and guardians and staff.

Possible questions to ask staff include

- Is the facility participating in any experimental research?
- If yes, what residents are involved? (Interview a sample of these residents.)[2]

Residents or guardians may be asked questions such as

- Are you participating in the__________study?
- Was this explained to you well enough so that you understand what the study is about and any risks that might be involved?[3]

Residents participating in research studies should fully understand the implications of the study. A nursing facility will not be found in compliance with the resident rights regulations if a resident consents to participate in a clinical study without full knowledge of the study.[4]

California has enacted legislation that protects the rights of research subjects and provides for fines and imprisonment if proper consent procedures are not followed. California Health & Safety Code §§24170–24179.5, 26668.4.

The court in *Blanton v. United States*, 428 F. Supp. 360 (D.C. 1977), held that where a "new drug" of unknown effectiveness was administered to a patient at a navy medical center, despite the availability of other drugs of known effectiveness, the hospital violated the accepted medical standards and its duty of due care, so that in the absence of the patient's consent to the experiment, the United States was liable for the resulting injury.

NURSING FACILITY LIABILITY

A nursing facility can be held liable if a medical procedure is performed without consent. It is the nursing facility's duty to protect a resident when it knows or should know of a resident's objections to a medical procedure. Under the doctrine of respondeat superior a nursing facility is liable for any wrongs of its employees while they are performing their duties. Treatment without consent is clearly a battery, and if performed by facility personnel the facility would be liable.

WHO MAY CONSENT

Consent of the resident is ordinarily required before treatment. However, when the resident is either physically unable or legally incompetent to consent and no emergency exists, consent must be obtained from a person who is empowered to consent on the resident's behalf. The person who authorizes the treatment of another must have sufficient information to make an intelligent judgment on behalf of the resident.

Competent Residents

A competent adult resident's wishes concerning his or her person may not generally be disregarded. The court in *In re Melideo*, 88 Misc. 2d 974, 390 N.Y.S.2d 523 (N.Y. Sup. Ct. 1976), held that every human being of adult years has a right to determine what shall be done with his or her own body and cannot be subjected to medical treatment without his or her consent. Where there is no compelling state interest that justifies overriding an adult resident's decision, that decision should be respected.

Only a compelling state interest will justify interference with an individual's free exercise of religious beliefs. If there is no compelling state interest to justify overriding a resident's intelligent and knowing refusal to consent to a medical procedure because of his or her religious beliefs, states are reluctant to override such a decision. The court in *In re Fosmire v. Nicoleau*, No. 267 (N.Y. January 18, 1990) took the position that citizens of the state have long had the right to make their own medical care choices without regard to their medical condition or status as parents. The court of appeals held that a competent adult has both a common law and statutory right to refuse life-saving treatment.

Consent of Minors

The question of whether the consent of a minor is sufficient, and if not from whom consent should be obtained, seems to be more applicable to hospitals than to nursing facilities. In those instances where minors are admitted to a nursing facility, the consent of the minor's parent or someone standing in loco parentis must be secured. Although parental consent should be obtained prior to the admission of a minor, specific parental consent should be sought for any non-routine services rendered to the minor. Parental consent is not necessary where the minor is married or otherwise emancipated. Most states have enacted statutes making it valid for married and emancipated minors to provide effective consent.

Some states have nursing facilities specializing in the care of minors. These states generally have special licensing requirements for such facilities.

Guardian

A guardian is an individual who by law is invested with the power and charged with the duty of taking care of a resident by protecting the resident's rights and managing the resident's estate. Guardianship is often necessary in those instances where a resident is incapable of managing or administering his or her private affairs due to physical and/or mental disabilities or because he or she is under the age of majority. Temporary guardianship can be granted by the courts if it is determined that such is necessary for the well-being of the resident.

Temporary guardianship was granted by the court in *In re Estate of Dorone*, 534 A.2d 452 (Pa. 1987), where the physician and administrator petitioned the court on two occasions for authority to administer blood. The patient's treatment required the administration of blood, which the parents would not consent to because of their religious beliefs. Following a hearing by telephone, the court of common pleas appointed the administrator as temporary guardian. The superior court affirmed the orders, and the parents appealed. The court held that the judge's decisions granting guardianship and the authority to consent to the administration of blood were considered absolutely necessary in light of the facts of the case. Nothing less than a fully conscious contemporary decision by the patient himself would have been sufficient to override the evidence of medical necessity.

See Chapter 13, "Euthanasia, Death, and Dying," for a discussion of living wills, health care proxies, and durable powers of attorney.

Consent of the Mentally Ill

A person who is mentally incompetent cannot legally consent to medical or surgical treatment. Therefore, the consent of the legal guardian must be obtained. Where no legal guardian is available, a court that handles such matters must be petitioned to permit treatment.

Subject to applicable statutory provisions, when a physician doubts a resident's capacity to consent, even though the resident has not been judged legally incompetent, the consent of the nearest relative should be obtained. If a resident is conscious and mentally capable of giving consent for treatment, the consent of a relative without the consent of the competent resident would not protect the physician from liability.

Incompetent Residents

The definition of legal incompetence varies from state to state. In most jurisdictions, the test utilized by the court to determine incompetence and the need for guardianship is either (1) the ability to make or communicate responsible decisions or (2) the ability to manage one's own property and/or care for oneself. The most frequently cited conditions indicative of incompetence are mental illness, mental retardation, senility, physical incapacity, and chronic alcohol or drug abuse. A number of states also include a spendthrift provision defining certain practices that waste the assets of the estate as evidence of incompetence. A handful of states permit the appointment of a guardian to protect mental incompetents. It should be noted that a resident who is not competent to manage his property may very well be competent to refuse medical care.

The ability to consent to treatment is a question of fact. The attending physician, who is in the best position to make the determination, should become familiar with his or her state's definition of legal incompetence. In any case where the physician doubts a patient's capacity to consent, the consent of the nearest relative should be obtained. If there are no relatives to consult, application should be made for a court order that would allow the procedure. It may be the duty of the court to assume responsibility of guardianship for a resident who is non compos mentis.

A resident who is mentally incompetent cannot legally consent to medical care. The consent of the resident's legal guardian must, therefore, be obtained. When the legal guardian is unavailable to authorize necessary treatment, a court may be requested to authorize the procedure.

IMPLIED CONSENT

Implied consent generally exists when immediate action is required to save a resident's life or to prevent permanent impairment of a resident's health. If it is impossible in an emergency to obtain the consent of the resident or someone legally authorized to give consent, the required procedure may be undertaken without liability for failure to procure consent. This privilege to proceed in emergencies without consent is accorded physicians because inaction at such times may cause greater injury to the resident and would be contrary to good medical practice.

Unconscious residents are presumed under law to approve treatment that appears to be necessary. It is assumed that such residents would have consented if they were conscious and competent. However, if a resident expressly refuses to consent to certain treatment, such treatment may not be employed after the resident becomes unconscious. Similarly, conscious residents suffering from emergency conditions retain the right to refuse consent. If a procedure is necessary to protect one's life or health, documentation justifying the need to treat prior to obtaining informed consent should be maintained.

Consent can also be implied in non-emergency situations. For example, a person may voluntarily submit to a procedure, implying consent, without any explicitly spoken or written expression of consent. In *O'Brien v. Cunard Steam Ship Co.*, 154 Mass. 272, 28 N.E. 266 (1891), a ship's passenger who joined a line of people receiving injections was held to have implied his consent to a vaccination. The rationale for this decision is that individuals who observe a line of people and who notice that injections are being administered to those at the head of the line should expect that if they join and remain in the line they will receive an injection. Therefore, the voluntary act of entering the line and the plaintiff's opportunity to see what was taking place at the head of the line were accepted by the jury as manifestations of consent to the injection. The O'Brien case contains all the elements necessary to imply consent from a voluntary act: the procedure was a simple vaccination, the proceedings were at all times visible, and the plaintiff was free to withdraw up to the instant of the injection.

Whether or not a resident's consent can be implied may be asked when the condition of a resident requires some deviation from an agreed-on treatment. If a resident expressly prohibits a specific treatment, consent cannot be implied.

Every effort must be made to document the medical need for proceeding with medical treatment without consent. It must be shown that the actual emergency situation actually constituted an immediate threat to life or health.

Many states have adopted legislation concerning emergency care that deals with consent. An emergency situation in most states eliminates the need for consent. When a resident's life is in jeopardy and he or she is clinically unable to give consent to a life saving emergency treatment, the law implies consent on the presumption that a reasonable person would consent to life saving emergency treatment.

When an emergency situation does arise, there may be little opportunity to contact the attending physician, much less a consultant. The resident's records must, therefore, be complete with respect to the description of his or her illness and condition, the attempts made to contact the physician as well as relatives, and the emergency measures taken and procedures performed. If a relative refuses to consent, it may be necessary to seek a court order. If time does not permit a court order to be obtained, a second medical opinion, when practicable, is advisable.

REFUSAL OF TREATMENT

Adult residents who are conscious and mentally competent have the right to refuse medical care to the extent permitted by law even when the best medical opinion deems it essential to life. Such a refusal must be honored whether it is grounded in religious belief or mere whim. Every person has the legal right to refuse to permit a touching of his or her body. Failure to respect this right can result in a legal action for assault and battery. If a resident refuses consent, every effort should be made to explain the importance of the procedure. Coercion through threat, duress, or intimidation must be avoided.

The patient's refusal should be noted on the medical record and a release form should be executed. The best possible care must be rendered to the resident at all times within the limits imposed by the resident's refusal. Such refusal is a defense to a lawsuit against the nursing facility and/or the physician for not administering necessary treatment.

When a resident refuses to consent for any reason, religious or otherwise, a release form should be completed to protect the facility and its personnel from liability. A notation should be placed on the resident's medical record when treatment (e.g., administration of medications) is refused. The completed release form provides documented evidence of a patient's refusal to consent to a recommended treatment. Should a resident refuse to sign the release form, this should be noted on the resident's medical record. It is advisable that the advice of legal counsel be sought in those cases where refusal of treatment poses a serious threat to a resident's health.

It is advisable that, with the advice of legal counsel, the nursing facility formulate a policy regarding treatment when consent has been refused. An administrative procedure should be developed to facilitate application for a court order when one is necessary and there is sufficient time to obtain one. Even though a signed consent form may not unequivocally constitute proof that informed consent was obtained from a resident, it does create a presumption that it was, thereby shifting the burden of responsibility to the resident to prove that it was not.

NOTES

1. 42 C.F.R. §483.10 (1989).
2. 42 C.F.R. §488.115 (1989).
3. *Id.*
4. *Id.*

Chapter 11

Resident Rights and Responsibilities

Every individual possesses certain rights guaranteed by the Constitution of the United States and its Amendments, including freedom of speech, religion, and association and the right not to be discriminated against on the grounds of race, color, creed, or national origin. The Supreme Court has interpreted the Constitution as also guaranteeing certain other rights not expressly mentioned, such as the right to privacy and the right to travel. Variations of these rights appear in the federal version and state versions of the resident's bill of rights. These rights are not automatically waived upon entering a health care facility.

Individuals also have responsibilities, such as the duty to obey the law and the duty to refrain from injuring others. Specific responsibilities of residents of health care facilities are discussed later in this chapter.

RESIDENT RIGHTS

The continuing trend of consumer awareness coupled with increased governmental regulations makes it advisable for every administrator and staff member to understand the scope of the resident's rights and how to ensure them. "OBRA 1987 made significant changes in federal oversight of state protection of nursing home residents. Facilities may no longer merely passively permit residents to exercise their rights, but must 'protect and promote' such rights."[1]

Persons entering a nursing home continue to have the same civil and property rights they had before entering the home. Nursing facilities participating in the Medicare and Medicaid programs must have established residents' rights policies. A large number of documents have been prepared on the national and state levels regarding resident rights. A suggested format for a "Resident's Bill of Rights" is included in Appendix C.

During a nursing facility survey, surveyors will determine whether a resident maintains, in so far as possible, those personal rights that are part of normal adult life, including the right to personal dignity. In the confusion surrounding admission to a facility and the extensive amount of information provided to a new resident and family, information transmitted at this time is often forgotten. As a result, the surveyors are asked to verify the resident's recollection of his or her rights through staff interview and record checks (e.g., admission records can be checked to determine whether the resident signed a document indicating receipt of resident rights upon admission, and social work records may indicate whether or not resident rights information were reviewed with the resident). Copies of residents' rights should be available to residents and visitors in such areas as resident lounges, lobbies, or other areas where residents and visitors could easily see and read them. The Health Care Financing Administration (HCFA) survey process may include the following questions by surveyors to residents regarding their rights:

- Did you receive a copy of the Resident's Bill of Rights? Was it explained to you?
- Were you told of any responsibilities you have in living here?
- Were you given a chance to ask questions?
- Did you receive a written copy of services provided by the facility and any additional costs for these services?
- If there are changes in services or costs, does someone explain these?[2]

The administrative staff may be asked such questions as:

- How do residents learn what is expected of them?
- How do they learn about any changes in the facility's procedures and/or costs?[3]

Residents' rights may be classified as either legal—those emanating from law—or human—statements of desirable principles, such as the right to health care or the right to be treated with human dignity. Both staff and residents should be aware and understand not only their own rights and responsibilities but also the rights and responsibilities of the other.

In recognition of the difficulties of self-regulation, the federal government and several state governments began taking steps to protect the rights of residents by including residents' rights in laws or regulations. The resident has a right to a dignified existence, self-determination, and communication with and access to persons and services inside and outside the facility. Each facility under federal regulations must protect and promote the rights of residents, including each of the following rights:

(a) Level B requirements: Exercise of rights.
(1) The resident has the right to exercise his or her rights as a resident of the facility and as a citizen or resident of the United States.
(2) The resident has the right to be free of interference, coercion, discrimination, or reprisal from the facility in exercising his or her rights.

(3) In the case of a resident adjudged incompetent under the laws of a state by a court of competent jurisdiction, the rights of the resident are exercised by the person appointed under State law to act on the resident's behalf.

(b) Level B requirement: Notice of rights and services.

(1) The facility must inform the residents both orally and in writing in a language that the resident understands of his or her rights and all rules and regulations governing resident conduct and responsibilities during the stay in the facility. Such notification must be made prior to or upon admission and during the resident's stay. Receipt of such information, and any amendments to it, must be acknowledged in writing;

(2) The resident has the right to inspect and purchase photocopies of all records pertaining to the resident, upon written request and 48 hours notice to the facility;

(3) The resident has the right to be fully informed in language that he or she can understand of his or her total health status, including but not limited to, his or her medical condition;

(4) The resident has a right to refuse treatment, and to refuse to participate in experimental research; and

(5) The facility must—

(i) Inform each resident who is entitled to Medicaid benefits, in writing, at the time of admission to the nursing facility, or when the resident becomes eligible for Medicaid of—

(A) The items and services that are included in nursing facility services under the State plan for which the resident may not be charged;

(B) Those other items and services that the facility offers and for which the resident may be charged, and the amount of charges for those services; and

(ii) Inform each resident when changes are made to the items and services specified in paragraphs (5)(i)(A) and (B) of this section.

(6) The facility must inform each resident before, or at the time of the admission, and periodically during the resident's stay, of services available in the facility and of charges for those services, including any charges for services not covered under Medicare or by the facility's per diem rate.

(7) The facility must furnish a written description of legal rights which includes—

(i) A description of the manner of protecting personal funds, under paragraph (c) of this section; and

(ii) A statement that the resident may file a complaint with the State survey and certification agency concerning resident abuse, neglect, and misappropriation of resident property in the facility.

(8) The facility must inform each resident of the name, speciality and way of contacting the physician responsible for his or her care.

(9) Effective October 1, 1990, the facility must prominently display in the facility written information, and provide to residents and potential residents oral and written information about how to apply for and use Medicare and Medicaid benefits, and how to receive funds for previous payments covered by such benefits.

(10) Notification of changes. (i) Except in a medical emergency or when a resident is incompetent, the facility must consult with the resident immediately and notify the resident's physician, and if known, the resident's legal representative or interested family member within 24 hours when there is—

(A) An accident involving the resident which results in injury;

(B) A significant change in the resident's physical, mental or psychosocial status;

(C) A need to alter treatment significantly; or

(D) A decision to transfer or discharge the resident from the facility as specified in Sec. 483.12(a).

(ii) The facility must also promptly notify the resident and, if known, the resident's legal representative or interested family member when there is—

(A) A change in room or roommate assignment as specified in Sec. 483.15(e)(2); or

(B) A change in resident rights under Federal or State law or regulations as specified in Sec. 483.10(b)(1).

(iii) The facility must record and periodically update the address and phone number of the resident's legal representative or interested family member.

* * *

(d) Level B requirement: Free choice.

The resident has a right to—

(1) Choose a personal attending physician;

(2) Be fully informed in advance about care and treatment and of any changes in that care or treatment that may affect the resident's well-being; and

(3) Unless adjudged incompetent or otherwise found to be incapacitated under the laws of the state, participate in planning care and treatment or changes in care and treatment.

* * *

(g) Level B requirement: Examination of survey results.

A resident has the right to—

(1) Examine the results of the most recent survey of the facility conducted by Federal or State surveyors and any plan of correction in effect with respect to the facility. The results must be posted by the facility in a place readily accessible to residents; and
(2) Receive information from agencies acting as client advocates, and be afforded the opportunity to contact these agencies.
(h) Level B requirement: Work.

The resident has the right to—

(1) Refuse to perform services for the facility;
(2) Perform services for the facility, if he or she chooses, when—
(i) The facility has documented the need or desire for work in the plan of care;
(ii) The plan specifies the nature of the services performed whether the services are voluntary or paid;
(iii) Compensation for paid services is at or above prevailing rates; and
(iv) The resident agrees to the work arrangement described in the plan of care.
(i) Level B requirement: Mail.

The resident has a right to privacy in written communications . . . .

* * *

(k) Level B requirement: Access and visitation rights.
(1) The resident has the right and the facility must provide immediate access to any resident . . . .

* * *

(l) Level B requirement: Telephone.
The resident has the right to have regular access to the private use of a telephone.
(m) Level B requirement: Personal property.
The resident has a right to retain and use personal possessions, including some furnishings, and appropriate clothing, as space permits, unless to do so would infringe upon the rights or health and safety of other residents.
(n) Level B requirements: Married couples.
The resident has a right to share a room with his or her spouse when married residents live in the same facility and both spouses consent to the arrangement.

(o) Level B requirement: Self-administration of drugs. Each resident has the right to self-administer drugs unless the interdisciplinary team, as defined . . . has determined for each resident that this practice is unsafe.[4]

Nearly every state has addressed one or more residents' rights issues in their licensing laws. The following excerpt from the New York State Nursing Home Code is generally consistent with documents regarding residents' rights in other states.

415.3 Residents' Rights

(a) The facility shall ensure that all residents are afforded their right to a dignified existence, self-determination, respect, full recognition of their individuality, consideration and privacy in treatment and care for personal needs and communication with and access to persons and services inside and outside the facility. The facility shall protect and promote the rights of each resident and encourage and assist each resident in the fullest possible exercise of these rights . . . The facility shall also consult with residents in establishing and implementing facility policies regarding residents' rights and responsibilities.

(1) The facility shall advise each member of the staff of his or her responsibility to understand, protect and promote the right of each resident as enumerated in this section.

(2) The facility shall fully inform the resident and the resident's designated representative both orally and in writing in a method of communication that the individuals understand the resident's rights and all rules and regulations governing resident conduct and responsibilities during the stay in the facility. Such notification shall be made prior to or upon admission and during the resident's stay. Receipt of such information, and any amendments to it, shall be acknowledged in writing. A summary of such information shall be provided by the Department and posted in the facility in large print and in language that is easily understood.

(3) The written information provided pursuant to paragraph (2) of this subdivision shall include but not be limited to a listing of those rights and facility responsibilities enumerated in subdivision (b) of this section. The facility's policies and procedures shall be provided to the resident and the resident's designated representative upon request.

(4) The facility shall communicate to the resident an explanation of his or her responsibility to obey all reasonable regulations of the facility and to respect the personal rights and private property of other residents.

(5) Any written information required by this part to be posted shall be posted conspicuously in a public place in the facility that is frequented by residents and visitors, posted at wheelchair height.[5]

Admission

At the time of admission, the resident should be informed, in writing, fully of his or her rights (see Appendix C for a sample copy of a resident's bill of rights) and responsibilities. This right to information is guaranteed by federal regulations governing nursing facilities receiving Medicaid funds. Federal regulations specify that the written statement of resident rights must include a copy of any state notice of the rights and obligations of residents under Medicaid.[6] If necessary, each resident has a right to have those rights explained to him/her.

(d) Level B requirement: Admissions Policy (effective October 1, 1990).

(1) The facility must—

(i) Not require a third party guarantee of payment to the facility as a condition of admission, or expedited admission, or continued stay in the facility;

(ii) Not charge, solicit, accept, or receive, in addition any amount otherwise required to be paid under the State plan, any gift, money, donation or other consideration as a precondition of admission, expedited admission or continued stay in the facility.

(2) A facility must—

(i) Not require residents or potential residents to waive their rights to Medicare or Medicaid;

(ii) Not require written or oral assurance that residents or potential residents are not eligible for, or will not apply for, Medicare or Medicaid benefits.

(3) States or political subdivisions may apply stricter admissions standards under State or local laws than specified in paragraphs (d)(1) and (2) of this section, to prohibit discrimination against individuals entitled to Medicaid benefits.

(4) A facility may require an individual who has legal access to a resident's income or resources available to pay for family care, to sign a contract, without incurring personal financial liability, to provide facility payment from the resident's income or resources.

(5) A nursing facility may charge a resident who is eligible for Medicaid for items and services the resident has requested and received, and that are not specified in the State plan as included in the term "nursing facility services."

(6) A nursing facility may solicit, accept or receive a charitable, religious or philanthropic contribution from an organization or from a person unrelated to the resident, or potential resident, but only to the extent that the contribution is not a condition of admission, expedited admission, or continued stay in the facility.[7]

Nursing facilities must not discriminate by reason of race, creed, color, sex, religion, or national origin. Those that do discriminate are in violation of constitutionally guaranteed rights. "State regulations requiring nursing homes to accept a reasonable number of indigent patients as a condition of licensure have been held constitutional." 52 A.L.R. 4TH 689, at 743 (1987). Discrimination in some states can be considered a misdemeanor and may also carry a civil penalty.

Most states have enacted laws to protect the civil rights of their citizens. Some of these statutes declare that life, liberty, and the pursuit of happiness should not be denied; others adhere closely to the language of federal civil rights legislation. State codes often provide regulations regarding the admission rights of residents. They may include such things as the prohibition of a third party guarantee of payment to the facility as a condition of admission, or expedited admission, or continued stay in the facility and the adherence to all pertinent state and local laws that prohibit discrimination against individuals entitled to Medicaid benefits.

Civil rights are rights assured by the United States Constitution and by the acts of Congress and the state legislatures. Generally, the term includes all the rights of each individual in a free society.

Discriminatory practices in health facilities have been dealt with by Congress and the federal courts. Discrimination in the admission of residents and segregation of residents on racial grounds are prohibited in any nursing facility receiving federal financial assistance. Pursuant to Title VI of the Civil Rights Act of 1964, the guidelines of the Department of Health and Human Services (HHS) prohibit the practice of racial discrimination by any health care facility or agency receiving money under any program supported by HHS. This includes all facilities that are "providers of service" receiving federal funds under Medicare legislation.

According to the Fourteenth Amendment to the Constitution, a state cannot act so as to deny any person equal protection of the laws. If a state or a political subdivision of a state, whether through its executive, judicial, or legislative branch, acts in such a way as to unfairly deny to any person the rights accorded to another, the amendment has been violated. If the state supports or authorizes an activity for the benefit of the public, it is possible that a private institution engaging in such activity will be considered to be engaged in state action and subject to the Fourteenth Amendment.

The acts of the executive, judicial, and legislative branches of government encompass the acts of government agencies as well, and state action has been extended to include activities of private entities under certain circumstances.

Considering the constitutional requirement together with HHS guidelines and the requirements of Title II of the Civil Rights Act of 1964, which prohibits discrimination in restaurants and other places of public accommodation and thus may include restaurants in a nursing facility, it is apparent that racial discrimination is prohibited in nursing facilities. The Civil Rights Act of 1964 specifies that health care workers, along with patients, be treated in a nondiscriminatory manner. Title VII makes it illegal to deny equal job opportunities on the basis of race, creed, color, religion, sex, or national origin; it also prohibits discrimination against patients, physicians, or employees.

Federal and state funds may be withheld from nursing facilities that practice discrimination. Most federal, state, and local programs specifically require, as a condition for receiving funds under such programs, an affirmative statement on the part of the facility that it will not discriminate. The Medicare and Medicaid programs specifically require affirmative assurances by health care institutions that no discrimination will be practiced.

Government Facilities

Whether a person is entitled to admission to a particular governmental institution depends on the statute establishing that institution. Governmental hospitals, for example, are by definition creatures of some unit of government; their primary concern is service to the population within the jurisdiction of that unit. In all cases, connection with the unit operating the hospital is necessary to entitle one to use the hospital facilities. Some of the statutes cover all inhabitants of the geographic area and, in addition, are broad enough to apply to any person within the area who falls ill or suffers traumatic injury and requires hospital care. However, many of the statutes limit use of the hospital facilities to patients of the governmental unit operating the hospital.

Placement of Residents

Placement of residents must be done in accordance with all federal and state statutes, rules, and regulations. The operator, of residential care facilities in *Murphy v. Senior Services Division*, 767 P.2d 104 (Ct. App. 1989), brought an action challenging rules of the Department of Human Resources, Senior Services Division and Mental Health Division, which require placement of residents according to their primary service needs. The operator claimed that the facilities he operated provided residential care to all persons in need of such care, regardless of age or diagnosis.

> The challenged rules restrict admissions to private residential care facilities, placing residents into separate facilities depending on their differing primary service needs. Exceptions are provided for individuals who can show that no space is available in a facility serving their primary service needs and that another facility is capable of providing adequate service. The effect of the regulations has been to restrict admissions at petitioner's Mt. Scott facility to elderly residents who are not mentally ill and at petitioner's Hoodview facility to those with severe mental or emotional disturbances.

Id. at 105. The court held that the rules were valid in that they complied with statutes on residential care facilities. In a previous decision by the court, it was held that "[t]he statutes, like the rules, clearly contemplated the establishment of different facilities under the auspices of different agencies to provide the services needed by persons with different problems." *Dempsey v. Senior Services Division*, 92 Or. App. 163, 167, 758 P.2d 367 (1988).

The individual needs of each resident should be taken into consideration when placing him or her within the facility. An alert resident should not be placed with a confused and noisy resident. A resident who is ill should be placed near the nursing station. Residents who do not share compatible life-styles and habits would not be a healthy match. For example, a chain-smoker and a non-smoker would not be considered compatible roommates.

Surveyors may ask residents during a long-term care survey:

- How well do you get along with your roommate?
- Have you ever been moved from one room to another? If yes, why?
- How were you involved in the decision to move?
- How much time was there between the time they told you that you were to be moved, and when you were moved?
- Have you asked for your room to be changed?[8]

Staff members may be asked:

- What are some of the reasons residents' rooms are changed?
- What are some of the reasons for discharge of residents or transfer to a hospital or LTC facility?
- How are residents involved in the decision to move?
- If a resident requests a room change, how is this handled?
- When a resident requests a room change, are the following areas of consideration presented and discussed?
  —cost factors
  —resident welfare
  —resident's reason for requesting the move
  —facility's assessment of whether the move would be beneficial or not for the resident[9]

Discharge and Transfer

Under OBRA requirements, the facility must permit each resident to remain in the facility, and may not transfer or discharge the resident from the facility unless:

> (i) The transfer or discharge is necessary for the resident's welfare and the resident's needs cannot be met in the facility;
> (ii) The transfer or discharge is appropriate because the resident's health has improved sufficiently so the resident no longer needs the services provided by the facility;
> (iii) The safety of individuals in the facility is endangered;
> (iv) The health of individuals in the facility would otherwise be endangered;

(v) The resident has failed, after reasonable and appropriate notice, to pay for (or to have paid under Medicare or Medicaid) a stay at the facility. For a resident who becomes eligible for Medicaid after admission to a facility, the facility may charge a resident only allowable charges under Medicaid; or

(vi) The facility ceases to operate.

(2) Documentation. When the facility transfers or discharges a resident under any of the circumstances specified in paragraphs (a)(1)(i) through (v) of this section, the resident's clinical record must be documented.

* * *

(3) Notice before transfer. Before a facility transfers or discharges a resident, the facility must—

(i) Notify the resident and if known, a family member or legal representative of the resident and of the transfer or discharge and the reasons;

(ii) Record the reasons in the resident's clinical record; and

(iii) Include in the notice the items described in paragraph (a)(5) of this section.

* * *

(b) Level B requirement: Notice of bed-hold policy and readmission (Effective October 1, 1990).

(1) Notice before transfer. Before a facility transfers a resident to a hospital or allows a resident to go on therapeutic leave, the facility must provide written information to the resident and a family member or legal representative that specifies—

(i) The duration of the bed-hold policy under the State plan, if any, during which the resident is permitted to return and resume residence in the facility; and

(ii) The facility's policies regarding bed-hold periods, which must be consistent with paragraph (b)(3) of this section, permitting a resident to return.

(2) Notice upon transfer. At the time of transfer of a resident to a hospital or for therapeutic leave, a nursing facility must provide written notice to the resident and a family member or legal representative, which specifies the duration of the bed-hold policy described in paragraph (b)(1) of this section.

(3) Permitting resident to return to facility. A nursing facility must establish and follow a written policy under which a resident whose hospitalization or therapeutic leave exceeds the bed-hold period under the State plan is readmitted to the facility immediately upon the first availability of a bed in a semi-private room if the resident—

(i) Requires the services provided by the facility; and
(ii) Is eligible for Medicaid nursing facility services.
(c) Level B requirement: Equal access to quality care (Effective October 1, 1990).
(1) A facility must establish and maintain identical policies and practices regarding transfer, discharge, and the provision of services under the State plan for all individuals regardless of sources of payment;
(2) The facility may charge any amount for services furnished to non-Medicaid residents consistent with the Medicaid requirement in Sec. 483.10(a)(5)(i) describing the charges; and
(3) The State is not required to offer additional services on behalf of a resident other than services provided in the State plan.[10]

A resident may not be detained in a nursing facility for inability to pay. An unauthorized detention of this nature could subject a facility to charges of false imprisonment.

An incompetent should be released in the care of an appropriate family member or guardian. At times residents will refuse discharge if they have no place to go. These cases should be handled on an individual basis and in consultation with counsel if necessary.

When discharging a resident, a physician should issue and sign all discharge orders. Residents in critical condition should be transferred to an appropriate facility for follow-up care.

Placement of residents outside the facility is just as important as placement within the facility. The health needs of a community are best served when it has at its disposal facilities that are capable of handling the health problems of its citizens, not only those acutely ill, but also those requiring recuperative and follow-up care. For this reason a complete health care program will include transfer agreements with both hospitals and extended care facilities.

In order to have the most comprehensive care given to residents and the most efficient use made of the facilities, it is necessary to have a coordinated plan for this utilization. This plan usually takes the form of a transfer agreement, which provides the basis for a working relationship between two or more health care institutions and establishes an atmosphere of cooperation between them.

OBRA requires that a nursing facility have in effect a written transfer agreement with one or more hospitals approved for participation under the Medicare and Medicaid programs that reasonably assures that residents will be transferred from the facility to a hospital when determined appropriate by the attending physician.[11] Generally speaking, a transfer agreement is a written document that sets forth the terms and conditions under which residents who no longer require the acute care furnished by the hospital may be transferred to a nursing facility. It also establishes procedures to admit residents of a facility into a hospital when their condition warrants a transfer.

It is important that the transfer agreement be written in compliance with and reflect the provisions of the many federal and state laws, regulations, and standards affecting health care institutions. The parties to a transfer agreement should be particularly aware of applicable federal and state regulations.

Regulations generally require that transfers between hospitals and nursing facilities are medically appropriate and that there will be an exchange of appropriate medical information between the sending and receiving institutions to assure continuity of care of the patient/resident.

Transfer agreements need not be limited to a single nursing facility and hospital. Every effort should be made to establish such agreements between groups of nursing facilities and hospitals, thus aiding in bringing about maximum utilization of the services of these facilities and assuring the best possible care for residents.

The basic elements that should be included in a transfer agreement are

- Identification of each party to the agreement, including the name and location of each institution to the agreement.
- Purpose of the agreement.
- Policies and procedures for transfer of patients/residents. Language in this section of the agreement should make it clear that the resident's physician makes the determination as to the patient/resident's need for the facilities and services of the receiving institution. The receiving institution should agree that, subject to its admission requirements and availability of space, it will admit the patient/resident from the transferring institution as promptly as possible.
- Institutional responsibilities in arranging and making the transfer. The transferring institution is generally responsible for making transfer arrangements. The agreement should specify who will bear the costs involved in the transfer.
- Exchange of information. The agreement must provide a mechanism for the interchange of medical and other information relevant to the patient/resident.
- Retention of autonomy. The agreement should make clear that each institution retains its autonomy and that the governing boards of each facility will continue to exercise exclusive legal responsibility and control over the management, assets, and affairs of the respective facilities. It should also be stipulated that neither institution assumes any liability by virtue of the agreement for any debts or obligations of a financial or legal nature incurred by the other.
- Procedure for settling disputes. The agreement should include a method of settling disputes that might arise over some aspect of the patient/resident transfer relationship.
- Procedure for modification or termination of the agreement. The agreement should provide that it can be modified or amended by mutual consent of the parties. It should also provide for termination by either institution upon notice within a specified time period.
- Sharing of services. Depending on the situation, cooperative use of facilities and services on an outpatient basis (e.g., lab and x-ray testing) may be an important element of the relationship between institutions. The method of payment for services rendered should be carefully described in the agreement.

- Publicity. The agreement should provide that neither institution will use the name of the other in any promotional or advertising material without prior approval of the other.
- Exclusive vs. non-exclusive agreement. In this age of patient/resident rights, it is advisable for institutions, when and where possible, to have transfer agreements with more than one institution. The agreement may include language to the effect that either party has the right to enter into transfer agreements with other institutions.

In addition to the actual agreement between the transferring and receiving facilities, there should be a written consent from the patient/resident indicating his or her agreement to the transfer. The right to choose a receiving facility must be honored when and where possible. Some state codes provide that, with the exception of a medical emergency, consultation with the resident, if competent, the resident's physician, and the resident's designated representative must be made aware within 24 hours of a decision to transfer or discharge a resident from the facility.[12]

The Medicaid resident in *Macleod v. Miller*, 612 P.2d 1158 (Colo. Ct. App. 1980), was found to be entitled to an injunction preventing his involuntary transfer from the nursing home. The resident had not been accorded a pre-transfer hearing as was required by applicable regulations. In addition, it was determined that the suffering from "transfer trauma" might result in irreparable harm to the resident. The appeals court remanded the case to the trial court with directions to enter an order enjoining the defendants from transferring the plaintiff pending exhaustion of his administrative remedies.

A 97-year-old resident in *Henson v. Department of Consumer and Regulatory Affairs*, 560 A.2d 543 (D.C. 1989), petitioned for review of a decision by the Department of Consumer and Regulatory Affairs to involuntarily discharge her from a "community residence facility." The resident had lived in the facility for eight years. The basis for the agency's decision was that the resident's discharge was "essential . . . to be in accordance with her prescribed level of care," pursuant to D.C. Code Section 32–1421(a). *Id.* at 544. The only evidence presented by the facility was three medical certification forms completed by Dr. Choisser, the treating physician, on March 2, 1987, on April 23, 1987, and again on August 25, 1987. The latter two forms indicated in an ambiguous check-off system that the resident required an intermediate level of care (ICF). This was contradicted by a letter written by Dr. Choisser on July 21, 1987, which stated, "I see no reason why she should not continue to reside in Chevy Chase House with complete safety . . . . It is my opinion that a change in her residence, at this stage in her life, would prove harmful to her emotionally and I strongly suggest that she be left as she is." *Id.* at 545. The court held that the need for the discharge was not proven by clear and convincing evidence.

Right To Die/Right To Choose

The Supreme Court's ruling in the Cruzan case (discussed in Chapter 13), which addresses right to die issues, has prompted nursing facility administrators to seek advance directives from residents in writing. Various communication tools that administrators have utilized to educate and acquaint residents with their rights include:

- brochures about living wills and durable powers of attorney (discussed more fully in Chapter 13), which should be made available to all residents
- lectures and current event meetings for residents that focus on treatment options
- periodic checks to update residents' wishes[13]

Financial Rights

Residents have financial rights, which include the safekeeping of their funds, reasonable access to their funds, and the right to be provided a copy of all bills and fees. Residents should be informed of the availability and cost of services which may or may not be covered by Medicare and Medicaid.

During an OBRA survey, residents may be asked:

- Are you able to take care of your own financial affairs?
- Does the facility keep some money for you that you can have when you request it?
- When you ask for this money, how quickly do you get it?
- Do you know the amount of money you have available at this time?
- If the facility pays bills for you, do they periodically provide an itemized listing of the transactions they have made?
- When did you receive the last itemized statement?
- Are you comfortable that your funds are taken care of correctly?
- If you deposit money or valuables with the facility, do you receive a receipt for this deposit?
- Are you or your family able to review your financial records when you request to do so?
- Have you ever had money or anything else stolen? If so, what was done about it?
- Does the home provide safe-keeping for valuables?[14]

The staff members may be asked during the survey:

- What is the procedure when residents lose personal belongings? When they lose valuables?
- How are resident personal funds handled?
- What is your procedure when a resident asks to get an accounting of his or her funds?[15]

Informed Consent

Residents of nursing facilities have a right to information, in terms they can understand, regarding their medical condition. Absent an emergency, no treatment may be given to a competent resident without his or her consent. This topic is fully discussed in Chapter 10, "Consent."

Right to Privacy

The right to privacy is implied in the Constitution, according to the Supreme Court. The right to privacy has traditionally been interpreted as the right to be free from unwarranted publicity or to live without having one's name, picture, or private affairs made public or published against one's will.

During a nursing home survey, surveyors will observe the interactions between staff and residents for indications that residents are treated with respect and consideration for their dignity and individuality. Surveyors should observe the following:

- How do staff members enter a resident's room or go behind a privacy curtain?
- Are privacy curtains used or doors shut when personal care needs and/or treatments are rendered?
- Are there areas for the residents to be alone or meet in private with visitors?[16]

State health codes generally cover resident's rights to privacy. New York, for example, provides:

> (d) Right to Privacy. Each resident shall have the right to:
>
> (1) personal privacy and confidentiality of his or her personal and clinical records which shall reflect:
> (i) accommodations, medical treatment, written and telephone communications, personal care, associations and communications with persons of his or her choice, visits, and meetings of family and resident groups. Resident and family groups shall be provided with private meeting space, and residents shall be given access to a private area for visits or solitude. Such requirement shall not require the facility to provide a private room for each resident; and
> (ii) the resident's right to approve or refuse the release of personal and clinical records to any individual outside the facility except when:
> (a) the resident is transferred to another health care institution; or
> (b) record release is required by law or third-party contract;
> (2) privacy in written communications, including the right to:
> (i) send and receive mail promptly that is unopened; and

(ii) have access to stationery, postage and writing implements at the resident's own expense; and

(3) regular access to the private use of a telephone that is wheelchair accessible and usable by hearing impaired and visually impaired residents;. . . [17]

Notice of Rights

A nursing facility has an obligation to inform each resident regarding its rules and regulations in a language that the resident understands. This includes making available large print texts of residents' rights, interpreters for hearing impaired residents, and written foreign language translations of residents' rights for those who speak a foreign language common in the nursing facility's locale. For languages less commonly encountered, a resident representative may sign a statement of residents' rights indicating that the resident's rights was interpreted to him or her.

Privacy in Care and Treatment

The right to privacy in care and treatment is one of the most difficult to protect in a health care setting. The limitations of space and finances have resulted in the need for sharing facilities by more than one resident. Nevertheless, the facility has a responsibility to provide as much privacy as is possible.

Confidentiality of Information

Residents have a right to expect that information regarding their care and treatment will be kept confidential. Facility staff must be careful not to discuss any aspect of a resident's case with others not involved in the case.

Violation and Enforcement

A violation of a resident's rights might constitute a violation of a state's requirements for licensure. With authority to decertify facilities from the Medicaid program, states have sufficient powers to pressure long-term care facilities into compliance with residents' rights provisions.

Treble damages were permitted under the Illinois Nursing Home Care Reform Act of 1979, Section 3-602, against those who violate a resident's rights. The purpose of this section was to punish those who violate a resident's rights and discourage future violations. Treble damages were found not to be abated by the resident's death in *Wills v. Dekalb Area Retirement Center*, 530 N.E.2d 1066 (Ill. Ct. App. Ct. 1988). The right to recover punitive damages passed on to the estate.

Grievances

Procedures must be implemented that provide residents with an opportunity to voice grievances without the fear of retribution. OBRA requirements provide:

> (f) Level B requirement: Grievances. A resident has a right to—
>
> (1) Voice grievances with respect to treatment or care that is, or fails to be furnished, without discrimination or reprisal for voicing the grievances; and
> (2) Prompt efforts by the facility to resolve grievances the resident may have, including those with respect to the behavior of other residents.[18]

RESIDENT RESPONSIBILITIES

Residents have responsibilities as well as rights. They must, for example, follow the reasonable instructions of their physicians and nurses. They have a duty to provide their physicians with accurate and complete information. Residents are expected to abide by the rules and regulations of the nursing facility and treat others with the respect and dignity they themselves would expect.

No constitutional right is absolute. Even the First Amendment rights to free speech will not protect a person who shouts "Fire" in a crowded room and causes injury to others. By analogy, it is necessary to periodically set specific policies for the welfare of all residents of the facility. One resident exercising his or her right to speak might disturb fellow residents. The right to speak is then conflicting with the right to privacy, which includes the right to peace and quiet. Because of the conflict of rights between residents, it is important to establish procedures to address such issues. For example, non-smokers should be placed with other non-smokers and smokers with other smokers.

Provision of Information

A resident has the responsibility to provide, to the best of his knowledge, accurate and complete information about present complaints, past illnesses, hospitalizations, medications, and other matters relating to his health. He or she has the responsibility to report unexpected changes in his or her condition to the responsible practitioner. A resident is responsible for making it known whether he or she clearly comprehends a contemplated course of action and what is expected of the resident.

Compliance Instructions

A resident is responsible for following the treatment plan recommended by the practitioner primarily responsible for his or her care. This may include following the instructions of nurses and allied health personnel as they carry out the coordinated plan of care and implement the responsible practitioner's orders, and as they enforce the applicable rules and regulations of the facility.

Refusal of Treatment

The resident is responsible for his or her actions if the resident refuses treatment or does not follow the practitioner's instructions.

Facility Charges

The resident is responsible for assuring that the financial obligations of his or her health care are fulfilled as promptly as possible.

Facility Rules and Regulations

The resident is responsible for following facility rules and regulations affecting resident care and conduct.

Respect and Consideration

The resident is responsible for being considerate of the rights of others and for assisting in the control of noise, smoking, etc. The resident is responsible for being respectful of the property of other persons and of the facility.

RESIDENT OMBUDSMAN

The concept of ombudsman originated in Sweden when it moved from a monarchy to a democratic form of government. "The Swedes felt the need for an agency or an office to be established to act as a go-between, between the average citizen and the government; someone who would be there to answer questions, to advocate on behalf of the citizens, someone who could receive and resolve complaints from the citizenry in regard to government policies and programs."[19]

The Swedish concept of ombudsman was adopted in the United States.

> The primary impetus for the program came from the Nixon Administration, and gradually the program has spread throughout the country. It was not until 1978 that the Older Americans Act Amendments (P.L. No. 95-478) mandated that every state have an ombudsman program and that a

> certain amount of the Older Americans Act funds from title III-B (the Social Services Section) had to be allocated to the ombudsman program.[20]

An ombudsman is a person who is designated to speak and act on behalf of a resident, especially in regard to his or her daily needs. Ombudsmen work for the Department of Aging. They deal with nursing facilities regarding resident abuse, neglect, etc. Current law has been expanded to require that the state long-term care ombudsman must be notified of any adverse action taken against a nursing facility. The ombusdman has a responsibility to receive complaints and serve as an advocate for nursing facility residents, as well as serve as a mediator between the residents and the facility. State survey agencies are required to enter into a written agreement with the office of the state long-term care ombudsman to provide for information exchange, case referral, and prompt notification of the office of any adverse action to be taken against a nursing facility under the enforcement section of nursing home reform law.[21]

Although ombudsman programs in nursing facilities have the potential to be a major force in quality assurance, their role to date has been ambiguous and variously interpreted from state to state. The skill and staffing levels around the country have been uneven. In 1985, there were only about 1,000 paid staff and 5,000 volunteers in ombudsman programs. Typically, nursing home ombudsmen have had little authority, sometimes not even enjoying clear access to facilities and/or records, and some programs have interpreted the role as a cross between a mediator and a personal service volunteer rather than as an advocate.[22]

Because nursing residents are often helpless and unable to speak for themselves, all caregivers, whether they are volunteers or paid staff, should consider themselves as resident advocates. Resident advocacy can be accomplished by caregivers providing quality day to day care in their particular areas of responsibility and expertise. Many states have established, by legislation, ombudsman programs.[23] Ombudsmen are responsible for the investigation of reports of resident abuse in nursing facilities.

NOTES

1. H.G. Collier, *Legal Issues in Long Term Care*, 1989 HEALTH LAW HANDBOOK 71 (1989).
2. 42 C.F.R. §488.115 (1990).
3. *Id.*
4. 42 C.F.R. §483.10 (1990).
5. N.Y. COMP. CODES R. & REGS. tit. 10, §415.3 (1991).
6. Key Medicare and Medicaid Legislation: 1990, OBRA 1990, Special Member Briefing, Chicago: American Hospital Association, January 1991, at 162.
7. 42 C.F.R. §483.12 (1990).
8. 42 C.F.R. §488.15 (1989).
9. *Id.*
10. 42 C.F.R. §483.12 (1990).
11. 42 C.F.R. §483.75 (1990).

12. N.Y. COMP. CODES R. & REGS. tit. 10, §415.3 (e)(1991).

13. *Nursing Homes Seek Advance Directives*, 64 HOSPITALS, November 20, 1990, p. 52.

14. 42 C.F.R. §488.115 (1990).

15. *Id.*

16. *Id.*

17. N.Y. COMP. CODE R. & REGS. tit. 10, §415.3(d) (1991).

18. 42 C.F.R. §483.10 (1990).

19. M. Wolff, *Long Term Care Ombudsmen: Training Role and Responsibility*, LONG TERM CARE AND THE LAW 191 (1983).

20. *Id.* at 192.

21. Key Medicare and Medicaid Legislation: 1990, OBRA 1990, Special Member Briefing, Chicago: American Hospital Association, January 1991, at 24.

22. A. MONK, L.W. KAYE, & H. LITWIN, RESOLVING GRIEVANCES IN THE NURSING HOME: A STORY OF THE OMBUDSMAN PROGRAM (1984).

23. CAL. WELF. & INST. CODE §51 et seq. (West 19); FLA. STAT. §415.106 (19); and MASS. GEN. LAWS ANN. ch. 19A, § et seq (West 19).

Chapter 12

Long-Term Care Records and Legal Reporting Obligations

Nursing facilities are required to maintain a medical record for each resident. Federal regulations under OBRA require that a nursing facility maintain clinical records on each resident in accordance with accepted professional standards and practices. The records must be complete, accurate, readily accessible, systematically organized, and retained in accordance with state law (or five years from the date of discharge when there is no requirement provided in state law and three years for a minor after the resident reaches legal age under state law).[1]

Medical records requirements are generally provided for in the public health laws of the various states. They generally have provisions requiring that each facility maintain a complete medical record for each resident that contains all pertinent information regarding the daily care and treatment of residents.

While many kinds of records are required to be maintained by nursing facilities (e.g., financial, personnel, and purchasing records), the primary emphasis here lies with medical records. Documentation of the facts of a resident's illness, symptoms, diagnosis, and treatment is one of the most important functions in furnishing modern long-term care services. Nurses and physicians are primarily charged with the responsibility of keeping accurate and up-to-date medical records.

Medical records are maintained primarily to provide complete information regarding the care and treatment of residents. They are the principal means of communication among health professionals in matters relating to resident care.

The major purposes of the medical record are to provide a planning tool for resident care; to record the course of a resident's treatment and the changes in a resident's condition; to document the communications between the practitioner responsible for the resident and any other health professional who contributes to the resident's care; to assist in protecting the legal interests of the resident, the nursing facility, and the practitioner; to provide a data base for use in statistical reporting, continuing education, and research; and to provide information necessary for third-party billing and regulatory agencies.

The nurse is generally the one medical professional the resident sees more than any other. Consequently, the nurse is in a position to keep constant watch over the resident's illness, response to medication, display of pain and discomfort, and general condition. Nursing assistants who have been properly trained and certified are responsible for reporting clinical information to nurses. The resident's care, as well as the nurse's observations, should be recorded fully, factually, and promptly.

CONTENTS OF THE MEDICAL RECORD

The medical record must be a complete, accurate, up-to-date report of the medical history, condition, and treatment of each resident. It is composed of at least two distinct parts, each of which is made up of several types of forms. The first part is compiled upon admission and includes

- the admission record, which describes pertinent data regarding the resident's age, address, reason for admission, social security number, marital status, religion, addresses, and any other information necessary to meet both federal and state requirements
- the general consent and authorization-for-treatment forms allowing the nursing facility to perform routine diagnostic testing, etc.

The second part, the clinical record, contains

- the medical history and physical examination, including diagnosis, and estimation of restoration potential
- discharge summary if the resident was admitted from a hospital
- diagnostic and therapeutic orders, including all medications, treatments, diet, and restorative and special medical procedures required for the safety and well being of the resident
- resident care and progress records describing significant changes in a resident's condition, written at the time of each visit
- nurse's notes containing observations made by the nursing personnel
- medication and treatment record including all medications, treatments, and special procedures performed for the safety and well-being of the resident
- temperature charts
- consultation notes and reports
- dental reports
- social service notes and reports
- recreational therapy notes and reports
- occupational therapy notes and reports
- physical therapy notes and reports
- activity therapy notes and reports

- dietary notes and reports
- resident care referral reports
- laboratory and x-ray reports
- fluid intake and output charts
- discharge summaries, etc.

Failure of a nursing facility to maintain a complete and accurate medical record reflecting the treatment rendered a resident may affect the ability of the facility to obtain third-party reimbursement. Under federal and state laws, the medical record must accurately reflect the treatment for which a facility seeks payment. Thus, the medical record is important to the facility for medical, legal, and financial reasons.

Various licensing regulations require prompt completion of records after the discharge of residents. Persistent failure to conform to a medical staff rule requiring the physician to complete records promptly can provide a basis for suspension of a staff member.

LEGAL REQUIREMENTS

Nursing facilities are required to maintain medical records under a variety of statutes and regulations. The scope and detail of record requirements vary from state to state. Licensure rules and regulations contained in state statutes generally describe the requirements and standards for the maintenance, handling, signing, filing, and retention of medical records. The court in *Koelbl v. Whalen*, 406 N.Y.S.2d 621 (N.Y. App. Div. 1978), held that regulations requiring that certain information be kept by the nursing home (e.g., chronological admission registers) were valid requirements.

In addition to state regulations, minimum standards for record keeping have been established by the federal government for nursing facilities receiving federal funding. In order to participate in federal programs, these minimum requirements must be met.

Medical records must be maintained for each resident admitted to a nursing facility in accordance with accepted professional principles. A separate record for each resident admitted must be maintained. All entries must be kept current, dated, and signed.

The medical records of all discharged residents must be completed promptly, filed, and retained in accordance with regulatory requirements. Policies should provide for the retention and safekeeping of each resident's records. If a resident is transferred to another health care facility, a copy of his or her record or an abstract thereof must accompany the resident.

The individual in charge of medical records must be sure that the facility complies with all regulations and amendments affecting medical records. If a nursing facility does not have a full or part time medical records librarian, an employee of the facility (generally a nurse or medical records coordinator) must be assigned the responsibility for assuring that records are maintained, completed, and preserved. The designated individual must be trained by and receive regular consultation from a certified medical records administrator.

The medical record should contain forms for certification and recertification pursuant to the requirements of Medicare. A special services form should be created that may constitute part of the resident's record. The form should indicate the kinds of services the resident receives. These services include such things as optometry, hair styling, podiatrist, etc. The service administered, as well as the title and signature of the person rendering the service shall be included on the form.

Records should be maintained on the physical, occupational, and speech therapy that the resident receives. Resident's outings should be reported and should show each time a resident leaves the facility, when he or she is expected to return, the signature of the person accompanying him or her, the relationship with the resident, and the signature of the charge nurse.

The nursing facility should receive from the referring institution the most complete record possible from that institution. This is necessary so that the facility will be aware of any and all conditions that affect the delivery of care to the resident while at the facility.

LEGAL PROCEEDINGS AND THE MEDICAL RECORD

The ever-increasing frequency of personal injury suits mandates that nursing facilities maintain complete, accurate, and timely medical records. Their importance as an evidentiary tool in legal proceedings cannot be overemphasized. The integrity and completeness of the medical record is extremely important in reconstructing the events surrounding any alleged negligence in the care of the resident. Medical records aid police investigations, provide information for determining the cause of death, and indicate the extent of injury in worker's compensation or personal injury proceedings.

When health professionals are called as witnesses in a proceeding, they are permitted to refresh their recollections of the facts and circumstances of a particular case by referring to the medical record. Courts recognize that it is impossible for a medical witness to remember the details of every resident's treatment. The record may therefore be used as an aid in relating the facts of a resident's course of treatment.

The medical record itself may be admitted into evidence in legal proceedings. In order for medical record information to be admitted into evidence, the court must be assured that the information is accurate, that it was recorded at the time the event took place, and that it was not recorded in anticipation of a specific legal proceeding. While it is recognized that witnesses may refresh their memories and that records may be admitted into evidence, there is nevertheless a need for assurance that the information is trustworthy.

When a medical record is introduced into evidence, the administrator must testify as to the manner in which the record was produced and the way in which it is protected from unauthorized handling and change. It should be noted that whether such records and other documents are admitted or excluded is governed by the facts and circumstances of the particular case, as well as by the applicable rules of evidence. Admission of a business record requires "the testimony of the custodian or other qualified witness." Federal Rules of Evidence 803(6).

> [A] writing is not admissible . . . merely because it may appear upon its face to be a writing made by a physician in the regular course of his practice. It must first be shown that the writing was actually made by or under the direction of the physician at or near the time of his examination of the individual in question and also that it was his custom in the regular course of his professional practice to make such a record.

Masterson v. Pennsylvania Railroad, 182 F.2d 793, 797 (3rd Cir. 1950).

The records purportedly relating to a patient's treatment in *Belber v. Lipson*, 905 F.2d 549 (1st Cir. 1990), were not admissible as business records since the witness who had possession of them had no personal knowledge of the circumstances under which the records were prepared.

Whatever the situation, it is clear that the record must be complete, accurate, and timely. If it can be shown that the record is inaccurate or incomplete, or that it was made long after the event it purports to record, it will not be accepted into evidence.

CONFIDENTIAL COMMUNICATIONS

The communications between a physician and his or her resident and the information generated during the course of the resident's illness are generally accorded the protection of confidentiality. Federal requirements under OBRA provide that a nursing facility must keep confidential all information contained in the resident's records.[2] "Patient confidentiality seems to have lost its meaning in the current health care environment, some experts say. Yet the dearth of litigation stemming from medical record disclosures clearly indicates that patients are not likely to sue over their loss of confidentiality."[3] Health professionals have a clear legal and moral obligation to maintain confidentiality. As noted above, medical records, with proper authorization, may be utilized for the purposes of research, statistical evaluation, and education. The information obtained from medical records must be dealt with in a confidential manner; otherwise, a nursing facility could incur liability. Disclosure may be required where a resident is the victim of a crime. A resident may also permit disclosure by his or her actions or words.

Participation in the Medicare and Medicaid programs is conditioned upon the adoption of a "Resident's Bill of Rights," which guarantees residents that their medical record will be treated confidentially and that they will have the right to control the release of their records to others.

OWNERSHIP AND RELEASE OF MEDICAL RECORDS

Ownership of medical records resides with the nursing facility. They are retained for the benefit of health care professionals in treating residents. Although medical records have generally been protected from public scrutiny by a general practice of nondisclosure, this practice has been waived under a limited number of specifically controlled situations.

Release of medical record information under OBRA may occur when requested by a facility to which a resident has been transferred, when required by law, under third party payment contract requirements, and when requested by the resident. A resident who asks to review his or her record must be permitted to have access to it. A copy must be provided, if requested, within 48 hours following such request.[4]

Resident Access

Health professionals and nursing facilities have generally held that all records are their exclusive property and have not as a rule released them to residents. However, residents have a legally enforceable interest in the information contained in their medical records. Under OBRA 90 regulations, access to clinical records is to be provided upon request within 24 hours (excluding hours during a weekend or holiday). Access is also to be provided to a resident's legal representative.[5] The courts have also taken a view that patients have a right to access to their medical records.

The New York Public Health Law, as amended on January 1, 1989, by adding Section 18, provides that patients may have access to review and obtain copies of their medical records. Access to information includes that maintained or possessed by a health care facility or a health practitioner who has treated or is treating a patient.

Nursing facilities can withhold records if it is determined that the information could reasonably be expected to cause substantial and identifiable harm to the resident.

Request by Third Parties

There are numerous reasons why a long-term care facility may disclose information without consent, such as disclosure to third party payors. Policies regarding the release of information to third parties should be formulated that address the rights of residents, insurance carriers processing claims, physicians and nursing facility staff, medical researchers and educators, governmental agencies, and the press.

The medical record is a peculiar type of property because there are several interests that are at times in competition for the information. The actual record belongs to the facility and the facility may restrict its removal from the institution.

Reproduction Charges

A reasonable charge for inspection and copies of medical records may be made, provided the charge does not exceed the costs incurred by the provider. The nursing facility in *XYZ Nursing Home, Inc. v. Kuriansky*, 552 N.Y.S.2d 438 (N.Y. App. Div. 1990), applied for an order directing the state to bear the costs of reproducing the original medical records that it had supplied to the state. The New York State Deputy Attorney General for Medicaid Fraud had obtained the original business records of the nursing home pursuant to a grand jury subpoena duces tecum. There was no effort by the state after four months of possession to return those records that did not bear upon the investigation. The trial court granted the facility's petition and the state appealed. The appellate court held that the state was required to provide the nursing home, at government expense, with photocopies of all subpoenaed documents as the facility might demand.

PRIVACY ACT OF 1974

The Privacy Act of 1974, codified at 5 U.S.C. §552a, et. seq., was enacted to safeguard individual privacy from the misuse of federal records, give individuals access to records concerning themselves that are maintained by federal agencies, and establish a Privacy Protection Safety Commission. A portion of the Privacy Act reads as follows:

> Sec. 2[a] The Congress finds that (1) the privacy of an individual is directly affected by the collection, maintenance, use, and dissemination of personal information by Federal agencies; (2) the increasing use of computers and sophisticated information technology, while essential to the efficient operations of the Government, has greatly magnified the harm to individual privacy that can occur from any collection, maintenance, use, or dissemination of personal information; (3) the opportunities for an individual to secure employment, insurance, and credit, and his right to due process, and other legal protections are endangered by the misuse of certain information systems; (4) the right to privacy is a personal and fundamental right protected by the Constitution of the United States; and (5) in order to protect the privacy of individuals identified in information systems maintained by Federal agencies, it is necessary and proper for the Congress to regulate the collection, maintenance, use, and dissemination of information by such agencies. [b] The purpose of this Act is to provide certain safeguards for an individual against an invasion of personal privacy by requiring Federal agencies, except as otherwise provided by law, to—(1) permit an individual to determine what records pertaining to him are collected, maintained, used, or disseminated by such agencies; (2) permit an individual to prevent records pertaining to

him obtained by such agencies for a particular purpose from being used or made available for another purpose without his consent; (3) permit an individual to gain access to information pertaining to him in Federal agency records, to have a copy made of all or any portion thereof, and to correct or amend such records; (4) collect, maintain, use, or disseminate any record of identifiable personal information in a manner that assures that such action is for a necessary and lawful purpose, that the information is current and accurate for its intended use, and that adequate safeguards are provided to prevent misuse of such information; (5) permit exemptions from the requirements with respect to records provided in this Act only in those cases where there is an important public policy need for such exemption as has been determined by the specific statutory authority; and (6) be subject to civil suit for any damages which occur as a result of willful or intentional action which violates any individual's rights under this Act.

COMPUTERIZED MEDICAL RECORDS

Because of the tremendous amount of paperwork required under OBRA regulations in caring for residents, computers have become an economic necessity. Problems associated with computerization include confidentiality, equipment failure, and questionable accuracy of input data by computer operators.

Nursing facilities undergoing computerization must determine user needs, design an effective system, select appropriate equipment, develop user training programs, develop a disaster recovery plan (e.g., provisions for backup files and electrical shutdowns), provide for data security, etc. Experienced computer consulting firms can save nursing facilities thousands of dollars with their expertise. Computers are not difficult to understand, but minor mistakes can cost major dollars.

MEDICAL RECORD BATTLEGROUND

The medical record must not be utilized as a battleground against another professional or the nursing facility. The medical record is a document that cannot be erased once a recording has been made. It should not be utilized as an instrument for registering a complaint against another health care professional or the institution. The health care professional who utilizes a resident's medical record unwisely may have vented his or her emotions for the moment, but may have at the same time provided the basis for having to justify his or her actions to another professional, to the institution, or to a jury. It should be remembered that comments written during a time of anger may have been based on inaccurate information, which in turn could be damaging to one's credibility and future statements.

FALSIFICATION OF RECORDS

All professionals should be aware that falsification of medical and business records is grounds for criminal indictment, as well as for civil liability for damages suffered. In *People v. Smithtown General Hospital*, 402 N.Y.S.2d 318 (N.Y. Sup. Ct. 1978), a motion to dismiss indictments against a physician and a nurse charged with falsifying business records in the first degree was denied. In each indictment it was charged that the defendant was in violation of a duty imposed on him or her by law or by the nature of his or her position. The surgeon was charged because he omitted to make a true entry in his operative report. The nurse was charged because she failed to make a true entry in the operating room log.

CHARTING—SOME HELPFUL ADVICE

The medical record is the most important document in a negligence action. Both plaintiff and defendant utilize it as a basis for their action and defense. The following advice on documentation should prove to be helpful in charting:

- The medical record describes how each resident is cared for in a facility. It should be sufficiently complete to allow those not treating a resident to review the record and assume his or her continuing care when necessary.
- Medical records entries should be legible, clear, and meaningful to each resident's course of treatment. Handwriting has long been a major problem in interpreting the events surrounding the care of residents. Illegible medical records not only damage one's ability to defend him or herself, but also can have an adverse effect on the credibility of other health professionals who read the record and act upon what they read.
- The medical record should be complete. This is often a problem with progress notes when there is little new information to report. Progress notes should describe the symptoms or condition being addressed, treatment rendered, resident response, and the resident's status at the time treatment is discontinued.
- Do not write long, defensive, or derogatory notes. Stick to the facts. Criticism, complaints, emotional comments, and extraneous remarks have no place in the medical record. Such remarks can in and of themselves precipitate a malpractice suit.
- Do not make erasures or use correction fluid to cover up entries, or tamper with the chart in any form. Draw a single line through a mistaken entry, enter the correct information, and then sign and date it. Tampering with records sends the wrong signal to jurors and can shatter one's credibility. Altered records can create a presumption of negligence. The court in *Matter of Jascalevich*, 442 A.2D 635, 182 N.J. Super. 455 (1982), held "... that a deliberate falsification by a physician of his patient's medical record, particularly

when the reason therefore is to protect his own interests at the expense of his patient's, must be regarded both as a gross malpractice endangering the health or life of his patient . . . ."

- Charts related to pending legal action should be placed in a separate file under lock and key. Legal counsel should be notified immediately of any potential lawsuit.
- A medical record has many authors. Do not ignore the entries made by others. Good resident care is a team effort and entries made by other health professionals provide valuable information in treating the resident.

RETENTION OF RECORDS

The length of time medical records must be retained varies from state to state. Administration, with the advice of an attorney, should determine how long records should be maintained, taking into account resident needs, statutory requirements, future need for such records, and the legal considerations of having the records available in the event of a lawsuit.

A California court revoked the license of a nursing facility for failure to keep adequate records (along with other violations of the law). In *Yankee v. State Department of Health*, 162 Cal. App. 2d 600, 328 P.2d 556 (1958), the facility claimed that the word "adequate" was unclear and therefore the requirement was invalid. The court stated the "the word 'adequate' is not so uncertain as to render a penal statute invalid."

Several jurisdictions recognize the principle that an individual has a right to privacy and to be protected from the mass dissemination of information pertaining to his or her personal or private affairs. The right of privacy generally is the right to be kept out of the public spotlight.

LEGAL REPORTING OBLIGATIONS

A society wishes the best possible environment for its members. It works through government to protect its people by health regulations and statutes. Only through reliable observations and reports can proper measures be instituted to safeguard the environment of society.

Of prime importance to the health professional are health statutes requiring that certain information be transmitted to the appropriate administrative bodies. Although most statutory reporting requirements do not contain an express immunity from suit for disclosure without the permission of the person affected, as a general rule a person making a report in good faith and under statutory command is protected.

Incident Reporting

Some state health codes provide that nursing facilities must investigate incidents regarding patient care and that certain incidents must be reported in a manner prescribed by regulation. Reportable incidents often include such things as those incidents that have resulted in a serious injury or resident's death, an event such as fire or loss of emergency electrical generator power, certain infection outbreaks, strikes by personnel, etc.

Although there are but a few cases dealing with incident reporting, nursing facility staff designated to report incidents must do so if required by a state's statute. The director of nursing at a nursing facility in *Choe v. Axelrod*, 534 N.Y.S.2d 739 (N.Y. App. Div. 1988), was fined $150 for failure to report an instance of patient neglect. An anonymous phone call had been placed with the Department of Health regarding two incidents of alleged patient neglect. In one incident a patient had been left unattended in a shower by an orderly, and the patient sprayed himself with hot water, which resulted in second degree burns on his forehead. On a second occasion, a similar incident occurred but no one was injured. Upon investigation by the Department of Health, a determination was made that both incidents constituted patient neglect, and that failure to report these incidents was a violation of Public Health Law Section 2803-d and Title 10, Section 81 of the Official Compilation of Codes, Rules & Regulations of the State of New York. Following a hearing by an administrative law judge, the charge in the first incident was sustained and the second incident was dismissed.

The director of nurses petitioned to annul the administrative determination. She contended that the Department of Health failed to establish a prima facie case of patient neglect and that the incident was an unavoidable accident and that the Department of Health's proof is based upon hearsay evidence. *Id.* at 741. The court held that evidence supported a finding that the director of nurses had failed to report an incident of patient neglect as required by statute. On the question of hearsay evidence:

> "It is now well established that an agency can prove its case through hearsay evidence . . . ." In the final analysis, the evidence showed that the patient was left unattended, albeit momentarily, O'Brien (the orderly) was disciplined for that act, and petitioner did not report the incident. The finding is thus supported by the "kind of evidence on which reasonable persons are accustomed to rely in serious affairs" . . . .

People ex rel. Vega v. Smith supra, 66 N.Y. 2d at 139, 495 N.Y.S.2d 332, 485 N.E.2d 997, quoting *National Labor Relations Board v. Remington Rand*, 2nd Civ., 94 7.2d 862, 873, cert. denied 304 U.S. 576, 585 Ct. 1046, 82, L. Ed. 1540. *Id.* at 741.

Although it may not always be clear as to when an incident report should be filed, appropriate procedures should be in place addressing how questionable events should be handled.

National Practitioner Data Bank

The Health Care Quality Improvement Act of 1986 (Title IV of P.L. 99-660), signed by President Reagan on November 14, 1986, was enacted to encourage greater efforts in professional peer review and to restrict the ability of incompetent practitioners who move from state to state attempting to avoid discovery of previous substandard performance or unprofessional conduct. The law established the National Practitioner Data Bank, to be operated under the authority of the Secretary of Health and Human Services. Responsibility for Data Bank implementation resides in the Bureau of Health Professions, Health Resources and Services Administration of HHS. The Act authorizes the Data Bank to be used to collect and release information on the professional competence and conduct of physicians, dentists, and other health care practitioners. Reporting and disclosure requirements for the National Practitioner Data Bank are also set out in regulations.[6]

After several delays and changes since it was mandated by Congress in 1986, the National Practitioner Data Bank became operational September 1, 1990. The regulations are intended to encourage good faith professional review activities. The Data Bank was established because: (1) there has been an increasing occurrence of medical malpractice and a need to improve the quality of medical care, both of which have become nationwide problems that warrant greater efforts than those that can be undertaken by any individual state; (2) there is a national need to restrict the ability of incompetent physicians to move from state to state without disclosure or discovery of the physician's previous damaging or incompetent performance; (3) there is a nationwide problem that can be remedied through effective professional peer review; (4) the threat of private money damage liability under federal laws, including treble damage liability under federal antitrust law, unreasonably discourages physicians from participating in effective professional peer review; and (5) there is an overriding national need to provide incentive and protection for physicians engaging in effective professional peer review.[7]

The Data Bank is responsible for collecting and releasing certain information related to the professional competence and professional conduct of physicians, dentists, and other health care practitioners.[8] Information gathered by the Data Bank will be maintained in computer format. Reports must be submitted on an "Adverse Action Report" form. An "Additional Information" form must be utilized in conjunction with an "Adverse Action Report" when the forms do not provide sufficient space for providing the information requested. (See Appendix D.)

Data Bank queries can be made by state licensing boards, hospitals, other health care "entities," and professional societies, which have entered or may be entering employment or affiliation relationships with a physician, dentist, or other health care practitioner who has applied for clinical privileges or appointment to the medical staff. A plaintiff's attorney is permitted to obtain information from the Data Bank when a malpractice action has been filed and the practitioner on whom information has been sought is named in the suit. A request for Data Bank information must be submitted on a "Request for Information Disclosure" form. When information is requested from the

Data Bank on more than one practitioner, the requesting body may utilize one or more "Request for Information Disclosure—Supplement" forms along with the "Request for Information Disclosure" form. The use of the Supplement form will save time in that the need to repeat certain information has been eliminated. (See Appendix D.)

The regulations establish reporting requirements applicable to hospitals; health care entities; boards of medical examiners; professional societies of physicians, dentists, or other health care practitioners that take adverse licensure or professional review actions (e.g., reduction, restriction, suspension, revocation, or denial of clinical privileges or membership in a health care entity of 30 days or longer); and individuals and entities (including insurance companies) making payments as a result of medical malpractice actions or claims. A medical malpractice action or claim has been defined as a written complaint or claim demanding payment based on a health care practitioner's provision of or failure to provide health care services, and includes the filing of a cause of action based on tort law, brought in any state or federal court or other adjudicative body.[9]

Hospitals or other health care entities that fail to report adverse professional review actions against the clinical privileges of physicians or dentists lasting more than 30 days can lose immunity protection provided by Title IV for a three-year period. Insurance carriers will be subject to a $10,000 penalty for each medical malpractice payment they make and fail to report on behalf of a physician, dentist, or other health practitioner.

Many nursing facilities are not eligible to participate in the Data Bank because they do not conduct professional review activities through a formal peer review process. For those health care providers who question whether or not they are covered under this law, the Department of Health and Human Services prefers to define the term "entity" broadly, rather than to attempt to focus on the myriad of health care organizations, practice arrangements, and professional societies, so as to ensure that the regulations include all entities within the scope of the statute.[10] The definition of health care entity is as follows:

> Health care entity means:
>
> (a) A hospital;
> (b) An entity that provides health care services, and engages in professional review activity through a formal peer review process for the purpose of furthering quality health care, or a committee of that entity; . . . .[11]

Health care practitioners include all health care practitioners authorized by a state to provide health care services by whatever formal mechanism the state employs (e.g., certification, registration, and licensure).[12] Examples of "other" health care practitioners are presented in Exhibit 12-1 below.

Under data-bank rules, Data Bank queries will cost $2 per request each time a physician and dentist apply for medical staff positions or for clinical privileges at their facilities. HHS's Health Resources and Services Administration (HRSA), which administers the Data Bank, hopes to keep the user fee to a minimum.

Exhibit 12-1 Examples of Other Health Care Practitioners

The following list of health care practitioners other than physicians and dentists is provided solely for illustrative purposes. The inclusion or exclusion of any health care occupational group in the list noted below should not be interpreted as a mandate or a waiver of compliance with National Practitioner Data Bank reporting requirements.

- Acupuncturists
- Audiologists
- Chiropractors
- Dental Assistants
- Dental Hygienists
- Denturists
- Dietitians
- Emergency Medical Technicians
- Home Health Aides
- Homeopaths
- Medical Assistants
- Medical Technologists
- Mental Health Counselors
- Midwives, Lay
- Naturopaths
- Nuclear Medicine Technologists
- Nurse Aides
- Nurse, Licensed Practical
- Nurse, Licensed Vocational
- Nurse Midwives
- Nurse Practitioners
- Nurse, Registered
- Nutritionists
- Occupational Therapists
- Occupational Therapy Assistants
- Ocularists
- Opticians
- Optometrists
- Orthotics/Prosthetics Fitters
- Pharmacists
- Pharmacists, Nuclear
- Physical Therapists
- Physical Therapy Assistants
- Physician Assistants
- Podiatric Assistants
- Professional Counselors
- Psychiatric Technicians
- Radiation Therapy Technologists
- Radiologic Technologists
- Rehabilitation Therapists
- Respiratory Therapists
- Social Workers, Clinical
- Speech/Language Pathologists

Source: National Practitioner Data Bank Guidebook, U.S. Department of Health and Human Services, Contracted by Unisys Corporation.[13]

Health care facilities must query the data bank every two years upon the renewal of staff privileges of physicians and dentists. The data bank will serve as a "flagging system" whose principal purpose is to facilitate a more comprehensive review of professional credentials. As a nationwide flagging system, it provides another resource to assist state licensing boards, hospitals, and other health care entities in conducting extensive independent reviews of the qualifications of health care practitioners they seek to license or hire, or to whom they wish to grant clinical privileges. Data Bank information can also be utilized for reviewing current medical staff members. As of November 30, hospitals had submitted 172,131 queries to the National Practitioner Data Bank.[14]

The National Practitioner Data Bank presents a number of challenges to health care institutions. A major one will be to educate the medical staff so that the Data Bank will not erode medical staff participation in risk management.[15] The purpose of the Data Bank is not punishment but prevention and deterrence.

Information reported to the Data Bank is considered strictly confidential. Individuals and entities who knowingly and willfully report to or query the Data Bank under false pretenses or fraudulently access the Data Bank computer directly will be subject to civil penalties.

> (a) Limitations on disclosure. Information reported to the Data Bank is considered confidential and shall not be disclosed outside the Department of Health and Human Services, except as specified in Sec. 60.10, Sec. 60.11 and Sec. 60.14. Persons and entities which receive information from the Data Bank either directly or from another party must use it solely with respect to the purpose for which it was provided. Nothing in this paragraph shall prevent the disclosure of information by a party which is authorized under applicable State law to make such disclosure.
>
> (b) Penalty for violations. Any person who violates paragraph (a) shall be subject to a civil money penalty of up to $10,000 for each violation . . . .[16]

Communicable Diseases

Most states have enacted laws that require the reporting of actual or suspected cases of communicable diseases. For example, the New York State Sanitary Code Chapter 1, Section 2.12 (1973), provides that

> When no physician is in attendance it shall be the duty of the head of a private household or the person in charge of any institution, school, hotel, boarding house, camp or vessel or any public health nurse or any other person having knowledge of an individual affected with any disease presumably communicable, to report immediately the name and address of such person to the city, council or district health officer.

The need for statutes requiring the reporting of communicable diseases is clear. If a state is to protect its citizens' health through its power to quarantine, it must ensure the prompt reporting of infection or disease.

Deaths

All deaths are reportable by statute. Death certificates must be signed by the physician pronouncing a death. Statutes requiring the reporting of deaths are necessary in order to maintain accurate census records. Census reports are of great importance to states seeking funding of federally sponsored programs, which often grant funds based on population statistics.

Suspicious Deaths

Greater than a state's interest in the recording of all births and deaths is the state's desire to review unnatural deaths that may be the result of some form of criminal activity. Unnatural deaths must be referred to the medical examiner for review. Such cases may include violent deaths, deaths caused by unlawful acts or criminal neglect, or deaths that may be considered suspicious or unusual (e.g., those involving a fracture within six months of death). The medical examiner may make an investigation of such cases and issue an autopsy report. The purpose of a medical examiner's investigation is to determine the actual cause of death and thereby provide assistance for any further criminal investigation that may be considered necessary.

NOTES

1. 42 C.F.R. §483.75 (1990).
2. 42 C.F.R. §483.75 (1990).
3. *Liability for Medical Record Disclosure Is Real But Rare*, HOSPITALS, August 20, 1990 at 32.
4. 42 C.F.R. §483.75 (1990).
5. Key Medicare and Medicaid Legislation: 1990, OBRA 1990, Special Member Briefing, Chicago: American Hospital Association, January 1991, at 162.
6. 54 Fed. Reg. 42,730 (1989) (to be codified at 45 C.F.R. §60.1).
7. Pub. L. No. 99-660 (1986) (codified at 42 U.S.C. §11101).
8. 54 Fed. Reg. 42,730 (1989) (to be codified at 42 C.F.R. §60.1).
9. 54 Fed. Reg. 42,723 (1989) (to be codified at 45 C.F.R. §60.3).
10. 54 Fed. Reg. 42,722, 42,723 (1989) (to be codified at 45 C.F.R. §60).
11. 54 Fed. Reg. 42,730 (1989) (to be codified at 45 C.F.R. §60.3).
12. 54 Fed. Reg. 42,723 (1989) (to be codified at 45 C.F.R. §60.3).
13. The Guidebook is meant to serve as a resource for the users of the National Practitioner Data Bank. It is one of a number of efforts to inform the U.S. health care community about the Data Bank and what is required to comply with the requirements established by Title IV of Public Health Law 99-660, the Health Care Quality Improvement Act of 1986. The Data Bank Help Line (1-800-767-6732) is a toll free telephone service that provides health care entities and health care practitioners with information about the Data Bank.
14. *Data-bank Officials Work to Allay Lawmakers' Fears*, 26(50) AHA News, December 24, 1990.
15. *Risk Managers See New Regulations as Boon and Burden*, HOSPITALS, September 20, 1990, at 48.
16. 54 Fed. Reg. 42,734 (1989), 45 C.F.R. §60.13.

Chapter 13

Euthanasia, Death, and Dying

The human struggle to survive and dreams of immortality have been instrumental in pushing mankind to develop means to prevent and cure illness. Advances in medicine and related technologies that have resulted from human creativity and ingenuity have indeed given society the power to prolong life. However, the process of dying can also be prolonged. Those victims of long-term pain and suffering, as well as patients in vegetative states and irreversible comas, are the most directly affected. Today, rather than watching hopelessly as a disease destroys a person or as a body part malfunctions, causing death to a patient, physicians can implant artificial body organs. In addition, exotic machines and antibiotics are new weapons in a physician's arsenal to help extend a patient's life. Such situations have generated vigorous debate. There seems to be an absence of controversy only when a patient who is kept alive by modern technology is still able to appreciate and maintain control over his or her life. However, when patients and their families see what they perceive as a deterioration of the quality of life and no end to unbearable pain, it is then that conflict arises between health care professionals who are trained to save lives and patients and their families who wish to end the suffering. This conflict centers around the concept of euthanasia and its place in the modern world.

From its inception, euthanasia has evolved into an issue with competing legal, medical, and moral implications, which continue to generate debate, confusion, and conflict. Currently, there is a strong movement advocating death with dignity, which excludes machines, monitors, and tubes.

DEFINING EUTHANASIA

Even the connotation of the word euthanasia has changed with time and those persons attempting to define it. Originating in the Greek language, euthanasia, meaning "good death," was accepted in situations where people had what were considered to be incurable diseases.[1] In the religions of Confucianism and Buddhism, suicide was an acceptable answer to unendurable pain and incurable disease. The Celtic people went a step farther, believing that those who chose to die of disease or senility, rather than committing suicide, would be condemned to hell.[2] Such acceptance began to change during the nineteenth century when Western physicians refused to lessen suffering by shortening a dying patient's life. Napoleon's physician, for example, rejected Napoleon's plea to kill plague-stricken soldiers, insisting that his obligation was to cure rather than to kill people.[3]

In the late 1870s writings on euthanasia began to appear, mainly in England and the United States. Although such works were, for the most part, written by lay authors, the public and the medical community began to consider the issues raised by euthanasia. Then defined as "the act or practice of painlessly putting to death persons suffering from incurable conditions or diseases,"[4] it was considered to be a merciful release from incurable suffering. By the beginning of the twentieth century, however, there were still no clear answers or guidelines regarding the use of euthanasia. Unlike in prior centuries when society as a whole supported or rejected euthanasia, different segments of today's society apply distinct connotations to the word, generating further confusion. Some believe euthanasia is meant to allow a painless death when one suffers from an incurable disease, yet is not dying. Others, who remain in the majority, perceive euthanasia as an instrument to aid only dying people in ending their lives with as little suffering as possible.

It has been estimated that of the "two million Americans who die each year, 80 percent die in hospitals or nursing homes, and 70 percent of those die after a decision to forego life-sustaining treatment has been made."[5] Although such decisions are personal in nature, and based upon individual moral values, they must comply with the laws applicable to the prolonging of the dying process. Courts have outlined the ways in which the government is allowed to participate in the decision-making process. The misconceptions and confusion regarding the topic have led to wide disparity among jurisdictions, both in legislation and in judicial decisions. As a result, the American Medical Association, the American Bar Association, legislators, and judges are actively attempting to formulate and legislate clear guidelines in this sensitive, profound, and as yet not fully understood area. In order to ensure compliance with the law, while serving the needs of their patients, it is incumbent upon health care providers to keep themselves informed of the legislation enacted in this ever-changing field.

CLASSIFYING EUTHANASIA

In order to properly address the topic of euthanasia, it is necessary to understand the precise meaning of the recognized forms. Rhetorical phrases such as "right to die," "right to life," and "death with dignity" have obfuscated, rather than clarified, the public's understanding of euthanasia.

Active or Passive

The labeling of euthanasia as active or passive is, for many, the most controversial distinction. Active euthanasia is commonly understood to be the commission of an act, such as giving a patient a lethal drug that results in death. The act, if committed by the patient, is thought of as suicide. Moreover, if the patient cannot take his or her own life, any person who assists in the causing of the death could be subject to criminal sanction for aiding and abetting suicide.

Passive euthanasia occurs when lifesaving treatment (such as a respirator) is withdrawn or withheld, allowing the patient diagnosed as terminal to die a natural death. Passive euthanasia is generally allowed by legislative acts and judicial decisions. *In re Estate of Brooks*, 32 Ill. 2d 361, 205 N.E.2d 435 (1965); *Superintendent of Belchertown State School v. Saikewicz*, 373 Mass. 728, 370 N.E.2d 417 (1977); *In re Quinlan*, 81 N.J. 10, 355 A.2d 647 (1976). These decisions, however, are generally limited to the facts of the particular case. The distinction between active and passive euthanasia are minor at best. The end result in both scenarios is the same.

The distinctions are important when considering the duty and the liability of a physician who must decide whether or not to continue or initiate treatment of a comatose or terminally ill patient. Physicians are bound to use reasonable care to preserve health and to save lives, so unless fully protected by the law, they will be reluctant to abide by a patient's or family's wishes to terminate life-support devices.

Although there may be a duty to provide life-sustaining machinery in the immediate aftermath of cardiopulmonary arrest, there is no duty to continue its use once it has become futile and ineffective to do so in the opinion of qualified medical personnel. Two physicians in *Barber v. Superior Court*, 147 Cal. App. 3d 1006, 195 Cal. Rptr. 484 (1983), were charged with the crimes of murder and conspiracy to commit murder. The charges were based on their acceding to requests of the patient's family to discontinue life-support equipment and intravenous tubes. The patient had suffered a cardiopulmonary arrest in the recovery room following surgery. A team of physicians and nurses revived the patient and placed him on life-support equipment. The patient had suffered severe brain damage that placed him in a comatose and vegetative state, from which, according to tests and examinations by other specialists, he was unlikely to recover. The patient, upon the written request of the family, was taken off life-support equipment. The patient's family (his wife and eight children) made the decision together after consultation with the physicians. Evidence had been presented that the patient, prior to his incapacitation, had expressed to his wife that he would not want to be kept alive by machine or "become another Karen Ann Quinlan." There was no evidence indicating that the family was motivated in their decision by anything other than love and concern for the dignity of their loved one. The patient continued to breathe on his own. Showing no signs of improvement, the physicians again discussed the patient's poor prognosis with the family. The IVs were removed, and the patient expired sometime thereafter.

A complaint was then filed against the two physicians. The magistrate who heard the evidence determined that the physicians did not kill the deceased, since their conduct was not the proximate cause of the patient's death. The superior court determined as a matter of law that the evidence required the magistrate to hold the physicians to answer and ordered the complaint reinstated. The court of appeal held that the physicians' omission to continue treatment, though intentional and with knowledge that the patient would die, was not an unlawful failure to perform a legal duty. The evidence amply supported the magistrate's decision. The superior court erred in determining that as a matter of law the evidence required the magistrate to hold the physicians to answer. The peremptory writ of prohibition to restrain the Superior Court of Los Angeles from taking any further action in this matter other than to vacate its order reinstating the complaint and to enter a new and different order denying the people's motion was granted.

Recently, however, other states are increasingly confronted with the question of whether it is ever right for a physician to provide a patient with aid in dying. On July 26, 1991, a Monroe County, New York, grand jury answered yes when it failed to indict Dr. Timothy Quill for giving a leukemia patient sleeping pills to enable her to take her own life. Dr. Quill, an associate chief of medicine at a hospital in Rochester, New York, wrote an article in the *New England Journal of Medicine* focusing on the suffering of terminal patients. Moreover, he discussed how doctors could relieve an individual's suffering. He is not alone in his support of physician-assisted suicide. Washington voters will be deciding in a referendum vote whether they want physician-assisted suicide legalized. In the bestselling book, *The Final Exit*, Derek Humphry, executive director of the Hemlock Society (a nationally known organization advocating the right to die) describes methods of self-assisted suicide for terminally ill people.

Voluntary or Involuntary

Both active and passive euthanasia may be either voluntary or involuntary. Voluntary euthanasia occurs when the suffering incurable makes the decision to die. To be considered voluntary, the request or consent must be made by a legally competent adult and be based on material information concerning the possible ramifications and alternatives available. The term legally competent was addressed in a right to refuse treatment case, *Lane v. Candura*, 6 Mass. App. Ct. 377, 376 N.E.2d 1232 (1979). The case involved a patient who twice refused to permit surgeons to amputate her leg in order to prevent gangrene from spreading. The patient's daughter sought to be appointed as a legal guardian to enable her to consent to her mother's surgery. The appellate court, finding no evidence indicating that Mrs. Lane was incapable of appreciating the nature and consequence of her decision, overturned the trial court's holding of incompetence. Therefore, even though Mrs. Lane's decision would ultimately lead to her death, she was found to be competent, and thus she was allowed to reject medical treatment.

The *Lane* court and others have defined legal competence as the mental ability to make a rational decision. A patient must exhibit perception and appreciation of all relevant facts and then make decisions based on those facts. In the active euthanasia context, the patient would be demonstrating that by voluntarily requesting euthanasia, he or she would be selecting death over life. *State Department of Human Services v. Northern*, 563 S.W.2d 197, 209 (Tenn. Ct. App.), appeal dismissed as moot, 436 U.S. 923 (1978).

In the case of *In re Lydia Hall Hospital*, 455 N.Y.S.2d 266 (N.Y. Sup. Ct. 1981), the patient, who was terminally ill and requiring dialysis, was taken off all medication to ensure that his mind would be clear when psychiatrists examined him to determine whether he was competent. Recent case law asserts that the standard of proof required for a finding of an incurable's incompetence is that of clear and convincing evidence. *In re Lydia E. Hall Hospital*, 455 N.Y.S.2d 706, 712 (N.Y. 1982) (quoting *In re Storar*, 438 N.Y.S.2d 266, 274 (N.Y. 1981)). This is a higher standard than the normal fair preponderance of the credible evidence required in civil proceedings.

Involuntary euthanasia, on the other hand, occurs when a person other than the incurable makes the decision to terminate an incompetent or an unconsenting competent person's life.[6]

The patient's lack of consent could be due to mental impairment or comatose unconsciousness. Important value questions face courts dealing with involuntary euthanasia: Who should decide to withhold or withdraw treatment? On what factors should the decision be based? Are there viable standards to guide the courts? Should criminal sanctions be imposed on a person assisting in ending a life? When does death occur?

CONSTITUTIONAL CONSIDERATIONS

In order to analyze the important questions regarding whether or not life-support treatment can be withheld or withdrawn from an incompetent patient, it is necessary to first consider what rights a competent patient possesses. Both statutory law and case law have presented a diversity of policies and points of view. Some courts point to common law and the early case of *Schloendorff v. Society of New York Hospital*, 105 N.E. 92 (N.Y. 1914), to support their belief in a patient's right to self-determination. The *Schloendorff* court stated: "Every human being of adult years has a right to determine what shall be done with his own body; and the surgeon who performs an operation without his patient's consent commits an assault for which he is liable for damages." *Id.* at 93. This right of self-determination was emphasized in *In re Storar*, 438 N.Y.S.2d 266 (N.Y. 1981), when the court announced that every human being of adult years and sound mind has the right to determine what shall be done with his own body. *Id.* at 272.

The Storar case was a departure from the New Jersey Supreme Court's rationale in the case of *In re Quinlan*, 81 N.J. 10, 355 A.2d 647 (1976). The Quinlan case was the first to significantly address the issue of whether euthanasia should be permitted where a patient is terminally ill.[7] The *Quinlan* court, relying on *Roe v. Wade*,

410 U.S. 113 (1973), announced that a patient's right to self-determination is protected by the constitutional right to privacy. The court noted that the right to privacy "is broad enough to encompass a patient's decision to decline medical treatment under certain circumstances, in much the same way as it is broad enough to encompass a woman's decision to terminate pregnancy under certain conditions." 81 N.J. at 40, 355 A.2d at 663.

The majority of cases today follow the right to privacy argument. The court, in reaching its decision, applied a test balancing the state's interest in preserving and maintaining the sanctity of human life against Karen Quinlan's privacy interest. It decided that, especially in light of the prognosis (physicians determined that Karen was in an irreversible coma), the state's interest did not justify interference with Karen's right to refuse treatment. Thus, Karen's father was appointed her legal guardian, and the respirator was shut off. Opponents of euthanasia argue that before the *Quinlan* decision, any form of euthanasia was defined as murder by our legal system. Although acts of euthanasia did take place, the law was applied selectively, and the possibility of criminal sanction against active participants in euthanasia was enough to deter physicians from assisting a patient in committing self-euthanasia.

In spite of intense criticism by legal and religious scholars, the *Quinlan* decision paved the way for courts to consider extending the right to decline treatment to incompetents as well. The United States Supreme Court has not yet addressed this issue, but state courts have; and even though the state courts recognize the right, they differ on how this right is to be exercised.

In the same year as the *Quinlan* decision, the case of *Superintendent of Belchertown State School v. Saikewicz*, 373 Mass. 728, 370 N.E.2d 417 (1977), was decided. There the court, utilizing the balancing test enunciated in *Quinlan*, approved the recommendation of a court-appointed guardian ad litem that it would be in Mr. Saikewicz's best interests to end chemotherapy treatment. Mr. Saikewicz was a mentally retarded, 67-year-old patient, suffering from leukemia. The court found from the evidence that the prognosis was dim, and even though a "normal person" would probably have chosen chemotherapy, it allowed Mr. Saikewicz to die without the treatment in order to spare him the suffering.

Although the court also followed the reasoning of the *Quinlan* opinion in giving the right to an incompetent to refuse treatment, based on either the objective "best interests" test or the subjective "substituted judgment" test, which it favored since Mr. Saikewicz had always been incompetent, the court departed from *Quinlan* in a major way. It rejected the *Quinlan* approach of entrusting a decision concerning the continuance of artificial life support to the patient's guardian, family, attending physicians, and a hospital "ethics committee." The *Saikewicz* court asserted that even though a judge might find the opinions of physicians, medical experts, or hospital ethics committees helpful in reaching a decision, there should be no requirement to seek out the advice. The court decided that questions of life and death with regard to an incompetent should be the responsibility of the courts, which would conduct detached but passionate investigations. The court took a "dim view of any attempt to shift the ultimate decision-making responsibility away from duly established courts of proper jurisdiction to any committee, panel, or group, ad hoc or permanent." *Id.* at 758, 370 N.E.2d at 434.

This major point of difference between the Saikewicz and Quinlan cases marked the emergence of two different policies on the incompetent's right to refuse treatment. One line of cases has followed *Saikewicz* and supports court approval before physicians withhold or withdraw life support. Advocates of this view argue that it makes more sense to leave the decision to an objective tribunal than to extend the right of a patient's privacy to a number of interested parties, as was done in *Quinlan*. They also attack the *Quinlan* method as being a privacy decision effectuated by popular vote.[8]

Six months after *Saikewicz*, the Massachusetts Appeals Court narrowed the need for court intervention in *In re Dinnerstein*, 6 Mass. App. Ct. 466, 380 N.E.2d 134 (1978), in finding that "no code" orders are valid to prevent the use of artificial resuscitative measures on incompetent terminally ill patients. The court there was faced with the case of a 67-year-old woman who was suffering from Alzheimer's disease. She was determined to be permanently comatose at the time of trial. Further, the court decided that *Saikewicz*-type judicial proceedings should take place only when medical treatment could offer "a reasonable expectation of effecting a permanent or temporary cure of or relief from the illness." 380 N.E.2d at 138.

The Massachusetts Supreme Judicial Court attempted to clarify its *Saikewicz* opinion with regard to court orders in *In re Spring*, 405 N.E.2d 115 (Mass. 1980). It held that such various factors as the patient's mental impairment and his or her medical prognosis with or without treatment must be considered before judicial approval is necessary to withdraw or withhold treatment from an incompetent patient. The problem in all three of these cases is that there is still no clear guidance as to exactly when the court's approval of the removal of life-support systems would be necessary. *Saikewicz* seemed to demand judicial approval in every case. *Spring*, however, in partially retreating from that view, stated that it did not have to articulate what combination of the factors it discussed, thus making prior court approval necessary. Recently, however, a Maine court ruled that it was within the scope of a guardian's powers and rights to request and instruct the treating physicians and hospital to stop all life support including food, water, and antibiotics—without prior court approval. *In re Hallock* (Kennebec County P. Ct. Sept. 26, 1988).

The inconsistencies presented by the Massachusetts cases have led the majority of courts since 1977 to follow the lead set by *Quinlan*, requiring judicial intervention. In cases where the irreversible nature of the patient's loss of consciousness has been certified by physicians, an ethics committee (actually a neurological team) could certify the patient's hopeless neurological condition. Then a guardian would be free to take the legal steps necessary to remove life-support systems. The major reason for the appointment of a guardian is to ensure that incompetents, like all other patients, maintain their right to refuse treatment. The majority of holdings indicate that since a patient has the constitutional right of self-determination, those acting on the patient's behalf can exercise that right when rendering their best judgment concerning how the patient would assert the right. This substituted judgment doctrine could be argued on standing grounds, whereby a second party has the right to assert the constitutional rights of another when that second party's intervention is necessary to protect the other's constitutional rights. Of course, the guardian's decision is more sound if based on the known desires of a patient who was competent immediately prior to becoming comatose.

Courts adhering to the *Quinlan* rationale have recognized that fact, and in 1984 the highest state court of Florida took the lead and accepted the living will as persuasive evidence of an incompetent's wishes. The Supreme Court of Florida, in *John F. Kennedy Memorial Hospital, Inc. v. Bludworth*, 452 So. 2d 925 (Fla. 1984), allowed an incompetent patient's wife to act as his guardian, and in accordance with the terms of a living will he executed in 1975, she was told to substitute her judgment for that of her husband. She asked to have a respirator removed. The court declined the necessity of prior court approval, finding that the constitutional right to refuse treatment that had been decided for competents in *Satz v. Perlmutter*, 362 So. 2d 160 (Fla. Dist. Ct. App. 1978), *aff'd*, 379 So. 2d 359 (Fla. 1980), extends to incompetents. The court required the attending physician to certify that the patient was in a permanent vegetative state, with no reasonable chance for recovery, before a family member or guardian could request termination of extraordinary means of medical treatment.

In keeping with *Saikewicz*, the decision maker would attempt to ascertain the incompetent patient's actual interests and preferences. Court involvement would be mandated only to appoint a guardian, or in one of the following cases: (1) if family members disagree as to the incompetent's wishes, (2) if physicians disagree on the prognosis, (3) if the patient's wishes cannot be known because he has always been incompetent, (4) if evidence exists of wrongful motives or malpractice, or (5) if no family member can serve as a guardian. *John F. Kennedy Memorial Hospital, Inc. v. Bludworth*, 452 So. 2d 925, 430 (Fla. 1984) (citing *In re Welfare of Colyer*, 99 Wash. 2d 114, 660 P.2d 738 (1983) where the court found prior court approval to be "unresponsive and cumbersome").

DEFINING DEATH

The decision in *John F. Kennedy Memorial Hospital v. Bludworth* increased the desire of the public, courts, and religious groups to know when a patient is considered to be legally dead and what type of treatment can be withheld or withdrawn at that point. Most cases dealing with euthanasia speak of the necessity that a physician diagnose a patient as being either of the following:

- in a persistent vegetative state, *Severns v. Wilmington Medical Center*, 425 A.2d 156 (Del. Ch. 1980) (incompetent's right to refuse medical treatment may be expressed through a guardian when the patient is in a chronic vegetative state); *Leach v. Akron General Medical Center*, 68 Ohio Misc. 1, 426 N.E.2d 809 (Ohio C.P. 1980) (right to privacy includes right of a terminally ill patient in a vegetative state to determine his or her own course of treatment)

- terminally ill, *Satz v. Perlmutter*, 379 So. 2d 359 (Fla. 1980) (constitutional right to privacy supports decision of a competent adult suffering from a terminal illness to refuse extraordinary treatment); *Superintendent of Belchertown State School v. Saikewicz*, 373 Mass. 728, 370 N.E.2d 417 (1977) (right to refuse medical treatment for terminal illness extended to incompetent patients).

This diagnostic role of the physician acts as a limitation on the decision-making role of the family or the guardian. Where death is actually present, of course, the termination of mechanical or other similar devices would be a consistent and permissible act.

Traditionally, the definition of death adopted by the courts has been the Black's Law Dictionary definition: "cessation of respiration, heartbeat, and certain indications of central nervous system activity, such as respiration and pulsation." *Schmitt v. Pierce*, 344 S.W.2d 120, 133 (Mo. 1961). At present, however, modern science has the capacity to sustain vegetative functions of those in irreversible comas. Machinery can actually sustain heartbeat and respiration even in the face of brain death. "With 10,000 patients existing in the twilight state at this time,"[9] every appellate court that has ruled on the question has recognized that the irreversible cessation of brain function constitutes death.

Further, ethicists who advocate the prohibition on taking action to shorten life agree that "where death is imminent and inevitable, it is permissible to forego treatments that would only provide a precarious and painful prolongation of life, as long as the normal care due to the sick person in similar cases is not interrupted."[10]

Relying on the 1968 Harvard Criteria set forth by the Ad Hoc Committee of the Harvard Medical School To Examine the Definition of Brain Death, the American Medical Association in 1974 accepted that death occurs when there is "irreversible cessation of all brain functions including the brain stem."[11] At least 38 states now recognize brain death by statute or judicial decision. New York, for example, in *People v. Eulo*, 482 N.Y.S.2d 436 (1984), in rejecting the traditional cardiopulmonary definition of death, announced that the determination of brain death need be made only according to acceptable medical standards in order to be valid. The court also repeated its holding in *In re Storar*, 438 N.Y.S.2d 266 (1981), that clear and convincing evidence of a person's desire to decline extraordinary medical care may be honored and that a third person may not exercise this judgment on behalf of a person who has not or cannot express the desire to decline treatment. Following the *Bludworth* logic, the court noted that health professionals acting within the cases should not face liability. Nearly half of the states, in response to cases since *Quinlan*, have enacted laws setting forth statutory guidelines that relieve courts of the burden of deciding on a case-by-case basis whether or not to terminate life support.

The clear and convincing evidence standard was recently more succinctly defined by the New York Court of Appeals in *In the Matter of Westchester County Medical Center ex. rel. O'Connor*, 72 N.Y.2d 517, 531 N.E.2d 607, 534 N.Y.S.2d 886 (1988). There the court determined that artificial nutrition could be withheld from

Mary O'Connor, a stroke victim who was unable to converse or feed herself. The court held that "nothing less than unequivocal proof of a patient's wishes will suffice when the decision to terminate life support is at issue." 534 N.Y.S.2d *Id.* at 891. The factors outlined by the court in determining the existence of clear and convincing evidence of a patient's intention to reject the prolongation of life by artificial means were

- the persistence of statements regarding an individual's beliefs,
- the desirability of the commitment to those beliefs,
- the seriousness with which such statements were made, and
- the inferences that may be drawn from the surrounding circumstances.

The Missouri Supreme Court has followed the Westchester ruling and has held that the family of a woman who has been in a persistent vegetative state since 1983 cannot order physicians to remove artificial nutrition. In 1983 Nancy Cruzan sustained injuries in a car accident, in which her car overturned, after which she was found face down in a ditch without respiratory or cardiac function. Although unconscious, her breathing and heartbeat were restored at the site of the accident. Upon examination at the hospital to which she was taken, a neurosurgeon diagnosed her as having suffered cerebral contusions and anoxia. It was estimated that she had been deprived of oxygen for from 12 to 14 minutes. After remaining in a coma for three weeks, Cruzan went into an unconscious state. At first she was able to orally ingest some food. Thereafter, surgeons implanted a gastrostomy feeding and hydration tube, with the consent of her husband, in order to make feeding her easier. She did not improve, and until December 1990, she lay in a Missouri state hospital in a persistent vegetative state that was determined to be "irreversible, permanent, progressive and ongoing." *Cruzan v. Harman*, 760 S.W.2d 408, 411 (Mo. 1988) (en banc). She was not dead, according to the accepted definition of death in Missouri, and physicians estimated that she could live in the vegetative state for an additional 30 years. Because of the prognosis, Cruzan's parents asked the hospital staff to cease all artificial nutrition and hydration procedures. The staff refused to comply with their wishes without court approval. The state trial court granted authorization for termination, finding that Nancy Cruzan had a fundamental right—grounded in both the state and federal constitutions—to refuse or direct the withdrawal of death prolonging procedures. Testimony at trial from a former roommate of Nancy Cruzan indicated to the court that Cruzan had stated that if she were ever sick or injured, she would not want to live unless she could live halfway normally. The court interpreted that conversation, which had taken place when Cruzan was 25, as meaning that she would not want to be forced to take nutrition and hydration while in a persistent vegetative state.

The case was appealed to the Missouri Supreme Court, which reversed the lower court decision. The court not only doubted that the doctrine of informed consent applied to the circumstances of the case, it moreover would not recognize a broad privacy right from the state constitution that would "support the right of a person to refuse medical treatment in every circumstance." *Id.* at 417, 418. Missouri is one of 37 states that recognize living wills,[12] and the court held that Cruzan's parents were not entitled to order the termination of her treatment, since "no person can assume that choice for an incompetent in the absence of the formalities required under Missouri's Living Will statutes or the clear and convincing, inherently reliable evidence absent here." *Id.* at 425. The court found that Cruzan's statements to her roommate did not rise to the level of clear and convincing evidence of her desire to end nutrition and hydration.

The United States Supreme Court, in June 1990, heard oral arguments and held that: "(1) the U.S. Constitution does not forbid Missouri from requiring that there be clear and convincing evidence of an incompetent's wishes as to the withdrawal of life sustaining treatment; (2) the Missouri Supreme Court did not commit constitutional error in concluding that evidence adduced at trial did not amount to clear and convincing evidence of Cruzan's desire to cease hydration and nutrition; (3) due process did not require the state to accept the substituted judgment of close family members, absent substantial proof that their views reflected those of the patient." *Cruzan v. Director, Missouri Department of Health*, 110 S.Ct. 2841 (1990).

In delivering the opinion of the Court, Justice Rehnquist noted that while most state courts have applied the common law right to informed consent, or a combination of that right and a privacy right when allowing a right to refuse treatment, the Supreme Court analyzed the issues presented in the Cruzan case in terms of a Fourteenth Amendment liberty interest, finding that a competent person has a constitutionally protected right grounded in the Due Process Clause to refuse lifesaving hydration and nutrition. The court, however, did not accept that an incompetent person has the same right, since he or she could not exercise the right based upon any informed and voluntary choice. Missouri provided for the incompetent by allowing a surrogate to act for the patient in choosing to withdraw hydration and treatment. Moreover, it put into place procedures to ensure that the surrogate's action conforms to the wishes expressed by the patient when he or she was competent. While recognizing that Missouri had enacted a restrictive law, the Supreme Court held that right-to-die issues should be decided pursuant to state law, subject to a due process liberty interest, and in keeping with state constitutional law. After the Supreme Court rendered its decision, the Cruzans returned to Missouri probate court, where on November 14, 1990, Judge Charles Teel authorized physicians to remove the feeding tubes from Nancy Cruzan. The judge determined that testimony presented to him early in November demonstrated to him clear and convincing evidence that Cruzan would not have wanted to live in a persistent vegetative state. Several of her co-workers had testified that she told them before her accident that she wouldn't want to live "like a vegetable." On December 26, 1990, two weeks after her feeding tubes were removed, Nancy Cruzan died.

Following the *Cruzan* decision, states have begun to rethink existing legislation and draft new legislation in the areas of living wills, durable powers of attorney, health care proxies, and surrogate decision making. Pennsylvania, which has not handled many right-to-die cases, and Florida were two of the first states to react to the *Cruzan* decision. The new Pennsylvania law is applied to terminally ill or permanently unconscious patients. The statute, the Advance Directive for Health Care Act,[13] deals mainly with individuals who have prepared living wills. It includes in its definition of life sustaining treatment the administration of hydration and nutrition by any means, if it is stated in the individual's living will. The statute mandates that a copy of the living will must be given to the physician, in order to be effective. Further, the patient must be incompetent or permanently unconscious. If there is no evidence of the presence of a living will, the Pennsylvania probate codes allow an attorney-in-fact who was designated in a properly executed durable power of attorney document to give permission for "medical and surgical procedures to be utilized on an incompetent patient." 20 Pennsylvania Consolidated Statutes Annotated §5602(a)(9) (1988). The Supreme Court stated in *Cruzan* that only 15 percent of the population has signed any living wills or other types of medical directives. In light of that, more states will have to address the problem of surrogate decision making for an incompetent. Legislation would not only have to include direction to consider evidence of an incompetent's wishes that had been expressed when he or she was competent, it would also have to include provisions for consideration and protection of an incompetent who never stated what he or she would want done if in a terminally ill or persistent vegetative state.

Unless there is some uniformity in the legislation nationally, patients and their families will shop for states that will allow them to have medical treatment terminated or withdrawn with as few legal hassles as possible. For example, on January 18, 1991, a Missouri probate court judge authorized a father to take his 20-year-old brain damaged daughter, Christine Busalacchi, from the Missouri Rehabilitation Center, to Minnesota for testing by a pro-euthanasia physician, Dr. Ronald Cranford. Cranford, who practices at the Hennepin County Medical Center, has been at the center of controversy in Minnesota. In January, 1991, Pro Life Action Ministries demanded Cranford's resignation, claiming that he "desires to make Minnesota the killing fields for the disabled."[14] He, however, views himself as an advocate of patients' rights. However the situation involving Dr. Cranford is resolved, it is clear that the main reason Mr. Busalacchi sought authorization to take his daughter to Minnesota is that he believed that he would have to deal with fewer legal impediments there in order to allow his daughter to die. Minnesota is in fact the state in which the courts are presently grappling with a right-to-die case where physicians and family members are on the sides opposite to their traditional positions on this issue. Helga Wanglie is an 87-year-old woman who is in a persistent vegetative state as a result of a heart attack that caused brain damage. Physicians have determined that she has no chance of recovery and that any further treatment would be meaningless to any recovery. They therefore have sought court permission to discontinue further life sustaining care. Wanglie's husband of 53 years asserted that his wife would not have wanted anything to shorten her life, and he is thus fighting to maintain life supporting treatment for her.[15]

Because of the continuing litigation concerning the right-to-die issue, it is clear that the public must be educated about the necessity of expressing their wishes concerning medical treatment while they are competent. Uniformity with regard to the legal instruments available for demonstrating what a patient wants should be a common goal of legislators, courts and the medical profession. If living wills, surrogates, and durable powers of attorney were to be enacted pursuant to national rather than individual state guidelines, the result should be a greater ease in resolving the myriad of conflicting issues in this area. Various states have addressed the problem by statutorily providing for these instruments, thereby enabling individuals to have a say in the medical care they should receive if they become unable to speak for themselves.

THE LEGISLATIVE RESPONSE

Chief Justice Dore of the Supreme Court of Washington voiced his opinion that a legislative response to right to die issues could be better addressed by the legislature. "The United States Supreme Court, in *Cruzan*, questioned whether a federally protected right to forgo nutrition and hydration existed. The *Cruzan* Court confronted the same philosophical issues that we face today and wisely recognized and deferred to the Legislature's superior policy-making abilities. As was the case in *Cruzan*, our legislature is far better equipped to evaluate this complex issue and should not have its power usurped by the court." *Farnam v. Crista Ministries*, 807 P.2d 830, 849 (Wash. 1991).

As a result of implementation of Section 4206 of the 1990 Omnibus Budget Reconciliation Act, nursing facilities participating in the Medicare and Medicaid reimbursement programs must deal with resident rights regarding life sustaining decisions and other advance directives. Nursing facilities will have a responsibility to explain to residents, staff, and families that residents do have a legal right to direct their own medical and nursing care as it corresponds to existing state law, including right-to-die directives. Those facilities which do not comply with a resident's directives or those of a legally authorized decision maker on treatment, are exposing themselves to the risk of a lawsuit.[16]

Until recently, the family of an incompetent patient was relied upon to assist the physician in making medical decisions for the patient. The courts were many times used to relieve a physician of any criminal or civil liability, if the physician withdrew or withheld life sustaining treatment. It became clear that the courts were not equipped to handle this type of medical–ethical conflict. Moreover, cases involving life sustaining decisions by their very nature demand immediate action. The taking of a case to court is an expensive and time consuming process.

The federal Council on the Aging, in its 1988 Annual Report to the President, stated that "Fair and realistic guardianship, living wills, powers of attorney, and trust standards must be a priority of all state legislatures, as well as the public in general, as increased longevity makes mental and physical incapacity more commonplace among the U.S. senior population."[17] At least 38 states have addressed this problem by enacting natural death, living will, or death with dignity statutes that grant statutory recognition to advance directives, wherein a patient, while competent, expressed his or her wishes with respect to life sustaining treatment. The currently recognized instruments are living wills, durable powers of attorney, and health care proxies.

Living Will

A "living will," also referred to in various states as a "directive" or "declaration," is the instrument or legal provision that enables others to carry out a person's wishes regarding the non-use of extreme life sustaining measures when he or she is no longer able to do so. Typically, a living will allows a person, when competent, to inform caregivers in writing of his or her wishes with regard to withholding and withdrawing life supporting treatment, including nutrition and hydration.

The living will should be signed and dated by two witnesses who are not blood relatives or beneficiaries of property. A living will should be discussed with the resident's physician and a signed copy should be placed in the resident's medical record. A copy should also be given to the individual designated to make decisions in the event the resident is unable to do so. A person who executes a living will when healthy and mentally competent cannot predict how he or she will feel at the time of a terminal illness. Therefore, it should be updated regularly so that it accurately reflects a resident's wishes.[18] The written instructions become effective when a resident is either in a terminal condition, permanently unconscious, or suffering irreversible brain damage. (See Appendix E for several examples of living wills.)

Forty-one states have enacted statutes that enable individuals to state their wishes in advance regarding the use of life sustaining procedures during a terminal illness.[19] California was the first state to enact what has been called a Natural Death or Living Will Act in 1976. Cal. Health & Safety Code Section 7185-95 (West 1983). California's legislation is typical of similar laws that exist in 38 other states that allow the creation of documents that provide a legally recognized way for competent adults to express in advance their desires regarding life-crucial medical decisions in the event they become terminally ill and death is imminent. Governor John D. Waihee of Hawaii has signed a bill that "would recognize the right to control a person's medical decisions as an 'unqualified right whose exercise requires no one else's approval, neither families, physicians, ethics committees, lawyers nor courts of law.'"[20]

Durable Power of Attorney

Power of attorney is a legal device that permits one individual known as the "principal" to give to another person called the "attorney-in-fact" the authority to act on his or her behalf. The attorney-in-fact is authorized to handle banking and real estate affairs, incur expenses, pay bills, and handle a wide variety of legal affairs for a specified period of time. The power of attorney may continue indefinitely during the lifetime of the principal so long as that person is competent and capable of granting power of attorney. If the principal becomes comatose or mentally incompetent, the power of attorney automatically expires just as it would if the principal dies.[21]

Because a power of attorney is limited by the competency of the principal, some states have authorized a special legal device for the principal to express intent concerning the durability of the power of attorney, to allow it to survive disability or incompetency.[22] The "durable power of attorney" is more general in scope and the patient does not have to be in imminent danger of death as is necessary in a living will situation. Although it need not specifically delineate desired medical treatment, it must indicate the identity of the principal's attorney-in-fact and that the principal has communicated his health care wishes to his attorney-in-fact. (See Appendix F for several examples of durable power of attorney forms.) Although the laws vary from state to state, all 50 states and the District of Columbia have durable power of attorney statutes. This legal device is an important alternative to guardianship, conservatorship, or trusteeship. Because a durable power of attorney places a considerable amount of power in the hands of the attorney-in-fact, it should be drawn up by an attorney in the state in which the client resides.

Health Care Proxy

A health care proxy allows a person to appoint a "health care agent" to make treatment decisions if he or she becomes unable to do so. (See Appendix G for examples of proxy forms.) Thirteen states authorize the appointment of health care proxies.[23] The agent must be made aware of the patient's wishes regarding nutrition and hydration to be allowed to make a decision concerning withholding or withdrawing them. In contrast to a living will, a health care proxy does not require a person to know about and consider in advance all situations and decisions that could arise. Rather, the appointed agent would know about and interpret the expressed wishes of the patient, and then make decisions about the medical care and treatment to be administered or refused. The *Cruzan* decision indicates that the Supreme Court views advance directives as clear and convincing evidence of a patient's wishes regarding life sustaining treatment.

While most of the statutes fail to cover incompetents, cases like *Quinlan* and *Saikewicz* created a constitutionally protected obligation to terminate the incurable incompetent's life when the doctrine of substituted judgment is used by guardians. Further, some states provide for proxy consent in the form of durable power of attorney statutes. Generally, these involve the designation of a proxy to speak on the incompetent incurable's behalf.[24] They represent a combination of the intimate wishes of the patient and the medical recommendations of the physicians.

Oral declarations are accepted only after the patient has been declared terminally ill. Moreover, the declarant bears the responsibility of informing the physician to ensure that the document becomes a part of the medical record. The California statute provides that the document be re-executed after five years. Other statutes differ in the length of time of effectiveness. The majority of states allow the document to be effective until revoked by the individual. To revoke, the patient must sign and date a new writing, destroy the first document himself or herself, direct another to destroy the first document in his or her presence, or orally state to the physician an intent to revoke.[25] The effect of the directive varies among the jurisdictions. However, there is unanimity in the promulgation of regulations that specifically authorize health care personnel to honor the directives without fear of incurring liability. The highest court of New York in *In re Eichner*, 52 N.Y.2d 363, 420 N.E.2d 64 (1981), complied with the request of a guardian to withdraw life support systems from an 83-year-old brain-damaged priest. The court reached its result by finding the patient's previously expressed wishes to be determinative.

Right-To-Die Tag

A Montana law allows the use of identification bracelets to alert health care providers, including ambulance crews, of their serious medical condition and their request not to be resuscitated. The ID bracelets will be made available through the Montana Health Department.[26]

Guardianship/Conservatorship

Guardianship or conservatorship is a legal mechanism by which the court declares a person incompetent and appoints a guardian. The court transfers the responsibility for managing financial affairs, living arrangements, and medical care decisions to the guardian.[27] A resolution by the federal Council on the Aging recommends the implementation of guardianship programs and laws for the benefit and protection of older Americans "as exemplified by the Statement of Recommended Judicial Practices adopted by the National Conference of the Judiciary on Guardianship proceedings for the Elderly."[28] The Statement of Recommended Judicial Practices is available from the American Bar Association, 1800 M Street, N.W., Washington, D.C.

The Patient Self-Determination Act of 1990

An attempt has been made on the federal level to establish unified mandates that specified health care providers must follow when dealing with patients in persistent vegetative states. Passed as part of the 1990 federal budget, the Patient Self-Determination Act of 1990 (PSDA) will require Medicare and Medicaid reimbursed hospitals, nursing homes, home health agencies, HMOs and hospices to comply with new obligations concerning advance directives of patients who lapse into a persistent vegetative state.

Some of the new requirements that go into effect on December 1, 1991 are:

- Every Medicare/Medicaid reimbursed institution must ask admitted patients if they have advance directives. If the patient does, then it must be documented in his or her medical chart.
- Patients must be advised of relevant state laws and their rights under those laws. Each state will assign an agency to review state laws, in order to assist providers in developing written information.
- To insure that patients, staff, and the community are made aware of the preparation and use of advance directives, institutions must provide education programs.
- Written policies and procedures about advance directives must be established and implemented.

Although the PSDA is being cheered as a major advancement in clarifying and nationally regulating this often hazy area of law and medicine, it has some problems that must be ironed out. For example, the act does not deal with how to advise patients admitted who are not able to take or understand instructions. There is no requirement that a copy of an advance directive be attached to a patient's medical record. Moreover, quadriplegic patients who are competent are not covered under the act, unless they become comatose and sustained on life support systems. Also, there are no specific mandates about how to handle emergency room patients. All of these concerns, however, may be addressed by the Health Care Financing Administration, which is in the process of drafting new provisions.

Now that there is increasing acceptance of the right to end what has been deemed extraordinary care for the terminally ill, a relatively new dilemma has emerged, "the insertion and/or withdrawal of feeding tubes."

FEEDING TUBES

Theologians and ethicists have long recognized a distinction between ordinary and extraordinary medical care. The theological distinction is based on the belief that life is a gift from God that should not be deliberately destroyed by humans. Therefore, extraordinary therapies that extend life by imposing grave burdens on the patient and family are not required. A patient, however, has an ethical and moral obligation to accept ordinary or life sustaining treatment.[29] Although the courts have accepted decisions to withhold or withdraw extraordinary care, especially the respirator, from those who are comatose or in a persistent vegetative state with no possibility of emerging, they have been unwilling until now to discontinue feeding, which they have considered ordinary care.

However, in 1985, the case of *In the Matter of Claire C. Conroy*, 486 A.2d 1209 (N.J. Sup. Ct. 1985), was heard by the New Jersey Supreme Court. The case involved an 84-year-old nursing home patient whose nephew petitioned the court for authority to remove the nasogastric tube that was feeding her. The court overturned the appellate division decision and held that life sustaining treatment, including nasogastric feeding, could be withheld or withdrawn from incompetent nursing home patients who will, according to physicians, die within one year, in three specific circumstances:

1. when it is clear that the particular patient would have refused the treatment under the circumstances involved (the subjective test)
2. when there is some indication of the patient's wishes (but he or she has not "unequivocally expressed" his or her desires before becoming incompetent) and the treatment "would only prolong suffering" (the limited objective test)
3. when there is no evidence at all of the patient's wishes, but the treatment "clearly and markedly outweighs the benefits the patient derives from life" (the pure-objective test based on pain)

A procedure involving notification of the state Office of the Ombudsman is required before withdrawing or withholding treatment under any of the three tests. The ombudsman must make a separate recommendation. *Id.* at 1232.

The court also found tubal feeding to be a medical treatment, and as such, it is as intrusive as other life sustaining measures are. The court in its analysis emphasized duty, rather than causation, with the result that medical personnel acting in good faith will be protected from liability. If physicians follow the *Quinlan/Conroy* standards and decide to end medical treatment of a patient, the duty to continue treatment ceases; thus, the termination of treatment becomes a lawful act.

Although *Conroy* presents case-specific guidelines, there is concern that the opinion will have far-reaching repercussions. There is fear that decisions to discontinue treatment will not be based on the "balancing of interests" test, but rather that a "quality of life" test similar to that used by Hitler will be utilized to end the lives of severely senile, very old, decrepit, and burdensome people.[30]

Those quality of life judgments would be most dangerous for nursing home patients where age would be a factor in the decision-making process. "Advocates of 'the right to life' fear that the 'right to die' for the elderly and handicapped will become a 'duty to die.'"[31] In both the Saikewicz and Spring cases, age was a determining factor weighing against life sustaining treatment. Further, in *In re Hier*, 464 N.E.2d 959, (Mass. 1984), the court found that Mrs. Hier's age of 92 made the "proposed gastrostomy substantially more onerous or burdensome . . . than it would be for a younger, healthier person." *Id.* at 964. Moreover, a New York Superior Court held that the burdens of an emergency amputation for an elderly patient outweighed the benefit of continued life. Finding that prolonging her life would be cruel, the court stated that life had no meaning for her. In *In re Beth Israel Medical Center*, 519 N.Y.S.2d 511, 517 (Sup. Ct. 1987), some courts are recognizing and other courts must address the difference between *Quinlan*-type patients and elderly, confined, and conscious patients who can interact, but whose mental or physical functioning is impaired.

However, at least in one recent situation, the New Jersey ombudsman denied a request to remove feeding tubes from a comatose nursing home patient.[32] In applying the *Conroy* tests, the ombudsman decided that Hilda Peterson might live more than one year, the period that *Conroy* used as a criterion for determining whether life support can be removed.

To further complicate this issue, on March 17, 1986, the American Medical Association changed its Code of Ethics on comas. Now physicians may ethically withhold food, water, and medical treatment from patients in irreversible comas or persistent vegetative states with no hope of recovery—even if death is not imminent.[33] While physicians can consider the wishes of the patient and family or the legal representatives, they cannot intentionally cause death. The wording is permissive, so those physicians who feel uncomfortable in withdrawing food and water may refrain from doing so. The AMA's decision does not comfort those who fear abuse or mistake in euthanasia decisions, nor does it have any legal value as such. There are physicians, nurses, and families who are unscrupulous and have their own, and not the patient's, interests in mind. Even with the *Conroy* decision and the American Medical Association's Code of Ethics change, the feeding tube issue is not settled.

On April 23, 1986, the New Jersey Superior Court ruled that the husband of severely brain damaged Nancy Jobes could order the removal of her life sustaining feeding tube, which would ultimately cause the 31-year-old comatose patient, who had been in a vegetative state in a hospice for the past six years, to starve to death. In *In re Jobes*, 108 N.J. 394, 403, 529 A.2d 434, 438 (1987), Dr. Fred Plum created and defined the term "persistent vegetative state" as one where

> the body functions entirely in terms of its internal controls. It maintains temperature. It maintains digestive activity. It maintains heart beat and pulmonary ventilation. It maintains reflex activity of muscles and nerves for low level conditioned responses. But there is no behavioral evidence of either self-awareness or awareness of the surroundings in a learned manner.

Medical experts testified that the patient could, under optimal conditions, live another 30 years. Relieving the nursing home officials from performing the act on one of its residents, the court ruled that the patient may be taken home to die (with the removal to be supervised by a physician and medical care to be provided to the patient at home).

The nursing home had petitioned the court for the appointment of a "life advocate" to fight for continuation of medical treatment for Mrs. Jobes, which, it argued, would save her life. The court disallowed the appointment of a life advocate, holding that case law does not support requiring the continuation of life support systems in all circumstances. Such a requirement, according to the court, would contradict the patient's right of privacy.

The court's decision applied "the principles enunciated in *Quinlan* and . . . *Conroy*" and the "recent ruling by the American Medical Association's Council on

Judicial Affairs that the provision of food and water is, under certain circumstances, a medical treatment like any other and may be discontinued when the physician and family of the patient feel it is no longer benefiting the patient."[34]

The Illinois Supreme Court in *In re Estate of Longeway*, 139 Ill. Dec. 780 (1989), agreed with the logic of the *Jobes* decision and other sister state rulings regarding the characterization of artificial nutrition and hydration as medical treatment. The Illinois court found that the authorized guardian of a terminally ill patient in an irreversible coma or persistent vegetative state has a common law right to refuse artificial nutrition and hydration. The court found that there must be clear and convincing evidence that the refusal is consistent with the patient's interest. The court also required the concurrence of the patient's attending physician and two other physicians. "Court intervention is also necessary to guard against the remote, yet real possibility that greed may taint the judgment of the surrogate decisionmaker." *Id.* at 790. Dissenting, Judge Ward said, "[t]he right to refuse treatment is rooted in and dependent upon the patient's capacity for informed decision, which an incompetent patient lacks." *Id.* at 793.

In addition, Elizabeth Bouvia, a mentally competent cerebral palsy victim, has won her struggle to have feeding tubes removed even though she is not terminally ill. *Bouvia v. Superior Court (Glenchur)*, 225 Cal. Rptr. 297 (Ct. App. 1986). The California Court of Appeals announced on April 16, 1986, that she can go home to die. The court found that Miss Bouvia's decision to "let nature take its course" did not amount to a choice to commit suicide with people aiding and abetting it. The court stated that it is not "illegal or immoral to prefer a natural, albeit sooner, death than a drugged life attached to a mechanical device." *Id.* at 306. The court's finding that it was a moral and philosophical question, not a legal or medical one, leaves one wondering if the courts are opening the door to permitting "legal starvation" to be used by those who are not terminally ill, but who do wish to commit suicide.

Unfortunately, there are those in the health care field who are using their knowledge to develop new instruments of death to assist those who are terminally ill and want to end their lives. Dr. Jack Kevorkian of Michigan announced in October 1989 that he had developed a device that will end one's life quickly, painlessly, and humanely.[35] He described his invention as a metal pole with bottles containing three solutions that feed into a common IV line. When the IV is inserted into the patient's vein, a harmless saline solution will flow to clean the line of air. The patient can then flip a switch causing an anesthetic to render the patient unconscious. Sixty seconds later, a lethal dose of potassium chloride will flow into the patient, causing heart seizure and death. The news of this invention motivated the medical community and society at large to repeat their fear that individuals would abuse the practice of euthanasia in spite of any safeguards that are in place. Dr. Kevorkian assisted Janice Adkins, a 54-year-old Alzheimer's disease patient in committing suicide on June 4, 1990. In December, he was charged with first degree murder, but the charge was dismissed since Michigan has no law against assisted suicide. He was ordered, however, not to help anyone else commit suicide, or to give advice about it. On February 6, 1991, he violated the court order by giving advice about the preparation of the drug to a terminally ill cancer patient.[36]

DO NOT RESUSCITATE ORDERS

Prior to the *Quinlan* decision, which began the focus on the withdrawal of life sustaining machines, the life sustaining treatment most discussed was cardio-pulmonary resuscitation, in terms of whether or not to issue a Do Not Resuscitate order (DNR).

Do not resuscitate orders are those given by a physician, indicating that in the event of a cardiac or respiratory arrest, no resuscitative measures should be employed to revive the patient. Such orders must be in writing, signed, and dated by the physician. In addition, appropriate consents must be obtained from the resident/patient or his or her family or a patient advocate, as appropriate. Many states have acknowledged the validity of DNR orders in cases involving terminally ill patients where no objections to such orders are made by the patient's family. New York law allows out-of-hospital do not resuscitate orders only for those individuals enrolled in a hospice program.[37]

Do not resuscitate orders should be of short duration and reviewed periodically in order to determine whether the patient's condition or other circumstances (e.g., change of mind by the patient or family) surrounding the no code orders have changed. Presently, it is generally accepted that if a patient is competent, the DNR order is considered to be the same as other medical decisions in which a patient may choose to reject life sustaining treatment. In the case of an incompetent, absent any advance written directives, the best interests of the patient would be considered. A lower court decision in favor of a physician was overturned by the Indiana Court of Appeals in *Payne v. Marion General Hospital*, 549 N.E.2d 1043 (Ind. Ct. App. 1990). The physician had issued a "no code" status on Mr. Payne in spite of evidence given by a nurse that up to a few minutes before his death Mr. Payne could communicate. The physician had determined that Mr. Payne was incompetent, thereby rendering him unable to give informed consent to treatment. Since there were no written directives left by Mr. Payne, the physician relied on one of Mr. Payne's relatives who asked for the DNR order. The court found that there was evidence that Mr. Payne was not incompetent, and should have been consulted before a DNR order was given. Further, the court reviewed testimony that one year earlier Mr. Payne had suffered and recovered from the same type of symptoms, leading to the conclusion that there was a possibility he could have survived if resuscitation had continued. There was no DNR policy in place at the hospital to assist the physician in making his decision. In order to avoid this type of problem, health care providers should adopt policies with respect to the issuance of "no code" orders.

HEALTH CARE ETHICS

The Oath of Hippocrates has been passed on to us as a living and workable statement of ideals to be cherished by the physician. This oath protects rights of the patient and appeals to the finer instincts of the physician without imposing sanctions or penalties. Other civilizations have developed written principles, but the Oath of Hippocrates has remained in Western civilization as an expression of ideal conduct for the physician. Adherence to professional medical ethics will go a long way in the prevention of lawsuits and the development of good physician–patient relationships.

The tremendous advances in technology and the resulting capability to extend life, beyond the point of what some may consider "a reasonable quality of life," has given rise to many ethical and moral as well as medical and legal issues for long-term care facilities and society in general. The issues of patient rights, when to transfer a resident to a health care facility providing a higher level of care than that available in the long-term care facility, when to maintain a resident and provide those medications and treatments necessary to keep the resident as comfortable as possible, euthanasia, when to connect or disconnect life support equipment, etc., are dilemmas for nursing facility residents, their families, health care professionals, religious communities, and various advocacy groups.

Public policy issues in the ethics arena include what percentage of the health care budget should the nation allocate to care for its aging population, who should have access to elder care, and whether insurance coverage should provide for unlimited care, which could negatively affect other important health care programs. These are difficult questions with no easy answers. Although there are no simple solutions to these dilemmas, a continuing effort must be made in search of the most acceptable solution.

Ethics Committees

An alternative to court litigation that has been considered to insure the safeguarding of a patient's interests is the institutional ethics committee. An ethics committee is a consultative committee whose role is to analyze ethical dilemmas and to advise and educate health care providers, patients, and families regarding difficult treatment decisions. Ethics committees have been formed in a variety of health care settings to deal with difficult ethical issues. They had their origins with the 1976 landmark Karen Ann Quinlan case. "Since then, ethics committees have continued to become more popular, having had a significant burst of interest in the early 1980's largely as a result of a series of well-publicized cases involving decisions to forego or terminate life sustaining treatment."[38]

The *Quinlan* court looked to the prognosis committee to verify Karen Quinlan's medical condition. It then factored in the committee's opinion with all other evidence before it in order to reach the decision to allow the withdrawing of her life support machine. To date, ethics committees, which are commonly comprised of religious leaders, health care professionals, attorneys, and ethicists, do not have sole surrogate decision-making authority. However, they play an ever-increasing role in developing policy and procedural guidelines to assist in resolving the ethical dilemmas inherent in a right to forego treatment case.

Ethics committees must take special care in resolving any dispute that involves the treatment of incompetent patients, especially where no family or friends are involved. In those situations, the committee must not fall victim to arriving at a decision too quickly without considering all available information and alternatives. The best interests of the patient standard must be applied to determine what treatment should be or not be rendered.

The elderly often are treated as though they are incapable of making their own treatment decisions. This faulty thinking must be corrected. They are very special people and every effort must be made to treat them as the adults that they are. Their age must not diminish the recognition and respect they rightfully deserve.

> Thus, a decisionally capable elderly patient has the right to be informed of the diagnosis, prognosis, proposed intervention, risks of that intervention, availability of other options and their risk, and consequences of not intervening at all. After receiving this information, he or she is legally empowered to either consent to or refuse the intervention, even if that refusal should lead to serious harm or death for the patient.[39]

Committee Composition

Ethics committees are often comprised of a multi-disciplinary group of individuals and have included religious leaders, health professionals not associated with the facility, legal counsel, etc. Noting that physicians are the practitioners of medicine, not health care institutions, their representation on ethics committees is considered extremely important. A comment made by George Annas, a medical ethicist, is appropriately applicable to all health care facilities providing medical care: "Hospitals are corporations that have no natural personhood, and hence are incapable of having moral or ethical objections to action . . . . Hospitals don't practice medicine, physicians do."[40]

Committee Function

The functions of ethics committees can be multifaceted and include the development of policy and procedure guidelines to assist in resolving ethical dilemmas, staff and community education, conflict resolution, individual case review and support, and consultation on specific cases. The degree to which an ethics committee serves each of these functions varies in different hospitals and nursing facilities.

Policy and Procedure Development. Nursing facility boards need to adopt policy and procedure guidelines that health care workers can look to in making difficult ethical decisions on issues that arise in the health care setting. Ethics committees can play a major role in the development of such guidelines. The guidelines should be available for public review and constructive input.

Educational Role. The most common and agreed upon role of ethics committees is staff education. There is a need to sensitize health care workers regarding the ethical issues and conflicts that arise in the health care setting.[41]

Support Role. Ethics committees can advise and provide support, when and where appropriate, with residents; their families, surrogates, or proxies; and those health care professionals responsible for their care.

> Most health care professionals are neither intellectually prepared to address all of the ethical issues that arise in the delivery of medical care, nor emotionally comfortable talking about them. Successful resolution of many of the ethical dilemmas arising in nursing facilities today demands calling on a wide range of perspectives. NFECs (Nursing Facility Ethics Committees) can bring a diversity of personal and community values, and moral and professional perspectives that lead to valuable insights and advice beyond the limits of individuals.[42]

Ethics committees weigh the various religious, ethical, and moral issues that pertain to a given situation. They strive to provide viable alternatives that will lead to the optimal resolution of the dilemmas confronting the continuing care of the resident. It is important to remember that an ethics committee functions in an advisory capacity and should not be considered a substitute proxy for the long-term care resident.

Consultation. The availability of consultation from ethics committees can be of tremendous value to health care workers faced with difficult ethical dilemmas. Ethics committees can serve as a forum for discussing and resolving ethical concerns regarding specific cases. Where ethics committees have been instituted, consultation services should be available to the staff, families, and patients to assist in making difficult treatment decisions.

There is a wealth of information available regarding the establishment of ethics committees. Long-term care facilities that are in the process of establishing such a committee should review the literature, as well as seek advice from those who have gone through the process of setting up their own committees.

CONCLUSION

Figures 13-1 and 13-2 illustrate and summarize the numerous ramifications of euthanasia, as discussed in this chapter.

Any discussion of euthanasia obliges a person to confront a human's greatest fear—death. The courts and legislatures have faced it and have made advances in setting forth some guidelines to assist decision makers in this area. However, more must be accomplished. Society must be protected from the risks associated with permitting the removal of life support systems. We cannot allow the complex issues associated with this topic to be simplified to the point where we accept that life can be terminated based on subjective quality-of-life considerations. The legal system must assure that the constitutional rights of the patient will be maintained, while at the same time protecting society's interests in preserving life, preventing suicide, and maintaining the integrity of the medical profession.

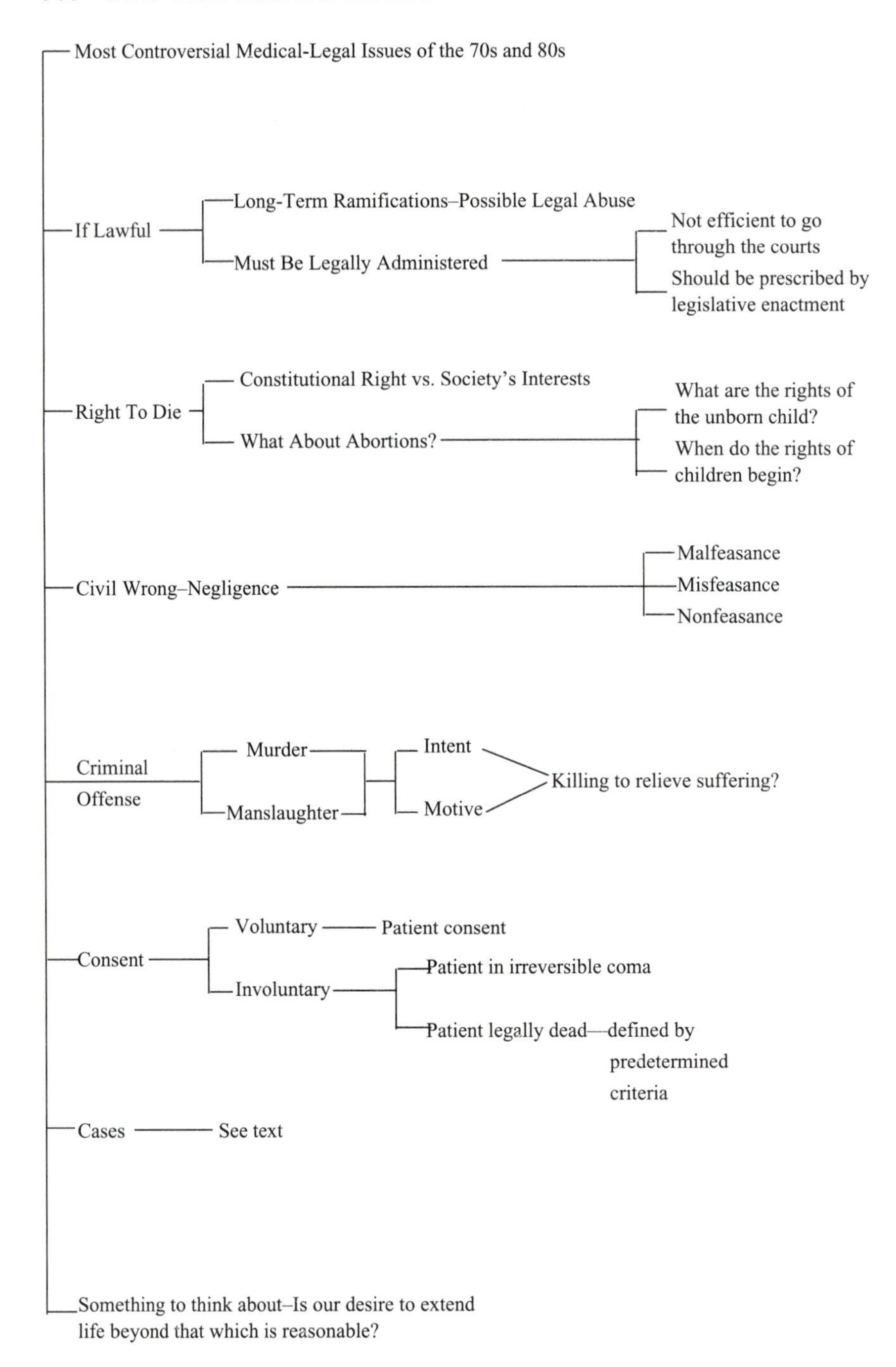

Figure 13-1 Legal Ramifications of Euthanasia

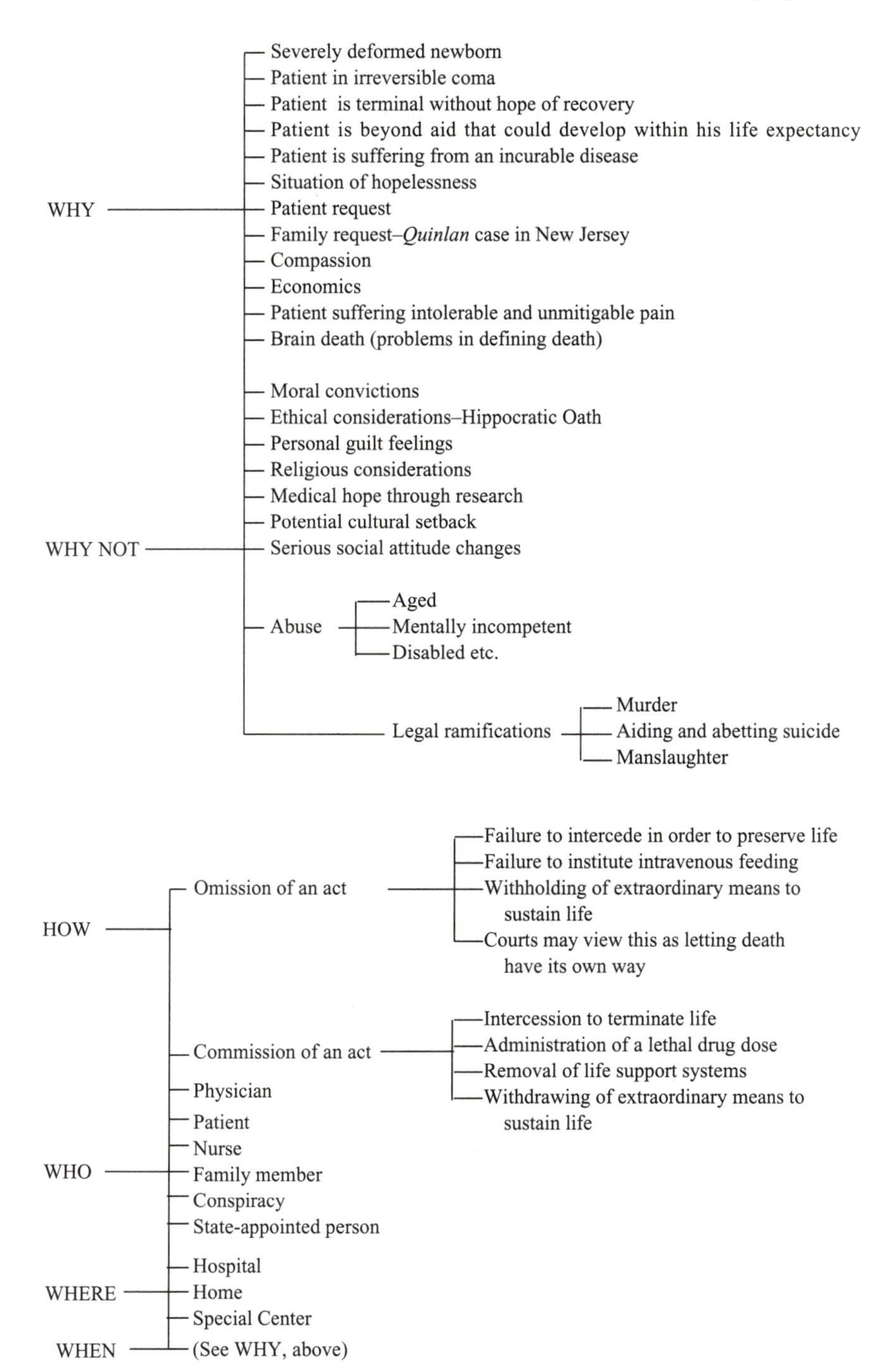

Figure 13-2 Considerations in Euthanasia

NOTES

1. R. GILLON, SUICIDE AND VOLUNTARY EUTHANASIA: HISTORICAL PERSPECTIVE IN EUTHANASIA AND THE RIGHT TO DEATH 173 (1969).

2. *Id.* at 182.

3. S. Reiser, *The Dilemma of Euthanasia in Modern Medical History: The English and American Experience*, ETHICS IN MEDICINE PERSPECTIVES AND MEDICAL CONCERNS 20 (1977).

4. WEBSTER'S THIRD NEW INTERNATIONAL DICTIONARY OF THE ENGLISH LANGUAGE UNABRIDGED 786 (1976).

5. Cruzan v. Director, Missouri Dept. of Health, 110 S.Ct. 2841, 2864 (1990).

6. Sherlock, *For Everything There Is a Season: The Right To Die in the United States*, B.Y.U. L. REV. 545 (1982).

7. Karen Ann Quinlan, at age 22, was in a coma due to an overdose of valium and alcohol. As a result, she was hooked up to a life supporting respirator.

8. Gelford, *Euthanasia and the Terminally Ill Patient*, 63 NEB L. REV. 741, 747 (1984).

9. Coyle, *Fast Furious Questioning Marks Session on Coma Case*, Nat'l L. J., Dec. 18, 1989, at 8; Wallis, *To Feed or Not To Feed*, Time (March 31, 1986), at 60.

10. Connery, *Prolonging Life: The Duty and Its Limits, Moral Responsibility in Prolonging Life's Decisions*, TO TREAT OR NOT TO TREAT 25 (1984).

11. AMA House of Delegates, Resolution 77, Statement of Medical Opinion Re: "Brain Death" (June 1974).

12. *Medical Care by Proxy*, 219, Estate Planning Review, March 31, 1989, at 17.

13. Pa. Senate Bill 646, Amendment A3506, Printer's No. 689, October 1, 1990.

14. *Hospital Wants to Let Wife Die*, Newsday, January 11, 1991, at 13.

15. *Id.*

16. *Advance Directives Linked to Residents' Rights Mandate*, 17(2) PROVIDER FOR LONG TERM CARE PROFESSIONALS, February 1991, at 32–34.

17. FEDERAL COUNCIL ON THE AGING, ANNUAL REPORT TO THE PRESIDENT (1988) 18.

18. U.S. DEPARTMENT OF HEALTH AND HUMAN SERVICES, OFFICE OF HUMAN DEVELOPMENT SERVICES, ADMINISTRATION ON AGING, WHERE TO TURN FOR HELP FOR OLDER PERSONS (1987), 27–28.

19. *Montana OKs Right-to-Die Tag*, Newsday (April 26, 1991), at 29.

20. *Hawaii: Living Will Legislation*, 27(23) AHA News, June 10, 1991, at 7.

21. *Id.* at 25.

22. *Id.* at 26.

23. Cruzan, *supra* note 5 at 2858.

24. *The Physician's Responsibility toward Hopelessly Ill Patients*, NEW ENGL. J. MED., Apr. 12, 1984, at 955.

25. Novak, *"Natural Death Acts": Let Patients Refuse Treatment*, HOSPITALS, Aug. 1, 1984, at 72.

26. Montana OKs Right-to-Die Tag, *supra* note 19, at 4, 29.

27. U.S. DEPARTMENT OF HEALTH AND HUMAN SERVICES, *supra* note 18, at 26.

28. FEDERAL COUNCIL ON THE AGING, *supra* note 17, at 11.

29. McCormick, *To Save or Let Die: The Dilemma of Modern Medicine*, 229 J.A.M.A. 172 (1974).

30. Wallis, *supra* note 9.

31. U.S. CONGRESS, OFFICE OF TECHNOLOGY ASSESSMENT, LIFE-SUSTAINING TECHNOLOGIES AND THE ELDERLY, PUB. NO. OTA-BA-306 (1987), at 48.

32. Sullivan, *Ombudsman Bars Food Tube Removal*, New York Times, March 7, 1986, at 82.

33. *AMA Changes Code of Ethics on Comas*, Newsday, Mar. 17, 1986, at 2.
34. *Man Wins Right To Let Wife Die*, Newsday, Apr. 24, 1986, at 3.
35. Fireman, *MD Invents Mercy Death Device*, Newsday, Oct. 27, 1989, at 6.
36. *Dr. Death at Work*, Newsday, February 7, 1991, at 12.
37. *Montana OKs Right-to Die Tag, supra* note 19, at 29.
38. M.D. Miller, *A Look at Long Term Care Ethics: Dilemmas and Decisions*, 16 PROVIDER 12 (1990).
39. U.S. CONGRESS, OFFICE OF TECHNOLOGY ASSESSMENT, *supra* note 31, at 107.
40. G.J. Annas, *Transferring the Ethical Hot Potato*, 17 HASTINGS CENTER REPORT 20, 21 (1987).
41. M.D. Miller, *supra* note 38, at 14.
42. *Id.* at 13.

Chapter 14

Autopsy and Donation

In the end stages of declining health, a resident of a nursing facility may require a higher level of care than it can offer to the resident. If a transfer becomes necessary, the receiving institution should be informed as to the resident's wishes with regard to the disposition of his or her body. It is important that each individual make informed choices about this most unpleasant task while he or she is competent to do so.

A resident often has specific wishes about burial arrangements and how a funeral service is to be conducted. Each individual has a right to choose only those arrangements he or she desires. Those wishes should be put in writing and left where they can be found easily by a responsible family member.

Should body or organ donations be requested by a resident, the receiving institution must be aware of the resident's wishes. The ever-increasing success of organ transplants and demand for organ tissue require the close scrutiny of each case, making sure that established procedures have been followed in the care and disposal of all body parts. Physicians, nurses, and other paramedical personnel assigned with this responsibility are often confronted with a variety of legal issues. Liability can be limited by complying with applicable regulations and adhering to procedures implementing these regulations.

A variety of responsibilities arise in long-term care facilities regarding the handling of dead bodies. Like any other aspect of facility operation, failure to fulfill these responsibilities can result in liability.

The legally protected interests of the surviving spouse or nearest relatives include the right to possession of the body and the right to bring suit and collect damages for injury or indignity to the body of a dead person.

The rule now uniformly recognized in the United States is that the person entitled to possession of a body for burial has certain legally protected interests. Interference with these rights can result in liability. Damages awarded in cases of liability through interference with the rights of a surviving spouse or near relative in the body of a decedent are based on the emotional and mental suffering that results from such interference. For damages to be awarded, the conduct of the alleged wrongdoer must be sufficiently disturbing to a person of ordinary sensibilities as to cause emotional harm. Cases involving the wrongful handling of dead bodies may be classified into four groups: mutilation of a body; unauthorized autopsy; wrongful detention; and miscellaneous wrongs such as unauthorized sale, refusal or neglect to bury, and unauthorized use or publication of photographs taken after death.

In many states, intentionally mutilating a dead body is a punishable crime as well as a basis for civil liability. Obviously, such acts could be said to cause substantial emotional suffering for those who loved and respected the decedent. Similarly, an unauthorized autopsy may disturb persons whose religious beliefs prohibit such a procedure as well as those persons who have a general aversion to the procedure. Where autopsies have been performed without statutory authorization and without the consent of the decedent, the surviving spouse, or an appropriate relative, liability may be imposed.

Refusal to deliver a dead body to a person who demands custody, and is entitled to receive it, may also result in liability. Unintentional as well as intentional conduct interfering with rights to a body can result in liability.

In order to limit lawsuits regarding the disposition of dead bodies, appropriate handling and release procedures should be established. Such procedures should be reviewed by legal counsel.

RIGHT OF SUIT FOR IMPROPER ACTION

Although several persons may suffer emotional stress and mental suffering because of indignities in the treatment of the body of the decedent, recovery for wrongful interference with the body and its proper burial has generally been limited to the person who has the right of possession of the body for burial. Some state statutes delineate an order of the duty to bury the decedent. Others set forth an order of persons authorized to give consent to autopsy, from which the order of devolution may be established. In states without either provision, case law must provide the guidelines. Generally, the primary right to custody of a dead body belongs to the surviving spouse. Where there is no spouse, the right passes to the adult children of the decedent, if any, and then to the decedent's parents.

The principal administrative question involves the effort the nursing facility must expend to discover and notify persons who have a duty to inhume the deceased. A reasonable effort should be made to locate the surviving spouse or closest kin. It is likely that a court would consider a release of a body to one person after a reasonably diligent search to be a satisfactory disposition, even though another with a superior claim might appear later.

AUTOPSY

Autopsies, or post-mortem examinations, are conducted to ascertain the cause of a person's death, which in turn may resolve a number of legal issues. An autopsy may reveal whether death was the result of criminal activity, whether the cause of death was one for which payment must be made in accordance with an insurance contract, whether the death is compensable under worker's compensation and occupational disease acts, or whether death was the result of a specific act or a culmination of several acts. Aside from providing answers to these specific questions, the information gained from autopsies adds to medical knowledge. As such, medical schools have an interest in autopsies for educational purposes.

Autopsy Consent Statutes

Recognizing both the need for information that can be secured only through the performance of a substantial volume of autopsies and the valid interests of relatives and friends of the decedent, most states have enacted statutes dealing with autopsy consent. Such legislation seems intended to have a two-fold effect: first, to protect the rights of the decedent's relatives, and second, to guide those performing autopsies in establishing procedures for consent to autopsy.

Most autopsy consent statutes can be classified in two groups. One group consists of the statutes that establish an order for obtaining consent to autopsy based on the degree of family relationship. The statutes of the second group contain provisions enumerating those persons from whom consent may be obtained, but they do not provide an order of priority among them. These laws say the consent is to be obtained from any one of the enumerated persons who has assumed custody of the body for burial. In some states with such statutes there are no additional statutes concerning the devolution of the duty to bury and the right to custody. Furthermore, the assumption of custody of the body by a person enumerated in the statutes must be clear before consent to an autopsy can be relied on.

In states that have autopsy consent statutes, as well as statutes specifying the order in which duty of burial and right to custody of the body devolve on the relatives of the decedent, the two statutes taken together indicate the proper person from whom consent is to be obtained. In states without autopsy consent statutes, other statutes regarding the duty to bury and the right to custody of a body for burial may prove helpful in determining which of the decedent's relatives may give effective authorization for autopsy.

Authorization by the Decedent

Most autopsy consent statutes provide that deceased persons may authorize an autopsy on their remains. Ordinarily such consent must be in writing. There may be legal as well as practical problems in obtaining authorization for an autopsy from a patient before death if the state does not provide by statute for such authorization. If an autopsy is desired, it would probably be simpler and more effective to obtain authorization from the relative or some other person who assumes the legal responsibility for burial, rather than from the patient before death.

In states where there is neither an autopsy consent statute nor a statute permitting donation that may be construed to include autopsy, it is unwise to rely exclusively on the authorization of a decedent to perform an autopsy. This is especially true where relatives of the deceased who assume custody of the body for burial object to an autopsy. Although many cases have upheld the wishes of the deceased with respect to the place of interment or the manner of disposition of the remains (i.e., by burial or cremation), it is possible that the courts will not afford the same weight to the decedent's wishes concerning autopsies. In such instances, compelling reasons presented by certain next of kin of the decedent, especially the surviving spouse, may prevail over the wishes of the decedent.

It is also possible that a patient would specifically request that no autopsy be performed on his or her body upon death. This request may stem from religious convictions or personal preference. Some state legislatures have specifically recognized this right to refuse an autopsy. For example, in New York, it is provided:

> Except as required by law, no dissection or autopsy shall be performed on the body of any person who is carrying an identification card upon his person indicating his opposition to such dissection or autopsy. To be valid, this card must be signed and dated by the person opposed to the dissection or autopsy and must be notarized.

New York Public Health Law Section 4209-a (1981).

Authorization by Person Other Than Decedent

Two closely related concepts concern the determination of who may authorize the performance of an autopsy. One of these has developed in litigation when a corpse has been mutilated and a person has been permitted to bring an action to recover damages. Such cases ordinarily determine an order of priority with respect to the person who may bring an action. The second concept—responsibility for burial of the deceased body—is the basis for the right of an individual to bring an action for mutilation of a dead body. The order of responsibility for burial is ordinarily the same as the order of preference for bringing an action for mutilation, since the latter arises from the former. The person on whom the duty to bury the deceased is imposed has the right to custody of the body and the right to recover for mutilation of the corpse; authority to perform an autopsy should be obtained from this person.

Where custody of the body has been assumed by the first person in the preference order, that person's consent is sufficient to authorize the autopsy and prevent liability for mutilation of the corpse. If consent to the autopsy is refused, performance of the autopsy could lead to liability even if some other relative of the deceased sought to authorize it. What if the first person in the order of preference is deceased or mentally incompetent, or is unwilling or unable to assume the responsibility for burial of the body, or fails to do so? It is then necessary to determine who has such responsibility and the concomitant right to authorize an autopsy. Fortunately, in many states the order of responsibility for burial is set forth in statutes, and the right to authorize an autopsy is given to the person who has assumed custody of the body for burial.

In the absence of statutes furnishing a preference order of responsibility for burial or for consent, the order usually followed is surviving spouse, adult children of the deceased, parents, adult brothers and sisters, grandparents, uncles and aunts, and finally cousins. A court may find that a surviving spouse's unwillingness to assume responsibility for burial is sufficient to permit the right to custody of the body to devolve on a relative who is willing to assume such responsibility.

Scope and Extent of Consent

Legal issues may arise as a result of an autopsy even if consent has been obtained from the person authorized by law to grant such consent. If autopsy procedures go beyond the limits imposed by the consent, or if the consent to an autopsy is obtained by fraud or without the formal requisites, liability may be incurred. It is a fundamental principle that a person who has the right to refuse permission for the performance of an act also has the right to place limitations or conditions on consent.

The principle involved in limiting the scope of an autopsy has been expressed as follows:

> One having the right to refuse to allow an autopsy has the right to place any limitations or restrictions on giving consent to such procedure, and one who violates such stipulations renders himself liable.[1]

Fraudulently Obtained Consent

It is a long-accepted principle that consent obtained through fraud or material misrepresentation is not binding and that the person whose consent is so obtained stands in the same position as if no consent had been given. This principle can apply to autopsies when facts are misrepresented to the person who has the right to consent in order to induce his or her consent.

ORGAN DONATIONS

Developments in medical science have enabled physicians to take tissue from persons immediately after death and use it for transplantation in order to replace or rehabilitate diseased or damaged organs or other parts of living persons. Progress in this field of medicine has created the problem of obtaining a sufficient supply of replacement body parts. Throughout the country there are eye banks, artery banks, and other facilities for the storage and preservation of organs and tissue that can be used for transplantation and for other therapeutic services.

Organs and tissues to be stored and preserved for future use must be removed almost immediately after death. Therefore, it is imperative that an agreement or arrangement for obtaining organs and tissue from a body be completed before death, or very soon after death, to enable physicians to remove and store the tissue promptly.

Persons aware of the shortage of dead bodies needed for medical education and transplantation may wish to make arrangements during their lifetime for the use of their bodies after death for such purposes. A surviving spouse may, however, object to such disposition. In such cases, the interest of the surviving spouse or other family member could supersede that of the deceased.

A Uniform Anatomical Gift Act drafted by the Commission on Uniform State Laws has been endorsed by the American Bar Association. This statute has been enacted by many states and has many detailed provisions that apply to the wide variety of issues raised in connection with the making, acceptance, and use of anatomical gifts. State statutes regarding donation usually permit the donor to execute the gift during his or her lifetime.

The right to privacy of the donor and his family must be respected. Information should not be disseminated regarding transplant procedures that publish the names of the donor or donee without adequate consent.

States have enacted legislation to facilitate donation of bodies and body parts for medical uses. Virtually all the states have based their enactments on the Uniform Anatomical Gift Act, drafted by the Commission on Uniform State Laws, but it should be recognized that in some states there are deviations from this act or additional laws dealing with donation.

Summary of the Uniform Anatomical Gift Act

Individuals who are of sound mind and 18 years of age or older are permitted to dispose of their own bodies or body parts by will or other written instrument for medical or dental education, research, advancement of medical or dental science, therapy, or transplantation. Among those eligible to receive such donations are any licensed, accredited, or approved hospitals; accredited medical or dental schools; surgeons or physicians; tissue banks; or specified individuals who need the donation for therapy or transplantation. The statute provides that when only a part of the body is donated custody of the remaining parts of the body shall be transferred to the next of kin promptly following removal of the donated part.

In cases of donation made by a written instrument other than a will, the instrument must be signed by the donor in the presence of two witnesses who, in turn, must sign the instrument in the donor's presence. If the donor cannot sign the instrument, the document may be signed by a person authorized by the donor, at the donor's direction and in the presence of the donor and the two signing witnesses.

Delivery of the document during the donor's lifetime is not necessary to make the donation valid. A donation by will becomes effective immediately upon the death of the testator, without probate, and the gift is valid and effective to the extent that it has been acted on in good faith. This is true even if the will is not probated or is declared invalid for testimonial purposes.

A donation by a person other than the decedent may be made by written, telegraphic, recorded telephonic, or other recorded consent. In the absence of a contrary intent evidenced by the decedent or of actual notice of opposition by a member of the same class or a prior class in the preference order, the decedent's body or body parts may be donated by the following persons in the order specified: (1) surviving spouse, (2) adult child, (3) parent, (4) adult brother or sister, (5) decedent's guardian, or (6) any other person or agency authorized to dispose of the body.

There are several methods by which a donation may be revoked. If the document has been delivered to a named donee, it may be revoked by a written revocation signed by the donor and delivered to the donee, an oral revocation witnessed by two persons and communicated to the donee, a statement to the physician attending during a terminal illness that has been communicated to the donee, or a card or piece of writing that has been signed and is on the donor's person or in the donor's immediate effects. If the written instrument of donation has not been delivered to the donee, it may be revoked by destruction, cancellation, or mutilation of the instrument. If the donation is made by a will, it may be revoked in the manner provided for revocation or amendment of wills. Any person acting in good faith reliance on the terms of an instrument of donation will not be subject to civil or criminal liability unless there is actual notice of the revocation of the donation.

The time of death shall be determined by a physician in attendance at the donor's death, or a physician certifying death, who shall not be a member of the team of physicians engaged in the transplantation procedure.

UNCLAIMED DEAD BODIES

Persons entitled to possession of a dead body must arrange for release of the body from the nursing facility, for transfer to an embalmer or undertaker, and for final disposal. The recognition by the courts of a quasi-property right in the body of a deceased person imposes a duty on the facility to make reasonable efforts to give notice to persons entitled to claim the body. When there are no known relatives or friends of the family who can be contacted by the facility to claim the body, the facility has a responsibility to dispose of the body in accordance with law.

Most states have statutes providing for the disposal of such bodies. Many administrative headaches can be avoided by maintaining current administrative policy and procedures regarding the disposal of dead bodies and current patient information files as to the nearest relative or appointed proxy.

Unclaimed bodies are generally buried at public expense; a public official, usually a county official, has the duty to bury or otherwise dispose of such bodies.

Most states have statutes providing for the disposal of unclaimed bodies by delivery to institutions for educational and scientific purposes. The public official in charge of the body has a duty to notify the government agency of the presence of the body. The agency then arranges for the transfer of the body in accordance with the statute. If no such agency exists under the statute, the nursing facility or the public official may be authorized to allow a medical school or other institution or person, designated by the statute as an eligible recipient of unclaimed dead bodies, to remove the body for scientific use.

Certain categories of persons are usually excluded from these provisions permitting the distribution of bodies for educational and scientific use. For public health reasons the statutes do not usually permit distribution of the bodies of persons who have died from contagious diseases.

While the majority of these statutes quite explicitly require notification of relatives and set time limits for holding the body to allow relatives an opportunity to claim the body, strict compliance with the statutory provisions is often impossible because of the very nature of the problems that arise in the handling of dead bodies and in the required procedures themselves. Noncompliance in such instances would not appear to cause liability. An example of such a provision is the requirement that relatives be notified immediately upon death and that the body be held for 24 hours subject to claim by a relative or friend. The procedure of locating and notifying relatives may consume the greater part of the 24-hour period following death; if relatives who are willing to claim the body are located, the body should be held for a reasonable time to allow them to arrange custody for burial. It should be recognized that literal compliance may prejudice the interests of relatives of the decedent.

NOTE

1. 22 Am. Jur. 2d *Dead Bodies* §64 (1988).

Chapter 15

Financing Long-Term Care

Spending in the United States for health care continues to rise. The nation expended 11.2 percent of its gross national product (GNP) on health in 1987. This represents a 3 percent increase over 1986.[1]

> In 1987 national health expenditures totaled $500 billion, an average of $1,987 per person. Between 1980 and 1987 the percent of health care dollars accounted for by hospital care decreased slightly from 41 to 39 percent, and the percent accounted for by physician services increased concomitantly from 19 to 21 and expenditures for nursing home care remained at 8% of the total. . . .[2]

The nation spent $604.1 billion on health care in 1989, according to a recent report of the U.S. Department of Commerce, *U.S. Industrial Outlook 1991*. This represents an 11.1 percent increase over 1988 levels. During the same period, the GNP grew 6.7 percent. Eight percent of the 1989 health care budget ($47.9 billion) was expended for nursing home care.[3]

Total expenditures for health care in 1990 are estimated to reach $675.5 billion once final figures have been compiled, with $54.1 billion having been expended for nursing home care.[4] Total health care expenditures for 1991 have been projected to rise to $756.3 billion, with $61.4 billion being spent on nursing home care.[5] The increase in expenditures for nursing home care appears somewhat modest in comparison to other health care expenditures (see Figure 15-1).

Long-term care can lead to catastrophic expenses for the nation's elderly. An extended stay in a nursing facility can literally force many of America's elderly into bankruptcy. Fifty percent of Americans over the age of 65 are expected to spend some time in a nursing home, according to some estimates.[6] A study conducted by the Employee Benefits Research Institute found that two thirds of single persons and one third of married persons exhausted all of their funds after just 13 weeks in a nursing home.[7]

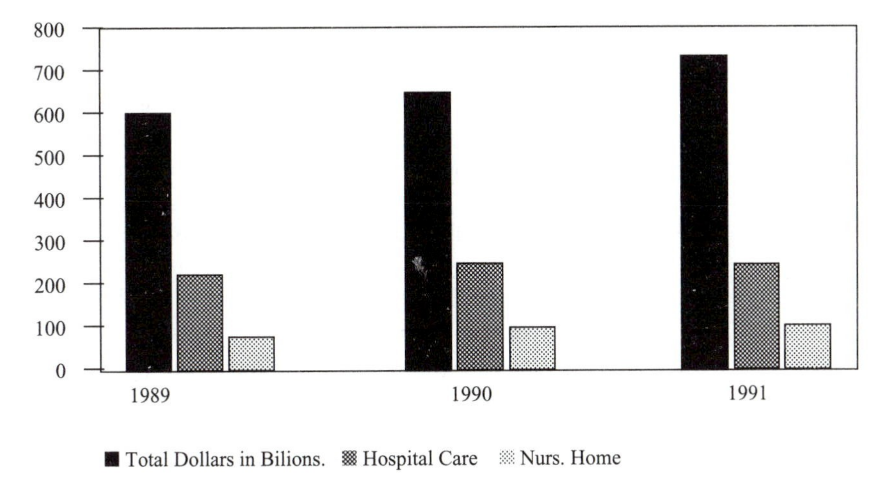

Figure 15-1 Selected Health Care Expenditures

The average cost of a year's stay in a nursing facility today is approximately $30,000. It can go much higher in big cities. "Very little of the tab—about 1.5 percent—is picked up by Medicare. And the private Medigap policies that some buy to coordinate with Medicare generally do not pick up the cost of long-term care either."[8]

Senior citizens tend to require more visits to physicians' offices. They also account for a greater percentage of discharges from hospitals.

> In 1981 the elderly averaged 1.75 more visits to physicians' offices and nearly twice as many hospital discharges per 1,000 compared to the population as a whole. On a per capita basis, the elderly typically spend approximately three times more on health care services than the rest of the population.[9]

Older age groups have both a lower income and a much greater need for health services and living assistance than do younger age groups. The age group that requires special attention and that will experience dramatic increases in numbers is the aged and very old. Less than 5 percent of the population was 75 or older in 1982; by 2030, almost 10 percent of the population is projected to be in that age group.[10] Because of the increasing number of persons who survive into their eighties, it is increasingly likely that older persons themselves will have a surviving parent.[11]

There is no doubt that long-term care is costly at 54.5 billion and has been increasing at a rate of 9–11 percent annually for several years, which is well above the general inflation rate.[12] "While the costs increase, the problems of inadequate staffing levels, high turnover rates, and poor quality nursing care are growing."[13]

By the year 2,000, there could be as many as 2.6 million nursing home residents. At the present rate of growth, expenditures for nursing home care could reach $90 billion.[14]

Table 15-1 presents the average total monthly charge of nursing home residents by source of payment.

Even with the wide variety of public and private sources for funding long-term care, families continue to pay the largest portion of nursing home expenses—$21.1 billion. Medicaid paid $17.3 billion, Medicare $.6 billion, and private insurance paid $.4 billion. Fewer than 1 percent of Medicare beneficiaries have supplemental insurance.[15] (See Figure 15-2 for distribution of nursing home expenditures by payor.)

Reimbursement for long-term care is often provided through private insurance. "[M]ost policies are bought by older people, worried about exhausting their assets or burdening their children."[16] The costs of long-term nursing home treatment are high, and the insurance protection available is minimal. Studies conducted by the Health Insurance Association of America revealed that 81 percent of out-of-pocket medical expenses for senior citizens were expended on nursing home care,[17] and, although 40 percent of elderly Americans can afford to purchase long-term care insurance, only 10 percent have done so.[18] A recent congressional report revealed that "Approximately one-half of the $6 billion spent annually on long-term insurance goes to agents as commission, according to the report, which was prepared by the House Aging and Small Business committees."[19]

A recent case, *Gust v. Pomeroy*, 466 N.W.2d 137 (N.D. 1991), illustrates how callous the insurance industry can be. An insurance agent appealed suspension of his license in a civil penalty imposed by the North Dakota Commissioner of Insurance for selling unnecessary or excessive insurance in violation of statute and administrative code. The Supreme Court of North Dakota held that the evidence supported

Table 15-1 Average Total Monthly Charge of Nursing Home Residents by Source of Payment

Residents by Age Group	*Average All Sources*	*Own Income or Family Support*	*Medicare*	*Medicaid Skilled*	*Medicaid Intermed.*
Under 45	1,443	1,211		1,928	1,485
45-54	1,351	1,047			1,247
55-64	1,360	1,168		1,938	1,285
65-69	1,304	1,301	1,544	1,896	1,193
70-74	1,415	1,463	1,802	1,913	1,258
75-79	1,481	1,455	2,059	1,941	1,310
80-84	1,458	1,437	2,576	1,869	1,281
85-89	1,492	1,486	2,585	1,861	1,299
90-94	1,489	1,526	1,215	1,886	1,281
95+	1,534	1,599	2,231	1,748	1,375

Source: The National Nursing Home Survey, 1985 Summary for the United States, Hyattsville, MD, U.S. Department of Health and Human Services, January 1969, at 26.

a finding that the insurance agent had sold unnecessary or excessive Medicare supplemental coverage. At the time of the sale the insured had four other policies that provided Medicare supplemental coverage and two other policies that provided nursing home coverage. Although the agent asserted that his two policies would replace the insured's other policies, this was not noted on the insured's application.

> As a licensed insurance agent, Gust is required to know the laws and rules and regulations governing the sale of insurance, for his license may be revoked for a violation of, or noncompliance with, an insurance law or lawful rules or orders of the Insurance Commissioner. . . . A licensed agent should have less trouble than a member of the general public in understanding what constitutes "unnecessary" or "excessive" insurance coverage.

Id. at 140.

The Federal Council on the Aging in its 1988 Annual Report to the President stated that there "will be staggering costs to the Federal government in the future if Congress does not work with the insurance industry now to draft legislation encouraging individuals to purchase on their own or through their employer plans to meet future long-term health care needs."[20] Under OBRA 90, the Secretary of HHS has been mandated to develop a proposal to modify the current system under which nursing facilities receive payments for extended care services under Part A of Medicare or a proposal to replace such system with a system under which payments would be made on the basis of prospectively determined rates. The Secretary was required to submit, by no later than April 1, 1991, any research studies to be used in developing the proposal to the Senate Committee on Finance and the House Committee on Ways and Means.[21]

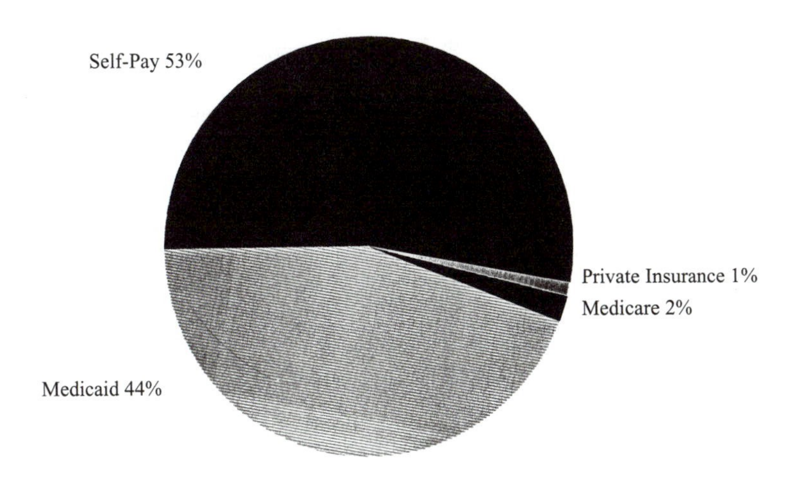

Figure 15-2 Nursing Home Expenditures by Payor

FEDERAL PROGRAMS FOR THE ELDERLY

The Medicare program was established by Public Law No. 89–97, which was effective July 30, 1965, also known as the Social Security Amendments of 1965. These amendments added two new titles to the Social Security Act of 1935, namely Title XVIII—Health Insurance for the Aged, generally known as Medicare, and Title XIX—Grants to States for Medical Assistance Programs, generally referred to as Medicaid. Title XX of the Social Security Act authorizes reimbursement to the states for social services via the Social Services Block Grant. The states have freedom to spend grant funds on state-identified needs (e.g., day care and home care services).

Title III of the Older Americans Act provides funds for services for the elderly (e.g., home delivered meals and senior citizens' centers). Title III financing totaled $669 million in 1985, serving some 654,000 elderly persons for homemaker services.[22]

MEDICARE

Medicare is a federally sponsored health insurance program for persons over 65 years of age and certain disabled persons. It has two complementary parts. Medicare Part A helps cover the costs of inpatient hospital care and, with qualifying preadmission criteria (e.g., three days in an acute care facility), up to 100 days per year in a "skilled nursing facility," home health care, and hospice care. Medicare Part B Medical Insurance helps pay for doctors' services, outpatient hospital services, etc.

It is funded through social security contributions (FICA payroll taxes), premiums, and general revenue. The program is administered through private contractors, referred to as "intermediaries" under Part A and "carriers" under Part B. The financing of the Medicare program has received much attention by Congress because of its rapidly rising costs (7.1 billion in 1970, 35.7 billion in 1980, and 70.5 billion in 1985) and drain on the nation's economy. Even though enormous benefits have been paid out under the Medicare program, the program requires substantial deductibles as well as coinsurance and, unfortunately, limits coverage for long-term care services.

The Health Care Financing Administration (HCFA) develops and implements policies, procedures, and guidance related to program recipients and the providers of services, such as hospitals, nursing homes, physicians, and the contractors who process claims. HCFA also coordinates with the states to develop departmental programs, activities, and organizations that are closely related to the Medicare program.[23] The Medicare program, as discussed below, differs from the Medicaid program in that Medicare is a program for social insurance, whereas Medicaid is a welfare program.

Assignment of Medicare Part B Claims

The Omnibus Budget Reconciliation Act of 1989, or OBRA89, which became effective September 1, 1990, provides that doctors are responsible for submitting the claim forms on all Medicare Part B claims—whether assigned or unassigned. "This is a change from the earlier practice, under which providers handled the paperwork for 'assigned claims,' and Medicare beneficiaries paid the care provider directly for 'unassigned claims' and then filed a claim for reimbursement with the carrier."[24] A 10 percent penalty of a provider's fee will be imposed for failure to submit a claim within a year of service. Failure to submit a claim can result in program actions as well as civil actions.[25]

Processing Medicare Part B Claims

The practice of charging a fee for processing Medicare claims is prohibited.

> Section 6102(g)(4) of OBRA89 states that for Medicare Part B services provided after Sept. 1, the physician (or other health care provider) is responsible for completing the standard Medicare form and submitting it to the carrier (the insurance company designated by the Health Care Finance Authority—HCFA—to handle claims processing). The care provider is allowed one year to do this and is not allowed to charge the beneficiary for processing the paperwork.[26]

A health provider who does ". . . impose a forbidden charge for claims processing, is subject to program and civil actions."[27]

Case Reviews

Case law continues to develop as benefit denials are challenged. As the following cases demonstrate, such challenges can lead to successful as well as unsuccessful lawsuits.

Rehabilitation Services

The decision of an administrative law judge to deny Medicare coverage for rehabilitative services provided to a 91-year-old resident following a shoulder fracture was reviewed in *Stenger v. Bowen*, 692 F. Supp. 1474 (E.D. N.Y. 1988). The administrative law judge had denied coverage based on his findings that the resident received mere custodial care. The judge was found to have failed to consider the resident's condition as a whole. The judge's determination that the resident had not received covered skilled rehabilitative services was not supported by substantial evidence in the record. The administrative law judge improperly relied exclusively on the opinion of a consulting physician who had never seen the resident, while at the same time ignoring numerous treating sources as well as evidence of actual treatment administered to the resident.

Benefit Denial

Extended care benefits for post-hospitalization were denied to a nursing facility resident in *Aurora v. Secretary of Health and Human Services*, 715 F. Supp. 466 (E.D. N.Y. 1989). The administrative law judge decided that the care rendered to the resident constituted custodial care, not skilled nursing care. The resident had been treated at a hospital for pain and swelling in her left knee. The services rendered to the resident were physical therapy, reassurance, medication for anxiety, and assistance in such daily activities as bathing and ambulation.

Reimbursement Denied for Punitive Damage Award

The provider of skilled nursing services in *American Medical Nursing Centers—Greenbrook v. Heckler*, 592 F. Supp. 1311 (1984), sought judicial review of a final decision of the Secretary of Health and Human Services denying Medicare reimbursement for punitive damages awarded in a malpractice suit. A malpractice judgment in the amount of $25,000 in compensatory damages and $750,000 in punitive damages was awarded based on actions and omissions by the facility and its employees that resulted in the death of a resident. The court held that the award of punitive damages and related costs was not a reimbursable loss under the Medicare program.

> The purpose of assessing punitive damages is "to punish the tort feasor . . . and to deter him and others from similar conduct." *City of Newport v. Fact Concerts, Inc.*, 453 U.S. 247, 101 S.Ct. 2748, 2759–60, 69 L.Ed.2d 616 (1981). That purpose would be ill served by reimbursement, which would shift the responsibility for paying the damages from Greenbrook to the Medicare trust fund, and ultimately to this nation's taxpayers who would bear the burden of plaintiff's wrongdoing.

Id. at 1313.

MEDICAID

The Medicaid program, Title XIX of the Social Security Act Amendments of 1965, is a government program administered by the states providing medical services (both institutional and outpatient services) to the medically needy. Federal grants, in the form of "matching funds," are issued to those states with qualifying Medicaid programs. In other words, Medicaid is jointly sponsored and financed by the federal government and the several states. Medical care for needy persons of all ages is provided under the definition of need established by each state. Each state has set its own criteria for determining eligibility for services under its Medicaid program. HCFA is responsible for working with the states to develop approaches toward meeting the needs of those who cannot afford adequate medical care.[28]

Because Medicaid has been designed for the poor, the elderly must often deplete a major part of their assets before they can become eligible for Medicaid benefits. Medicaid benefits provide for a variety of long-term care services for the elderly that are limited or not provided under Medicare regulations.

Day Care Centers

Medicaid is currently the main source of funding for adult day care, according to a recently completed national adult day center census commissioned by the Health Care Financing Administration and the American Association of Retired Persons.

> States most commonly pay for adult day care under Medicaid through a program created by Congress in 1981. It allows state Medicaid programs to apply for waivers to provide a range of home- and community-based services for those who otherwise would require institutionalization.
>
> * * *
>
> States that choose this option have the right to make such services available to specific populations in certain geographic areas, rather than extending the home- and community-based services to all Medicaid-eligible recipients. Adult day care is one of several such services, which also may include personal care, rehabilitation, and homemaker services.
>
> States can also claim matching federal Medicaid funds for adult day care under the auspices of another authorized Medicaid service, such as outpatient hospital care or clinical services. In this case, the adult day care provided would have to be strictly medical versus under the waiver, where there's more latitude for social day care.
>
> * * *
>
> Nonetheless, Zawadski, of the University of California, San Francisco, says the census indicates that Medicaid funding for adult day care centers has increased "dramatically, threefold in the last five years."
>
> Statistics bear this out. In the 1989 adult day care center census, Medicaid funding represented 29 percent of center revenues. But when all Medicaid related programs were taken into account, Medicaid funding

equaled 41 percent of center revenues. In 1985, income from Medicaid equaled 23 percent of total center revenues, according to Hart, of the National Institute on Adult Daycare.*

Case Reviews

Case law continues to develop as reimbursement methodologies and benefit denials are challenged. As the following cases demonstrate, such challenges can lead to successful as well as unsuccessful lawsuits.

State Reimbursement Rates Challenged

Privately owned nursing facilities and a resident of one facility brought an action to declare invalid Oregon's plan reducing Medicaid reimbursement rates effective July 1, 1986. The trial court invalidated the plan and ordered the Department of Human Resources to reimburse the defendants under the previous plan and the defendants appealed. *Volk v. Dept. of Human Resources*, 799 P.2d 658 (Or. App. 1990). When Medicaid was enacted in 1965, the Secretary of Health, Education and Welfare (now the Department of Health and Human Services) was responsible for the adoption of standards for reimbursement. Federal law required that nursing facilities be reimbursed for their "reasonable costs." In 1972, Congress gave more flexibility to the states in developing reimbursement with the proviso that reimbursement continue to be based on reasonable costs. In 1980, the Boren amendment further reduced the government's role in determining and reviewing reimbursement rates by assigning that role to the states. The states were to determine annually that reimbursement rates were reasonable and adequate and that such assurances were to be submitted to the Secretary when making any substantial changes in reimbursement rates. *Id.* at 660. The respondents alleged that the Medicaid plan amendments were not reasonable and were adopted because of the state's budgetary problems. *Id.* at 661. The Court of Appeals of Oregon held that the Medicaid reimbursement rates were invalid. The plaintiffs were entitled to be reimbursed in accordance with the prior promulgated plan for the entire time during which the invalid plan was in effect and until a new plan was promulgated.

Inadequate Base Report/Rate Reconsideration Granted

A nursing facility was entitled to an increased Medicaid rate where the base report used for computing the reimbursement rate was grossly inadequate and prepared by the facility's accountant. *Department of Social Services v. Our Lady of Mercy*, 803 S.W.2d 72 (Mo. Ct. App. 1990). The nursing facility had hired a new accounting firm, which determined that the facility's base report resulted in insufficient Medicaid reimbursement to the facility. As a result of the information provided by the accounting

---

**Source*: Reprinted from *Hospitals*, Vol. 64, No. 21, by permission, November 5, 1990, Copyright 1990, American Hospital Publishing, Inc., at 34.

firm, the nursing facility applied for informal rate reconsideration with the director of the Department of Social Services. The director determined that an increase was warranted and recommended an increase to the rate advisory committee. The Department of Social Services, however, rejected the advisory committee's recommendation. Upon appeal to the Administrative Hearing Commission, an increase in the reimbursement rate was granted. The Department of Social Services, not satisfied with the decision, made an appeal to the Circuit Court, which reversed the decision of the Administrative Hearing Commission. The nursing facility then appealed to the Court of Appeals, which determined that the nursing facility's economic loss due to grossly prepared and inadequate base reports constituted significant and extraordinary circumstances that warranted an increase in the facility's Medicaid reimbursement rate.

License Revoked/Recovery of Payments Sought

The Pennsylvania Department of Public Welfare (DPW) sought to recover approximately $250,000 for the care of Medical Assistance patients at a skilled nursing facility for a five-month period in 1984, during which time the appellant's participation in the Medicare program had been terminated, in *Chester Extended Care Center v. DPW*, 586 A.2d 379 (Pa. 1991). The Commonwealth of Pennsylvania, Department of Health (DOH) had revoked the appellant's license to operate as a skilled nursing facility on January 6, 1984. The Department of Health and Human Services (HHS) had notified the appellant on January 18, 1984, that the nursing facility would be terminated from participation in the Medicare program as of February 15, 1984. DPW notified the appellant on February 7, 1984, that termination from the Medicare program automatically resulted in the appellant's termination from the state's Medical Assistance program and that all payments to the appellant would cease as of March 16, 1984. The appellant appealed the decision to the DOH, the state's survey agency for Medicare and Medical Assistance, and requested a resurvey of the facility. DOH, following resurvey of the facility, granted the appellant a six month provisional license, and on March 8, 1984 recommended to HHS that the appellant continue to participate in the federal programs. On April 17, 1984, HHS informed DOH that the appellant's participation in the federal programs was terminated as of February 15, 1984. The appellant was not notified of this decision. DOH again recommended, on May 2, 1984, support of the appellant's application for readmission into the Medicare program. On November 8, 1984, HHS once again denied the request and notified both DOH and the appellant. DPW notified the appellant on November 13, 1984 that it was not eligible to receive Medical Assistance payments as of February 15, 1984 and that recovery for Medical Assistance payments after February 15, 1984 was being sought.

Upon appeal to the Supreme Court of Pennsylvania, the Commonwealth was estopped from recovering Medical Assistance payments made to the appellant,

> Although it is a general rule that estoppel against the government will not lie where the acts of its agents are in violation of positive law . . ., this rule cannot be slavishly applied where doing so would result in a fundamental

> injustice. It would clearly be a fundamental injustice to hold appellant herein responsible for the cost of caring for its Medical Assistance patients. The agencies that administer the welfare programs in this Commonwealth have a duty to deal fairly and justly with those who assume the task of caring for our indigent citizens.

Id. at 383.

Case Mix

The nursing facility in *Monroe County Nursing Home District v. Missouri Department of Social Services*, 778 S.W.2d 721 (Mo. Ct. App. 1989), was granted an increase in its reimbursement rate due to a change in its case mix. There was evidence that Medicare regulations caused hospitals to release patients in worse physical condition than in prior years. As a result, the nursing facility received residents who required additional nursing care and incurred additional expenses in responding to a more demanding caseload.

Wage Increases

The court in *Westhampton Nursing Home v. Whalen*, 413 N.Y.S.2d 244 (N.Y. App. Div. 1979), held that Medicaid reimbursement rates should have included wage increases granted to the union. The court held that the refusal to consider the actual wage increases was arbitrary and capricious. "In determining reimbursement to be allowed to nursing home which participated in medicaid program, refusal to consider increase in wage rates which nursing home was required to pay to its employees under terms of agreement settling strike in August of certain year was arbitrary and capricious." *Id.* at 245. The Commissioner of Health, however, acted properly in refusing to reimburse the nursing facility for all the salaries of its owners as well as the facility's alleged automobile expenses.

Employee Benefits

The nursing facility in *Monroe County Nursing Home District v. Missouri Department of Social Services*, discussed above, was granted an increase in its reimbursement rates as a result of the facility's institution of a health insurance benefit program for its employees. The nursing facility's purchase of medical insurance constituted significant and extraordinary costs for which it was entitled to reimbursement. The program had been established as a means for decreasing employee turnover, thus limiting the cost of training new employees. The facility had to compete with other employers who were already providing employees with health insurance benefits.

Depreciation

The state in *Hoodkroft Convalescent Centers v. State of New Hampshire, Division of Human Services*, 701 F. Supp. 17 (D. N.H. 1988), was entitled to repayment of Medicaid reimbursement for depreciation after the nursing home was sold for a gain. Because the facility had been sold for a gain, it had not actually incurred the costs of depreciation, even though its assets had suffered wear and tear. Medicaid providers had been put on notice that their depreciation expense would be subject to recapture if they sold a nursing home at a profit. They did not have a valid expectation that they were entitled to keep depreciation expense reimbursement, so as to make recapture an interference with a constitutionally protected property right. *Id.* at 18.

Historical Costs

South Carolina's implementation of a new Medicaid reimbursement policy of reimbursing nursing homes for lease costs on the basis of the owner's historical costs could not be considered as violating the federal "reasonable reimbursement" requirement in *Anco, Inc. v. Human Services Finance Commission*, 388 S.E.2d 780 (S.C. 1989). Evidence did not support the contention that the reimbursement policy was an arbitrary cutback based entirely upon budgetary considerations. "[I]mpetus for the policy was desire for expenditure of more money on patient services rather than facility costs." *Id.* at 781. Voluntary participation in the Medicaid program foreclosed the possibility that the change in the reimbursement policy could be construed as the taking of private property.

Indirect Costs

The nursing facility in *Silver Lake Nursing Home v. Axelrod*, 549 N.Y.S.2d 210 (N.Y. App. Div. 1989), was not entitled to a Medicaid rate increase for increases in its indirect care services staff. The nursing facility had filed a rate appeal requesting a revision of its Medicaid reimbursement rates to cover the costs of an additional 13 full time equivalent employees (FTEs). Documentation submitted on appeal indicated that the revision was required solely because of an increase in the number of employees entitled to the maximum annual leave under the facility's union contract. The appeal was approved for 8.7 FTEs providing "direct care" nursing services. The remaining 4.3 FTEs employed as relief personnel were denied on the grounds that they provided "indirect care" nursing services, and that only those employees providing "direct care" nursing services were entitled to be included in the total of allowable additional staff coverage. In finding for the state, the court reasoned that the pertinent issue is not whether the nursing facility experienced increased labor costs, but whether it was entitled to reimbursement under the prevailing regulations.

> It is fundamental that courts will defer to an agency's interpretation of its own regulations if not irrational . . . In this case, we do not find respondent's (Department of Health) distinction between direct care nursing and indirect care services . . . to be unreasonable or irrational.

Id. at 211.

Legal Fees

The government was not liable for costs and fees where its decisions denying benefits to a nursing home resident in *Behnke v. Department of Health and Social Services*, 430 N.W.2d 600 (Wis. Ct. App. 1988), had been substantially justified even though the resident's medical assistance application was eventually approved on appeal. The record indicated that prior to entering the nursing facility the resident's granddaughter had been given $17,000 from the resident for alleged care provided to the resident during the preceding five years. The payment was made in a lump sum and not in monthly payments as was called for in a written agreement with the resident. The circumstances surrounding the case provided reasonable justification for the initial denial of benefits.

Nonresident Coverage

The owner-operator of nursing facilities in *State v. Stuckey Health Care, Inc.*, 375 S.E.2d 235 (Ga. Ct. App. 1989), brought an action against the state of Georgia and the Department of Medical Assistance to recover payment for long-term care patients pursuant to its provider agreement. Thirty-three patients at South Carolina State Hospital had relocated in August of 1982 to Georgia and were placed in the appellee's nursing facility. At the time of the transfer, Georgia and South Carolina had a reciprocal interstate agreement providing Medicaid coverage for long-term care placements. The agreement between the two states was terminated on March 1, 1983, and thereafter the appellants refused to reimburse the appellee for the care of these patients, claiming that they were not obligated to do so since the patients were not Georgia residents. The trial court granted summary judgment for the owner-operator and the state appealed. The appeals court held that the appellants were required to provide Medicaid coverage for out-of-state patients who expressed their desire to remain in the state.

Ruling for Treatment of Mental Patient Overturned

In *State of Connecticut, Department of Income Maintenance v. Heckler*, 731 F.2d 1052 (2nd Cir. 1984), a federal district court found that Middletown Haven Rest Home was improperly denied reimbursement on the grounds that it was an institution for mental disease. On appeal to the Second Circuit, the court held that the intent of Congress was to exclude the use of Medicaid funds for custodial care and treatment of the mentally ill under the age of 65, regardless of the type of facility in which care and treatment are provided. The Department of Health and Human Services, therefore, properly disallowed medicaid payments to Connecticut for services provided to those under 65.

Supplemental Payments

No valid claim was stated against a guarantor of supplemental payments for a private room in excess of Medicaid reimbursement in *Voa Autumnwood Care Center v.*

Shiff, 542 N.E.2d 1121 (Ohio Mun. 1988). Although the daughter of a nursing facility resident had orally agreed to pay an amount in addition to the amount paid by Medicaid so that her mother could remain in a private room after the mother's resources had been exhausted, the nursing facility did not have a valid claim against the daughter for supplemental payments for an optional private room, where the nursing facility did not comply with Ohio Admin. Code §5101:3–3–52(C) in view of facts that there had been no specific written request for a private room and that supplemental charges had not been computed so that true cost was evident to the resident or her daughter, as guarantor for her mother.

Eligibility

Eligibility for the Medicaid program is determined for the individual or family according to the statutes and regulations of the individual states. These statutes and regulations vary from state to state. Qualifications for individual coverage are generally based on an applicant's savings and current income. The program is administered by the states and is financed in part by the federal government. Unfortunately, eligibility for Medicaid is usually met after one has reached the poverty level by spending his or her life savings. "Within one year of entering a nursing home, more than 90 percent of these elderly are impoverished."[29]

Medicaid Patient Quotas for Nursing Homes

An action was brought by a not-for-profit membership corporation challenging regulations of the public health council setting quotas for Medicaid patients in nursing homes in *New York State Health Facilities Association, Inc. v. Axelrod*, 155 App. Div. 208, 554 N.Y.S.2d 352 (1990). The corporation consisted of approximately 230 nursing facilities. The trial court held that the regulations were invalid and an appeal was taken. The appellate court found that the public health council's regulations setting quotas for Medicaid patients in nursing homes overstepped the bounds of the council's lawfully delegated legislative authority. The regulations had been based on the socioeconomic status of patients rather than on their health needs. There had been no legislative directive to the council to adopt a Medicaid admissions quota. The council acted in an area in which the legislature had repeatedly tried and failed to reach agreement.

PRIVATE INSURANCE

Long-term care policies, marketed by private insurance companies, are written to help pay for long-term care at home or in a long-term care facility. These policies are generally too expensive for many of the nation's senior citizens. However, expanding consumer education efforts and the encouragement of individuals to buy long-term care insurance at an earlier age could help to protect elderly Americans from high health costs during a period of government funding cutbacks.[30] "Policies typically offer indemnity benefits ranging from $10 to $100 per day—with up to four years of coverage. Premiums, which range from $100 to $2,000 annually, are based on age and vary by the indemnity level and waiting period chosen."[31]

Day Care Centers

> A December 1989 Health Insurance Association of America (HIAA) survey shows that of 15 of the top-selling companies of long-term care insurance policies, which account for 75 percent of all the long-term care products sold in 1989, seven provided an adult day care benefit, an HIAA spokesman says.
>
> * * *
>
> Although insurance companies may be increasing their entry into the long-term care market, still "insurance plays a relatively small role" in terms of funding for adult day care, says Zawadski, of the University of California, San Francisco.
>
> For the future, he says, without Medicare to pave the way for long-term care financing, growth on private sector initiatives to pay for adult day care will be constrained by cost while Medicaid will continue to expand its role.*

Medigap Insurance Policies

"Medigap" insurance policies are provided by private insurance carriers to supplement services not covered under Medicare. Due to the fact that policies vary widely from state to state, it is important that senior citizens review them closely prior to purchase. Approximately 20 million elderly people in the United States spend more than a total of $15 billion on medigap policies annually.[32]

Because of widespread reports of abuse in the sales and marketing of Medigap policies, Congress implemented a voluntary certification program in 1980.[33] The abuses continued and Congress, as part of the deficit-reduction bill (H.R. 5835—H. Rptr. 101-964), expanded federal regulations of private insurance plans offering Medigap policies. The regulations will replace the voluntary program with one which

---

**Source*: Reprinted from *Hospitals*, Vol. 64, No. 21, by permission, November 5, 1990, Copyright 1990, American Hospital Publishing, Inc., at 38.

- requires that all policies be approved by either the state or the federal government before they may be sold
- provides civil penalties for selling policies that duplicate Medicare benefits
- limits the number of policies
- calls for standardization of all Medigap policies so that they can be easily compared by prospective customers prior to purchase[34]

Because of unscrupulous insurance practices in the offering of Medigap policies, as well as a mandate from Congress, the National Association of Insurance Commissioners have designed nine benefit packages to be used as standards for Medigap policies.[35] Such standardization is expected to make it easier for consumers to evaluate which policy is best for them. Fewer policies should help to eliminate the costly duplicative policies that senior citizens often carry.

LIFE CARE CONTRACTS

Reimbursement arrangements in some types of long-term care facilities can take the form of a "life care contract," under which the resident is provided a home for the remainder of his or her life in exchange for an entrance fee and the assignment of certain of a prospective resident's assets to the facility. Residents are generally required to sign a formal contract upon admission. Some of the more common legal issues related to life care contacts are discussed in the following paragraphs.

Mutual Obligation

In order for a contract to be legally effective, it must be agreed upon by all parties to the contract. Unless the parties to a contract are mutually bound, there is no contract.

In order for a contract to be binding, there must be consideration, which may be defined as an act (e.g., provide a service) or a promise to act, offered by one party to another, in return for an act (e.g., payment for the service). The consideration in a nursing facility contract is the type of service offered or to be given in return for the fee to be paid by the resident for the service.

Fraud

Fraud may be defined as a misrepresentation or deception, by words or by conduct, or by the concealment of something that should have been disclosed, to induce another to act in reliance thereon to his or her legal injury or detriment. Misrepresentations by a resident might include misrepresenting age, financial situation, or other matters pertaining to a prospective resident's eligibility for admission to the facility.

Illegality—A Gambling Contract

The courts have dismissed the contention sometimes raised that a contract requiring the applicant to transfer his or her property to the home in exchange for lifetime care is against public policy because it amounts to a wager, which would make it an illegal contract.

Unconscionable Contract

The point has been raised that to require a prospective resident to assign his present and future property to a facility is unfair, even unconscionable. This type of contract has been upheld, even where the applicant expired within several days following admission to the facility. Courts generally go to great lengths to uphold contracts favoring institutions or agencies whose work is for the benefit or welfare of the public.

The reasoning that motivates the courts in upholding these kinds of contracts is well expressed in *Stiegelmeier v. West Side Deutscher Frauen Verein*, 20 Ohio Op. 2d 368, 178 N.E.2d 516 (Ohio Ct. App. 1961), in which the court stated that the public welfare is better served by upholding contracts of this kind, because institutions that care for the aged tend to relieve the public of this burden.

Termination of Contract

The courts have held that, when a resident terminates his stay at a facility during the probationary period, he or she is entitled to a refund of all the funds and property conveyed to the home in anticipation of his or her lifetime stay, less a deduction for the expenses incurred by the facility during the stay of the resident. Facilities that admit prospective life residents on a probationary basis should set a fixed rate sufficient to assure recovery of the costs expended to care for the resident during his or her stay.

Death of Resident during Probationary Period

The courts have generally held that the property transferred to a facility must be returned to the resident's estate in the event the resident expires during the probationary period. The death of a resident during the probationary period makes it impossible for him or her to elect whether or not to remain as a permanent resident at the facility and also prevents the facility from making a similar decision.

A facility could consider the advisability of including in its contract a clause to the effect that should the resident expire during the probationary period of the contract, the property conveyed to the facility shall remain its property. It should be noted, however, that prospective residents may be reluctant to sign such a contract.

Inability To Perform Contract

The resident in *Stocking v. Hall*, 81 R.I. 168, 100 A.2d 408, *rehearing denied*, 81 R.I. 176, 100 A.2d 850 (1953), who had paid $3,000 for life care services in a convalescent home, recovered a judgment of $2,450 where, subsequent to the contract, the resident was committed to a mental hospital. The court held that the resident was entitled to this recovery because the contract had become impossible to perform through no fault of either party.

Breach of Contract Because of Medical Care Costs

Occasionally, a long-term care facility is put in a position where it has to expend extraordinary costs for medical care for one of its residents because of conditions not contemplated at the time the resident was admitted to the facility. In those situations where a facility has agreed to provide medical services and the resident has turned over his or her life's holding as consideration, the facility is bound by the contract. The resident of a retirement home in *Bruner v. Oregon Baptist Retirement Home*, 208 Or. 502, 302 P.2d 558 (1956), brought suit against the home for performance of the home's contract with the resident and damages. The contract, which was executed on August 16, 1948, provided that

> The Oregon Baptist Retirement Home of Portland, Oregon, hereby agrees to receive the party of the second part into its Home as guest for life and will provide the said, second party (a) a good comfortable lodging, (b) board, (c) the needed care by the Home nurse, medical treatment by the physician of the home in case of ordinary or usual disease, except insanity, (d) ward care in a hospital as supervised by the home physician, (4) [sic] laundry,
>
> * * *
>
> The party of the second part hereby agrees to make consideration in the amount of Thirty-eight Hundred and Seventy-five dollars ($3,875.00) less the sum of Two Hundred Sixty dollars ($260.00) heretofore paid in monthly installments. Balance due Thirty Six Hundred and Fifteen Dollars ($3,615.00), which shall become the absolute property of the first.

Id. at 559.

The resident injured her leg on or about December 5, 1951. She was later, on December 10, 1951, transferred to Emanuel Hospital for treatment. Following her discharge from the hospital, the patient was transferred to Wildwood Rest Home because of her bedridden condition (the defendant home was not licensed to care for bedridden residents). The defendant paid for the resident's care up to approximately October 1, 1955, after which Oregon Baptist refused further liability for the resident's care. The resident brought legal action and the trial court held for the resident. On appeal by the defendant, the Supreme Court of Oregon also found for the resident.

> In our opinion, the provisions of this contract are definite, certain, and wholly unambiguous.
>
> * * *
>
> It is thus apparent that the defendant has lost money under its contract with plaintiff, but that fact is wholly unimportant insofar as the issues in this case are concerned. However, it might be well to point out that the money paid by each person entering defendant's home immediately becomes the property of defendant and is retained by the defendant even though the guest should live but a week or two after entering the home. In other words, many who enter the home do not live out their life expectancy as contemplated by the agreement, and the unused funds of those persons become available to make up the deficiency arising in the accounts of those who live beyond their life expectancies or suffer disability requiring hospital care, as did the plaintiff.

Id. at 560.

FINANCIAL OBLIGATIONS OF THE SPOUSE

Although a spouse is generally responsible for the other's cost of medical care, there are exceptions to this general rule. The spouses of Medicaid recipients receiving nursing home care cannot be held accountable beyond their financial means. The court in *Conrad v. Hackett*, 562 N.Y.S.2d 331, 332 (N.Y. Sup. Ct. 1990), held that the Department of Social Service's interpretation of regulations to require that a non-institutionalized spouse's resources totaling $10,000 be reduced to a minimal medical assistance level of $3,250 before she was eligible for support from her institutionalized spouse was arbitrary and capricious, irrational, and had no basis in law. The petitioners prevailed in securing a federally guaranteed right by setting forth a conflict between state practice and a specific federal mandate prohibiting complete divestment of a spouse's resources in order to become eligible for medical benefits.

> Significantly, the 1989 level of the retainable assets was set at $60,000.00 to "enable the working poor to qualify for benefits, and eliminate much of the administrative court costs associated with evaluating marginally eligible elderly and disabled persons, forcing liquidations of modest holdings,

> and obtaining court ordered divisions of property" (1989 McKinney's Session Laws of New York, c. 558, Memorandum of State Executive Department, p. 2203). In approval, the Governor commented that "(o)ur senior citizens should not live their golden years in the shadow of impoverishment. Until this bill, the possibility of long-term care has carried such a threat. This bill removes that threat . . . (1989 McKinney's Session Laws of New York, c. 558, Executive Memorandum, p. 2415).

Id. at 335.

AVOIDING LEGAL PITFALLS

Because of the opportunity for lawsuits regarding the financial arrangements between long-term care facilities and their residents, careful attention should be given when drafting the language of agreements with prospective residents. Special attention should be given to the following:

- termination during the probationary period
- payment required during the probationary period
- notice of intent to terminate
- death during the probationary period
- assignment of after acquired property
- transfer to another institution

DRGs AND NURSING FACILITIES

Diagnostic related groups (DRGs) refer to a methodology developed by professors at Yale University for classifying patients in categories according to age, diagnosis, and treatment resource requirements. It is the basis for the Health Care Financing Administration's prospective payment system (PPS), which is contained in the 1983 Social Security Amendments for reimbursing inpatient hospital costs for "Medicare" beneficiaries. Under this system, cost reduction could be accomplished either by reducing length of stay or by decreasing utilization of ancillary services, such as physical therapy.

The key source of information for determining the course of treatment of each patient and the proper DRG assignment is the medical record. Reimbursement is based on pre-established average prices for each DRG. As a result of this reimbursement methodology, poor record keeping can precipitate financial disaster. The major purpose of the amendments is to hold down the rise in Medicare expenditures before the social security system experiences serious deficits. The potential financial savings for Medicare are substantial. Under this system of payment, if hospitals can provide quality patient care at a cost under the price established for a DRG, they may keep the excess dollars paid. This is an incentive for hospitals to keep costs under control. There is, however, a fear that patients may, to their detriment, be discharged too early for financial reasons. This in turn could lead to costly malpractice suits for hospitals.

The early release of Medicare patients from hospitals under the DRG methodology of payment can be costly for nursing facilities. Early and sometimes premature discharge of patients from hospitals often results in sicker residents being admitted to nursing facilities. This scenario can increase a facility's costs, exposure, and risks of negligence suits.

The nursing facility in *Monroe County Nursing Home District v. Missouri Department of Social Services*, 778 S.W.2d 721 (Mo. Ct. App. 1989), received certification to participate in the state administered Medicaid program. The facility's initial reimbursement rate was set at $25.20, based on its total allowable resident care expenses divided by resident days. A formula allows increases in the rate of reimbursement based on the original rate. At the time of the hearing, Monroe received a per diem rate of $32.15. Monroe had made application to the Department of Social Services for an adjustment in its reimbursement rate for "changes in costs due to changes in the level of care or case mix . . . ." *Id.* at 722. Ms. Gritton, the nursing facility administrator, testified that changes in "Medicare" regulations have caused hospitals to release elderly patients earlier, and consequently in a more debilitated physical state. The poorer condition of new residents placed additional demands on the nursing facility. As a result of those demands, the nursing facility had to adjust staff hours, add nurses, and develop a physical rehabilitation department. The Department denied the request for an increase in the reimbursement rate. The Administrative Hearing Commission granted $1.25 per diem increase in the facility's Medicaid reimbursement rate, finding that there was a substantial change in its resident case mix. On appeal, the circuit court reversed the Commission's order providing an increase in Monroe's reimbursement rate. Upon further appeal, the Missouri Court of Appeals held that the evidence supported the Commission's finding of a changed case mix, warranting an increase in the reimbursement rate.

Important to Monroe's case was evidence detailing the various time-consuming diagnoses of newly admitted residents. The importance of accurate and meaningful record keeping cannot be over-emphasized. In this instance, it provided the necessary documentation leading to a successful financial ending.

RUGS—THE CASE MIX REIMBURSEMENT SYSTEM

A new case mix reimbursement system for payment of nursing home care for Medicaid patients was implemented in New York State on January 1, 1986. The overall objective of the system is to provide a prospective reimbursement methodology that employs case mix measures, allowing for reimbursement of facilities based on the characteristics of the residents in the facility. The more extensive the care required by residents, the higher the reimbursement rate. Even though private pay patients are not covered by Medicaid, they are included in the methodology for determining the overall case mix of a facility. This system is currently referred to as Resource Utilization Groups or (RUGs). The purpose of RUGs is to

1. provide a reimbursement system that reflects individual needs
2. reduce the number of hospital patients awaiting nursing home placement by providing financial incentives to nursing facilities that accept residents needing a higher level of care
3. encourage the utilization of rehabilitative services by paying more for them.[36]

The Resource Utilization Groups

Residents are classified into one of the five major groups based on their medical conditions and care needs. The five categories and a brief description of each follows.

- Heavy rehabilitation—Residents in this group receive physical or occupational therapy services at least five days a week. Their therapy is seen as having restorative goals.
- Special care—Residents in this group have a need for heavy care. Characteristics of residents in this category may include coma, quadriplegia, multiple sclerosis, stage 4 decubiti (severe breakdown of the skin involving muscle and bone), nasal-gastric feeding, parenteral feeding, suctioning, etc.
- Clinically complex—This group has extensive medical problems requiring physician care at least once a week. Characteristics of residents in this group will include one or more of the following: cerebral palsy, hemiplegia, urinary tract infection, dehydration, internal bleeding, stasis ulcer, late stages of terminal illness, oxygen therapy, wound/lesion care, chemotherapy, transfusions, dialysis, etc.
- Severe behavioral problem—Residents in this group have a high frequency and severity level of one or more of the following behavioral problems: physical aggression; verbal abuse; hallucinations; and disruptive, infantile, and socially inappropriate behavior.
- Reduced physical functioning—Residents who do not fit into one of the above groups are included in this group. These residents have problems with activities of daily living as the only problem requiring care.

Residents are further classified into one of 16 subgroups based on their medical conditions and Activities of Daily Living (ADL) scores, which are based on eating, toileting, and transferring difficulties (e.g., bed to wheelchair). The ADL scores range from 3 to 10. The higher the score the greater the assistance needed for daily living. Reimbursement is higher for those residents requiring more extensive medical care and staff time.

The state sets an average, minimum, and maximum price for each RUG category. That is, the state pays a fixed per diem for the direct cost (e.g., nursing services, activities, social services, and various therapies) portion of the resident care within each RUG category. Each price is set in advance so that the facility knows in advance how much it will get for each resident it admits. Facilities are encouraged to spend less than the minimum and maximum prices set.

- If a facility is able to spend less than the minimum price set for each category, it will be allowed to keep the difference. This will result in a profit.
- If a facility spends more than the maximum price set for each category, it will pay the difference between the maximum price and its actual costs. This will result in a loss.
- If a facility spends anywhere between the minimum and maximum price set, it will have repaid all its costs and will break even.[37]

The direct cost is not the total cost of reimbursement the nursing home receives, but rather those costs due to providing care to the resident. The other factors used to determine total reimbursement include indirect costs (e.g., housekeeping, laundry, maintenance, medical records, and security), non-comparable costs (e.g., the costs of services that may vary from facility to facility, such as, laboratory and radiology services), and capital costs (e.g., depreciation on buildings and major equipment). Various states are currently reviewing the New York State RUGs system of prospective payment of nursing facility care for possible implementation.

NOTES

1. NATIONAL CENTER FOR HEALTH STATISTICS, HEALTH, UNITED STATES 1989, (1990) at 4.

2. *Id.*

3. *Health Care Expenditures Estimated To Be $756 Billion in 1991*, 27(3) AHA News, January 21, 1991, at 3.

4. *Id.*

5. *Id.*

6. *The Long-Term Care Quagmire*, CXL(48, 388), The New York Times, October 14, 1990, Sec. 3, at 16F.

7. *Id.*

8. *The Long-Term Care Quagmire, supra* note 6, at 16F.

9. P.R. Willging, *Introduction*, DIRECTORY OF NURSING HOMES (3rd ed., 1988) at x.

10. America in Transition: An Aging Society, U.S. Department of Commerce, Bureau of the Census (1983), at 3.

11. *Id.*

12. *Educating and Licensing Nursing Home Administrators: Public Policy Issues*, 30 THE GERONTOLOGIST, October 1990, at 581.

13. *Id.*

14. *Id.*

15. THE ROBERT WOOD JOHNSON FOUNDATION, FACTSHEET ON THE ELDERLY IN THE UNITED STATES AND THE NEED FOR LONG-TERM CARE INSURANCE 2 (1988).

16. *The Long Term-Care Quagmire, supra* note 6, at 16F.

17. FEDERAL COUNCIL ON THE AGING, ANNUAL REPORT TO THE PRESIDENT 1988, at 14.

18. *Strong Government Role in LTC Insurance Prescribed*, 27(3) AHA News, January 21, 1991, at 2.

19. *House Panel's Probe Finds Misrepresentation of Some LTC Policies*, 27(26) AHA News, July 1, 1991, at 2.

20. FEDERAL COUNCIL ON THE AGING, *supra* note 17, at 19.

21. Key Medicare and Medicaid Legislation: 1990, OBRA 1990, Special Member Briefing, Chicago: American Hospital Association, January 1991, at 25.

22. R.A. KANE & R.L. KANE, LONG-TERM CARE: PRINCIPLES, PROGRAMS AND POLICIES 78 (1987).

23. NATIONAL CENTER FOR HEALTH STATISTICS, *supra* note 1, at 307–308.

24. P.J. Strauss, *Law and the Aging*, 20 NEW YORK L. J., (1990).

25. *Id.*

26. *Id.*

27. *Id.*

28. NATIONAL CENTER FOR HEALTH STATISTICS, *supra* note 1, *Health, United States 1989*, at 308.

29. P.R. Willging, *supra* note 9.

30. *Prepare Elderly for Cost of LTC, House Panel Urged*, 26(44) AHA News, November 5, 1990, at 2.

31. P.R. Willging, *supra* note 9, at x–xi.

32. *Congress Making Progress on "Medigap" Regulations*, 26(43) AHA News, October 29, 1990, at 2.

33. *101st Congress Leaves Behind a Ream of Health Measures*, XX THE NATION'S HEALTH, December 1990, at 11.

34. *Id.*

35. *NAIC Proposes Nine Medigap Plans as Standards*, 27(15) AHA News, April 15, 1991, at 1.

36. C. RUDDER, REIMBURSEMENT AND THE NURSING HOME RESIDENT 3 (1988).

37. *Id.* at 10.

Chapter 16

Malpractice Insurance

> I never was ruined but twice—once when I gained a lawsuit, and once when I lost one.
>
> *Francois Marie de Voltaire* (1694–1778)

The cost of malpractice insurance continues to be a major concern for the health care industry due to the large number of malpractice claims and exorbitant jury awards. Malpractice became a major problem for the health care industry in the 1960s. The rise in the occurrences of malpractice claims has resulted in unwieldy malpractice insurance rates for both physicians and health care organizations.[1] According to 1,100 doctors from New York and Long Island responding to a Newsday survey on "What Bothers Doctors," 17.4 percent of physicians consider insurance to be today's main health care problem.[2] A $3.1 million, 1,100 page Harvard Medical Practice Study, commissioned by the state of New York because of sharply increasing malpractice rates, showed that "The risk of sustaining an adverse event increased with age. Persons over 65 had twice the chance of being injured by health practitioners than patients between 16 and 44.[3]

Nursing facilities are increasingly being sued for malpractice on the grounds of poor or substandard care. The incidence of nursing home malpractice suits is likely to increase with the implementation of various cost containment strategies that will result in nursing facilities caring for sicker residents.[4]

The medical professional insurance marketplace is relatively small in comparison with other lines of insurance. A handful of standard insurance companies offer medical professional liability insurance, excluding statewide association programs.

Medical professional insurance, as all insurance, is subject to the cyclical nature of the insurance market. Further problems intrinsic in malpractice insurance include the uncertainty of our legal system, the effects of inflation on ultimate claim values, emerging technology treatments, and diseases.[5]

Health care facilities and professionals of the mid-seventies and mid-eighties experienced difficult times in obtaining medical liability insurance coverage. Competition between insurers was minimal, with adequate umbrella coverage difficult to obtain, and premiums were high. Between those hard markets was a soft market that brought steady premium reduction and greater availability of coverage.[6] Since 1986 there has been another softening of the market. In 1988 insurers of medical professional liability coverage provided increased flexibility of programs, premium reductions, and broadened coverage. The short-term outlook is good. Additional insurers and additional capacity are becoming available. Costs may not be reduced, but large increases were not seen in 1989 and 1990 premiums. On a long-term basis, the cyclic underwriting pattern of the insurance industry might very well result in a return once again to a crisis in the medical malpractice insurance market.[7]

Malpractice insurance rates have significantly affected the availability as well as the cost of insurance. Many commercial insurance carriers discontinued writing professional liability coverage since the middle to late 1970s. As a result, some states required insurance carriers to join a consortium of insurance companies in order to underwrite medical malpractice insurance. These consortiums were referred to as joint underwriting associations. According to one study, there were only 12 such consortiums in 1986.[8] Concern regarding insurance industry practices is strong on the federal level for some public officials. Senator Jay Rockefeller, in an interview by American Hospital Association staff regarding his health agenda for 1991, stated

> Insurance reform is right up there. Unless the private insurance industry can demonstrate that they are about the business of managing and controlling costs in health care and not just avoiding them, which is what they do now, I predict that they will not survive this decade.[9]

THE INSURANCE POLICY

Insurance is a contract that creates legal obligations on the part of both the insured and the insurer. It is a contract in which the insurer agrees to assume certain risks of the insured for consideration, or payment of a premium. Under the terms of the contract, also known as the insurance policy, the insurer promises to pay a specific amount of money if a specified event takes place. An insurance policy contains three necessary elements: (1) identification of the risk involved, (2) the specific amount payable, and (3) the specified occurrence.

A risk is the possibility that a loss will occur. The major function of insurance is to provide security against this loss. Insurance does not prevent or hinder the occurrence of the loss, but it does compensate for the damages.

An insured individual may be exposed to three categories of risk: (1) risk of property loss or damage, (2) risk of personal injury or loss of life, and (3) risk of incurring legal liability. Property risk is the possibility that an insured's property may be damaged or destroyed by fire, flood, tornado, hurricane, or other catastrophe. Personal risk is the possibility that the insured may be injured in an accident or may become ill; the possibility of death is a personal risk covered in the typical life insurance plan. Legal liability risk is the possibility that the insured may become legally liable to pay money damages to another, and includes accident and professional liability insurance. The various types of policies include (1) occurrence policies, which cover all incidents that arise during a policy year, regardless of when they are reported to the insurer, and (2) claims-made policies, which cover only those claims made or reported during the policy year, regardless of when they occurred.

Insurance companies are required by the laws of the various states to issue only policies that contain certain mandated provisions and to maintain certain financial reserves to guarantee to policyholders that their expectations will be met when the coverage is needed. The basic underlying concept of insurance is the spreading of risk. By writing coverage for a large enough pool of individuals, the company has determined actuarially that a certain number of claims will arise within that pool, and if the premium structure has been established correctly and the prediction of claims made accurately, the company ought to be able to meet those claims and return a profit to its shareholders.

LIABILITY OF THE PROFESSIONAL

A nurse or a physician who provides professional services to another person may be legally responsible for any harm the person suffers as a result of negligence and subject to a loss of money in the form of legally awarded damages. Many professionals protect themselves from their exposure to a legal loss by acquiring a professional liability insurance policy. The court in *Jones v. Medox, Inc.*, 413 A.2d 1288, 430 A.2d 488 (D.C. 1981), held that only the nurse's insurance carrier, Globe Insurance, was liable for injuries sustained by the plaintiff while at Doctors Hospital; these injuries resulted from an injection administered by the nurse. Ms. Jones was employed by Medox, Inc., a corporation providing temporary medical personnel to Doctors Hospital. Following settlement of the claim against the nurse, the hospital, and the nurse's employer, the nurse and her insurer brought an action against Doctors Hospital, Medox, Inc., and their insurers. The trial court granted summary judgment in favor of the hospital and its insurer and dismissed the claim against Medox, Inc., and its insurer.

The Supreme Court of New Jersey in *American Nurses Association v. Passaic General Hospital*, 98 N.J. 83, 484 A.2d 670 (1984), held that the nurse's insurance policy was primary with respect to the first $100,000 of a settlement that resulted from a malpractice action against the nurse. The National Fire Insurance Company had issued an insurance policy covering the contractual obligation of the American Nurses Association to its members. The court also held that the judgment against the nurse in excess of $100,000 was properly apportioned equally between the hospital's liability insurer and the nurses association's liability insurer.

The potential for liability is not limited to licensed professionals. Students engaged in learning a profession and paraprofessionals such as therapists, etc., who engage in activities involving the care and treatment of others face potential liability for their acts. For this reason, these individuals often obtain personal insurance coverage or assure themselves of such coverage through the institution in which they are employed or the institution in which they are enrolled to obtain their education. The process by which an institution provides coverage by pledging its assets to the defense and payment for claims against its employees or agents is known as indemnification.

An example of the necessity of insurance coverage for a licensed professional is provided by the private duty nurse. A private duty nurse is not an employee of an institution, but rather is engaged by the patient (or the patient's family) to provide services to that patient. As such, the nurse should obtain personal coverage. In fact, the patient engaging the nurse would be well advised to ask about the availability of such coverage, as would the institution in which the nurse is providing professional care for that patient.

LIABILITY INSURANCE

A nursing facility, nurse, physician, and other health practitioners who are covered by an insurance policy must recognize the rights and duties inherent in the policy. The professional should be able to identify the risks that are covered, the amount of coverage, and the conditions of the contract.

Although the policies of different insurance companies may vary, the standard policy usually says the insurance company will "pay on behalf of the insured all sums which the insured shall become legally obligated to pay as damages because of injury arising out of malpractice error, or mistake in rendering or failing to render professional services."

A standard liability insurance policy has five distinct parts: (1) the insurance agreement, (2) defense and settlement, (3) the policy period, (4) the amount payable, and (5) conditions of the policy.

Insurance Agreement

The insurer, under the terms of the policy, has a legal obligation to pay any sum that has been agreed to or determined by a court, up to the policy limit, including legal fees. It will not pay or respond merely because the insured professional feels a moral obligation toward an injured party.

Under a professional liability policy, the professional is protected from damages arising from rendering or failing to render professional services. Thus, a professional who performs a negligent act resulting in legal liability or who fails to perform a necessary act (thereby incurring damages) is personally protected from paying an injured party. The actual payment of the legal money damages to the injured party is made by the insurance company.

Defense and Settlement

In the defense and settlement portion of the insurance policy, the insured and the insurance company agree that the company will defend any lawsuit against the insured arising from performance or non-performance of professional services and that the company is delegated the power to effect a settlement of any claims as it deems necessary. A policy stating that the insurer will provide a defense of all lawsuits guarantees such a defense in any suit including those that are groundless, false, or fraudulent. In the case of a professional liability policy, the duty of the insurer under this clause is limited to the defense of lawsuits against the insured that are a consequence of professional services.

The insurance company fulfills its obligation to provide a defense by engaging the services of an attorney on behalf of the insured. The obligation of the attorney is to the insured directly, since the insured is the attorney's client. Of course, there is to some extent a divided loyalty since the attorney looks to the insurance company to obtain business. Nevertheless, the attorney–client relationship exists only between the attorney and the insured, and the insured has the right to expect the attorney to fulfill the requirements of such relationship.

If an insurance company has established the right to obtain a settlement of any claim before trial, the company's only obligation is to act reasonably and not to the detriment of the insured. According to a study by the U.S. General Accounting Office, nearly 90 percent of medical malpractice claims were settled prior to trial.[10]

Policy Period

The period of the policy is always stated in the insurance contract. Under the "occurrence" form of coverage the contract provides protection only for claims that occur during the time frame within which the policy is stated to be in effect. Any incident that occurs before or after the policy period would not be covered under the insuring agreement. A "claims-made policy" provides coverage for only those claims instituted during the policy period. Occurrence policies provide coverage for all claims that may arise out of a policy period. The actual reporting time has no bearing on the validity of the claim, as long as it is filed before the applicable statute of limitations runs out. While the reporting time has no bearing on the validity of the claim from the standpoint of coverage under the policy, the conditions of the policy will require notice within a specified time. Failure to provide such notice could void the insurer's obligation under the policy if it can be demonstrated that the carrier's position was compromised as a result of the late report or filing of a claim.

Coverage—The Amount Payable

The amount to be paid by the insurer is determined by the amount of damage incurred by the injured party. This determination may be made by a trial jury, or the insurance company and the injured party may reach a settlement before the lawsuit comes to trial or before the jury has determined the amount of damages.[11] In any event, the insurance company will pay the injured party no more than the maximum limit stated in the insurance policy. The insured professional must personally pay any damages that exceed the policy limit.

Under a policy with maximum coverage of $1 million for each claim and $3 million for aggregate claims, the aggregate claim figure is the total amount payable to all injured parties. Thus, the insured is protected on each individual claim up to $1 million and will not pay more than $3 million in a policy period.

Punitive Damages

A claim for punitive damages awarded in a malpractice suit was submitted to a facility's insurance carrier for payment but was subsequently denied by the carrier. The insurance carrier cited Florida public policy, which prohibits coverage of punitive damage awards. *American Medical Nursing Centers—Greenbrook v. Heckler*, 592 F. Supp. 1311, 1312 (D.D.C. 1984).

Obligation To Defend

The insurer of a nursing facility in *Hartford Accident & Idemnity v. Regent Nursing Home*, 413 N.Y.S.2d 195 (N.Y. App. Div. 1979), was found to have an obligation to defend the nursing facility despite an exclusion for malpractice coverage in the policy. The "complaint in primary action gave sufficient notice that alleged breach of duty may have encompassed ordinary negligence as well as professional malpractice . . . ." *Id.* at 195.

Intentional Torts

An action was brought by a comprehensive liability insurer for declaratory judgment as to its duty to defend insureds in civil actions alleging slander, interference with business relations, and violations of the federal antitrust laws in *St. Paul Insurance Companies v. Talladega Nursing Home*, 606 F.2d 631 (5th Cir. 1979). The federal district court ruled for the defendants and the nursing facility appealed. The Fifth Circuit held that the insurer has no duty to defend or provide coverage for alleged intentional torts. Under Alabama law, all contracts insuring against loss from intentional wrongs are void as being against public policy.

Conditions of the Policy

Each insurance policy contains a number of important conditions. Failure to comply with these conditions may cause forfeiture of the policy and nonpayment of claims against it. Generally, insurance policies contain the following conditions:

- Notice of occurrence—When the insured becomes aware that an injury has occurred as a result of acts covered under the contract, the insured must promptly notify the insurance company. The form of notice may be either oral or written, as specified in the policy.
- Notice of claim—Whenever the insured receives notice that a claim or suit is being instituted, prompt notice must be sent by the insured to the insurance company. This provides the insurance company with an opportunity to investigate the facts of a case. The policy will specify what papers are to be forwarded to the company. The mere failure to timely advise may be in and of itself a breach of the insurance contract, entitling the insurer to decline coverage. It may not matter that the insurer has in no way been prejudiced by the late notification. The mere fact that the insured has failed to carry out obligations under the policy may be sufficient to permit the insurer to avoid its obligations. Where the insurer has refused to honor a claim because of late notice and the insured wishes to challenge such refusal, an action can be brought asking a court to determine the reasonableness of the insurer's position.
- Assistance of the insured—The insured must cooperate with the insurance company and render any assistance necessary to reach a settlement.
- Other insurance—If the insured has pertinent insurance policies with other insurance companies, the insured must notify the insurance company in order that each company may pay the appropriate amount of the claim.
- Assignment—The protections contracted for by the insured may not be transferred unless permission is granted by the insurance company. Because the insurance company was aware of the risks the insured would encounter before the policy was issued, the company will endeavor to avoid protecting persons other than the policyholder.
- Subrogation—This is the right of a person who pays another's debt to be substituted for all rights in relation to the debt. When an insurance company makes a payment for the insured under the terms of the policy, the company becomes the beneficiary of all the rights of recovery the insured has against any other persons who may also have been negligent. For example, if several nurses were found liable for negligence arising from the same occurrence and the insurance company for one nurse pays the entire claim, the company will be entitled to the rights of that nurse and may collect a proportionate share of the claim from the other nurses.
- Changes—The insured cannot make changes in the policy without the written consent of the insurance company. Thus, an agent of the insurance company ordinarily cannot modify or remove any condition of the liability contract. Only the insurance company, by written authorization, may permit a condition to be altered or removed.
- Cancellation—A cancellation clause spells out the conditions and procedures necessary for the insured or the insurer to cancel the liability policy. Written notice is usually required. The insured person's failure to comply with any

terms of the policy can result in cancellation and possible nonpayment of a claim by the insurance company. As a legal contract, failure to meet the terms and conditions of an insurance policy can result in a breach of contract and voidance of coverage.

MEDICAL LIABILITY INSURANCE

The fundamental tenets of insurance law and their application to the typical liability insurance policy are pertinent to the provisions of medical professional liability insurance as applied to individuals and institutions. Professional liability policies vary in the broadness, the exclusions from coverage, and the interpretations a company places on the language of the contract.

There are three medical professional liability classes:

1. Individuals including (but not limited to) physicians, surgeons, dentists, nurses, osteopaths, chiropractors, opticians, physio-therapists, optometrists, and various types of medical technicians. This category may also include medical laboratories, blood banks, and optical establishments.
2. Health care institutions, such as extended care facilities, homes for the aged, institutions for the mentally ill, sanitariums, and other health institutions where bed and board are provided for patients or residents.
3. Clinics, dispensaries, and infirmaries where there are no regular bed or board facilities. These institutions may be related to industrial or commercial enterprises; however, they are to be distinguished from facilities operated by dentists or physicians, which are usually covered under individual professional liability contracts.

The insuring clause will usually provide for payment on behalf of the insured if an injury arises from either of the following:

- malpractice, error, or mistake in rendering or failing to render professional services in the practice of the insured's profession during the policy period
- acts or omissions on the part of the insured during the policy period as a member of a formal accreditation or similar professional board or committee of a nursing facility or a professional society

While injury is not limited to bodily injury or property damage, it must result from malpractice, error, mistake, or failure to perform acts that should have been performed.

The most common risks covered by medical professional liability insurance are (1) negligence, (2) assault and battery as a result of failing to obtain consent to a medical or surgical procedure, (3) libel and slander, and (4) invasion of privacy for betrayal of professional confidences. Coverage may vary from company to company, but standards of policy coverage are generally followed. The premium rates are generally approved by state insurance departments as filed by insurance companies. Rates will differ for individuals by profession and specialty and by type of health care facility (e.g., nursing facility and hospital).

MEDICAL MALPRACTICE INSURANCE ASSOCIATIONS

The difficulty that health care facilities and physicians had in obtaining malpractice insurance in a number of states during the early '80s resulted in the formation of medical malpractice insurance associations. The purpose of these associations is to provide a market for institutions or physicians who are unable to obtain medical malpractice insurance in the open market at a reasonable price. Legislation was introduced requiring all insurance carriers engaged in writing personal liability insurance within a particular state to provide malpractice coverage through these associations (similar to "assigned risk" pools for problem automobile drivers).

> Most physician-owned liability insurance companies are not-for-profit enterprises. In general, their policies are set by physician boards of directors, but their business operations are managed by professional insurance executives. Most of these companies were established by and retain close ties to medical societies. Most physician-owned companies were established in order to maintain access to malpractice insurance when commercial insurers withdrew from the market in the late 1970's.[12]

SELF-INSURANCE

Skyrocketing medical malpractice insurance premiums have often produced situations in which the premium cost of insurance has approached and, on occasion, actually reached the face amount of the policy. Due to the extremely high cost of maintaining such insurance, some institutions have sought alternatives to this conventional means of protecting against medical malpractice. One alternative that is becoming increasingly popular is self-insurance. When a health care facility self-insures its malpractice risks, it no longer purchases a policy of malpractice insurance, but instead periodically sets aside a certain amount of its own funds as a reserve against malpractice losses and expenses. An institution that self-insures generally retains the services of a self-insurance consulting firm and of an actuary to determine the proper level of funding that the institution should maintain.

A self-insurance program need not involve the elimination of insurance coverage in its entirety. A health care facility may find it prudent to purchase excess coverage whereby the institution self-insures the first agreed-on dollar amount of risk and the insurance carrier insures the balance. For example, in a typical program the facility may self-insure the first $1 million of professional liability risk per year. Since the vast majority of claims will be disposed of within such limitation, the cost of excess insurance may be quite reasonable.

Before a corporation makes a decision to self-insure, not only must it determine the economic aspects of such a decision and the necessary funding levels to maintain an adequate reserve for future claims, but it also must determine whether there are any legal impediments to such a program. A corporation that has obtained funding from governmental sources or that has issued bonds or other obligations containing certain covenants may find itself unable to self-insure because of these prior commitments. Nursing facilities are urged to consult their counsel to review appropriate and applicable documentation before making the self-insurance decision.

OTHER INSURANCE COVERAGES

Besides insurance coverage for liability risks, a nursing facility is typically involved in numerous other insurance situations. For example, it provides fringe benefits to its employees that may include health insurance, disability insurance, life insurance, and a pension or other retirement plan also involving insurance. These programs require appropriate administration and create rights and obligations on the part of the facility and its personnel. Such issues as eligibility for coverage, coverage for particular circumstances, termination of coverage, etc., can give rise to substantial legal problems and possibly even litigation.

Other insurance coverages in which a facility will be involved include coverages for the facility's physical plant, motor vehicles, and, where applicable, construction projects. In the course of a construction project, appropriate insurance coverages for liability risks, fire risks, and other similar hazards must be considered. In addition, the requirement that contractors obtain a payment and performance bond to ensure the completion of their work and the payment of all subcontractors and material suppliers is important. Substantial litigation can arise during the course of or at the conclusion of a construction project involving large sums of money because of inappropriate construction or the failure to complete construction, or because of the failure to follow plans or specifications, to live up to expectations, or to adhere to schedules.

TRUSTEE COVERAGE

Health care facility trustees should be covered by liability insurance just as physicians and other health professionals. In *Lynch v. Redfield Foundation*, 9 Cal. App. 3d 293, 88 Cal. Rptr. 86 (1970), a California bank refused to honor corporate drafts unless all trustees concurred. They could not agree, and the non-interest bearing account continued to grow in principal from $4,900 to $47,000 over a five-year period. Although two trustees did try to carry on corporate functions despite the dissident trustee, their good faith did not protect them from liability in this case. The money could have been transferred to at least an interest-bearing account without the third trustee's signature. The trustees were held jointly liable to pay to the corporation the statutory rate of simple interest.

Before an insurer writing trustees' coverage (generally known as directors' and officers' liability insurance) will respond to defend or pay on behalf of a trustee, it must be shown that the trustee acted in good faith and within the scope of his or her responsibilities. Ordinarily, coverage would not be afforded where a trustee is accused of acting improperly in his or her relationship with the corporation. In addition, insurance coverage for officers' and directors' liability generally excludes as a covered event the failure to obtain insurance. Thus, if a nursing facility is held liable in an instance where insurance coverage normally would have been available and the facility has failed to procure such coverage, the facility cannot take action against its trustees and through the mechanism of the officers' and directors' liability policy hope to avail itself of such coverage.

MANDATED MEDICAL STAFF INSURANCE COVERAGE

Physicians are often required by health care institutions to carry their own malpractice insurance. A federal district court in New Orleans has ruled that a hospital has the legal right to suspend a staff physician for failing to comply with its requirement that physicians carry medical malpractice insurance coverage. The decision resulted from a suit brought against Methodist Hospital in New Orleans by a physician whose staff privileges were suspended because he failed to comply with a newly adopted hospital requirement that all staff physicians provide proof of malpractice coverage of at least $1 million. The court rejected the physician's charges that the requirement violated his civil rights and antitrust laws in *Pollack v. Methodist Hospital*, 392 F. Supp. 393 (E.D. La. 1975).

The court in *Wilkinson v. Madera Community Hospital*, 144 Cal. App. 3d 436, 192 Cal. Rptr. 593 (1983), held that a Health and Safety Code provision providing that a health facility may require every member of its medical staff to have professional liability insurance as a condition to being on staff was not an unconstitutional delegation of legislative authority to hospitals as insurance companies. Dr. Wilkinson was refused reappointment because he failed to maintain malpractice insurance with a "recognized insurance company" as required by the hospital.

INVESTIGATION AND SETTLEMENT OF CLAIMS

An injured party may request settlement of a claim before instituting legal action. The majority of malpractice claims are settled before reaching the courtroom. A study by the U.S. General Accounting Office indicates that approximately 90 percent of malpractice claims are settled in this manner.[13]

As a first step toward settlement of a claim, the insurance carrier may send an investigator to interview a claimant regarding the details of the alleged occurrence that led to the injury. Itemization of damages (e.g., lost wages and medical expenses) and a request for a physical examination may be made by the insurance company. Following an investigation, the insurance company may agree to a settlement if liability is questionable and the risks of proceeding to trial are too great. Should settlement negotiations fail, an attorney may be employed by the injured party to negotiate a settlement. If the attorney fails to obtain a settlement, either the claim is dropped or legal action is commenced. If the claim is settled, a general release is signed by the plaintiff, surrendering the right of action against the defendant. Should the claimant be married, a general release must also be obtained from the spouse, since there may be a cause of action because of loss of the injured spouse's services, such as companionship. A parent's release surrenders only a parental claim. Approval of the court is necessary to release a child's claim. Release by a minor may in some instances be repudiated by the minor upon reaching majority.

Intoxication, the influence of drugs, shock, or extreme pain can prevent sufficient understanding of a general release and therefore prevent or void its execution. The same may apply in cases where the signer of a general release does not understand the language, has not had the opportunity to obtain appropriate legal consultation, or has been subjected to mental or physical duress. Misrepresentation or fraud can void an agreement. Those who are mentally incompetent cannot give a valid release. In this instance, a court-appointed guardian is required to execute a release on behalf of a mental incompetent, and a court must pass on the terms of any settlement.

RISK MANAGEMENT

Risk management is "a systematic program designed to reduce preventable injuries and accidents and minimize the financial severity of claims."[14] Liability insurers have been strong proponents of risk management, in many cases insurers have cut premiums for doctors and health care facilities who adopt sanctioned risk management practices.

In nursing facilities risk management must include a heightened sensitivity to the emotional needs of residents. The input of the provider-patient relationship cannot be overemphasized, especially in the nursing home setting where the provider-resident relationship is intense and inescapable. It is individuals, not incidents, who bring lawsuits.[15] Also, in nursing homes good relationships with the residents are very important in preventing malpractice suits. Public relations for health care professionals is a challenge. It is not only good medical practice "but it is at the very core of the problem of medical malpractice."[16]

A risk management program in a nursing facility should include the following:

- insurance education for all staff
- identification and investigation of specific incidents of resident injuries and, where possible, intervention

- generation and maintenance of a risk data base from which hazardous trends and areas may be identified and corrected

---

NOTES

1. U.S. DEPARTMENT OF HEALTH AND HUMAN SERVICES, TASK FORCE ON MEDICAL LIABILITY AND MALPRACTICE 3 (1987); AMERICAN MEDICAL ASSOCIATION, SOCIOECONOMIC MONITORING SYSTEM SURVEY (1986).

2. R.F. Clay, *What Bothers Doctors*, THE NEWSDAY MAGAZINE, January 13, 1991, at 15.

3. Zinman, *Study Finds Hospitals "Harm" Some*, 50(177) Newsday, March 1, 1990, at 17.

4. M. Kapp, *Preventing Malpractice Suits in Long Term Care Facilities*, QRM MONTHLY, March 1986, at 109.

5. American Society for Healthcare Risk Management Proceedings, Risk Financial Management Mechanism, Orlando, Fla., 1989, at 35.

6. *Id.*

7. The Robert Wood Johnson Foundation, *Profile: Walter Wadlington, LLB, Director, RWJF Medical Malpractice Program*, ADVANCES, Spring 1991, at 4.

8. NATIONAL ASSOCIATION OF INDEPENDENT INSURERS, REPORT OF THE FINANCIAL SOLVENCY OF STATE MEDICAL MALPRACTICE JUAS TO THE NAII LAWS COMMITTEE (1986).

9. M. Burke, *Congressional Leaders Outline Their Health Agendas: Sen. Jay Rockefeller*, 65(1) HOSPITALS, January 5, 1991, at 26.

10. U.S. DEPARTMENT OF HEALTH AND HUMAN SERVICES, TASK FORCE ON MEDICAL LIABILITY AND MALPRACTICE 114 (1987).

11. Some states have provisions mandating that, prior to any settlement of a negligence claim, consent of the court or, in the alternative, a medical malpractice panel to any proposed resolution must be obtained in order to best protect the minor's interests.

12. U.S. DEPARTMENT OF HEALTH AND HUMAN SERVICES, *supra* note 10, at 147.

13. U.S. GENERAL ACCOUNTING OFFICE, MEDICAL MALPRACTICE, CHARACTERISTICS OF CLAIMS CLOSED IN 1984 (1987).

14. J. Showalter, *Quality Assurance and Risk Management: A Provider of Two Important Monuments*, J. LEGAL MEDICINE 497 (Sept. 1984).

15. *Press I, The Predisposition to File Claims: The Patient Perspective*, LAW, MEDICINE AND HEALTH CARE 53 (April 1984).

16. R.R. Sanderson, *Medical Practice and Malpractice*, LEGAL ASPECTS OF MEDICAL PRACTICE 45 (June 1987).

Chapter 17

Labor Relations

The relationship between employers and employees is regulated by both state and federal laws (and, to a lesser extent, local laws). Nursing facilities are not exempt from the impact of these laws and therefore are required to take into account such matters as employment practices (wages, hours, and working conditions), union activity, worker's compensation laws, occupational safety and health laws, and employment discrimination laws.[1]

Federal or state regulation generally pervades all areas of employer–employee relationships. The trend is toward greater involvement of the federal government in matters of labor relations. The most significant piece of federal legislation dealing with labor relations is the National Labor Relations Act. While federal laws generally take precedence over state laws where there is a conflict between the state and the federal laws, state laws are applicable and must be considered, especially where the state standards are more stringent than those mandated by the federal government.

Professional and occupational associations, such as state nurses associations, historically known for their social and academic efforts, have involved themselves in collective bargaining for their profession. Union activity has been successful most often in those geographical areas in which unions have been active in other industries. As a result, labor relations has become an important factor in the operation of long-term care facilities.

UNIONS AND NURSING FACILITIES

The health care employee is likely to be more concerned with labor relations than is a person who is privately employed. Through the mid–1930s, union organizational activity in the health care industry was minimal, and it continued that way with relatively slow growth until the late 1950s. However, unions now play a significant role in employee relations.

A variety of labor organizations are now heavily involved in attempts to become the recognized collective bargaining representatives in health care facilities. There are craft unions, which devote their primary organizing efforts to skilled employees such as carpenters and electricians; industrial unions and unions of governmental employees, which seek to represent large groups of unskilled or semiskilled employees; and professional and occupational associations and societies, such as state nurses associations, which are interested in representing their members. To the extent that the professional organizations seek goals directly concerned with wages, hours, and other employment conditions and engage in bargaining on behalf of employees, they perform the functions of labor unions.

FEDERAL LABOR ACTS

National Labor Relations Act

The National Labor Relations Act (NLRA)[2] was enacted in 1935. It defines certain conduct of employers and employees as unfair labor practices and provides for hearings on complaints that such practices have occurred. This act was modified by the Taft–Hartley amendments of 1947 and the Landrum–Griffin amendments of 1959.

Jurisdiction

Nearly all proprietary nursing facilities have, for some time, been subject to the provisions of the NLRA. The National Labor Relations Board (NLRB), which is entrusted with enforcing and administering the act, has jurisdiction over matters involving proprietary and not-for-profit health care facilities with gross revenues of at least $250,000 per year and nurses associations and health-care-related facilities with gross revenues over $100,000 per year.[3] Butte Medical Properties, 168 NLRB Dec. (CCH) ¶226 (1967).

The NLRB's basic method of operation is to investigate claims or complaints of unfair practices submitted by either the employer or employees or both. The Board reviews the claim, determining whether in fact there have been unfair labor practices, and recommends a remedy.

Most questions submitted to the Board involve claims by employees that their rights to self-organization or the choosing of their collective bargaining representative have been interfered with by the employer. Employers may also submit complaints to the NLRB (e.g., where two unions are seeking recognition and one of them intimidates employees by making allegations that a sweetheart relationship exists between the employer and the competing union in an effort to disrupt the certification process).

An exemption for governmental institutions was included in the 1935 enactment of the National Labor Relations Act, and charitable health care institutions were exempted in 1947 by the Taft–Hartley Act amendments to the NLRA.[4] However, a July 1974 amendment to the National Labor Relations Act extended coverage to employees of nonprofit health care institutions that had previously been exempted from its provisions. In the words of the amendment, a health care facility is "any hospital, convalescent hospital, health maintenance organization, health clinic, nursing home, extended care facility, or other institution devoted to the care of the sick, infirm or aged."[5]

The amendment also enacted unique, special provisions for employees of health care facilities who oppose unionization on legitimate religious grounds. These provisions allow a member of such an institution to make periodic contributions to one of three non-religious charitable funds selected jointly by the labor organization and the employing institution, rather than paying periodic union dues and initiation fees. If the collective bargaining agreement does not specify an acceptable fund, the employee may select a tax-exempt charity.

Elections

The NLRA sets out the procedures by which employees may select a union as their collective bargaining representative to negotiate with health care facilities over employment and contract matters.[6] A health care facility may choose to recognize and deal with the union without resorting to the formal NLRA procedure. If the formal process is adhered to, the employees vote on union representation in an election held under NLRB supervision.[7] If the union wins, it is certified by the NLRB as the employees' bargaining representative.

The NLRA provides that the representative, having been selected by a majority of employees in a bargaining unit, is the exclusive bargaining agent for all employees in the unit. *Montgomery Ward & Co.*, 137 NLRB Dec. (CCH) ¶346, 50 L.R.R.M. (BNA) 1137 (1962). The scope of the bargaining unit is often the subject of dispute, for its boundaries may determine the outcome of the election, the employee representative's bargaining power, and the level of labor relations stability.

When the parties cannot agree on the appropriate unit for bargaining, the NLRB has broad discretion to decide the issue. But the NLRB's discretion is limited to determining appropriate units for only those employees who are classified as professional, supervisory, clerical, technical, or service and maintenance employees when they are included in units outside their particular category. This is the case unless there has been a self-determination election in which the members of a certain group vote, as a class, to be included within the larger bargaining unit. For example, nurses and other professional employees can be excluded from a bargaining unit composed of service and maintenance employees unless the professionals are first given the opportunity to choose separate representation and reject it. Supervisory nurses have also been held to be entitled to a bargaining unit separate from the unit composed of general duty nurses.[8] *St. Francis Hospital*, 265 NLRB Dec. (CCH) ¶1025 (1982).

While the NLRA does not require employee representatives to be selected by any particular procedure, the act provides for the NLRB to conduct representation elections by secret ballot. The NLRB may conduct such an election only when a petition for certification has been filed by an employee, a group of employees, an individual, a labor union acting on the employees' behalf, or an employer. When the petition is filed, the NLRB must investigate and direct an election if it has reasonable cause to believe a question of representation exists. After an election, if any party to it believes that certain conduct created an atmosphere that interfered with employee free choice, that party may file objections with the NLRB.[9]

The National Labor Relations Board has held in *N.L.R.B. v. Woodview–Calabasas Hospital*, 112 L.R.R.M. (BNA) 3290 (9th Cir. 1983), that strikers are eligible to vote in a decertification election even though they may be employed elsewhere during the strike.

Unfair Labor Practices

The NLRA prohibits nursing facilities from engaging in certain conduct classified as employer unfair labor practices.[10] For example, discriminating against an employee for holding union membership is not permitted. The NLRA stipulates that the employer must bargain in good faith with representatives of the employees; failure to do so constitutes an unfair labor practice. *NLRB v. Reed & Prince Manufacturing Co.*, 205 F.2d 131 (1st Cir.), *cert. denied*, 346 U.S. 887 (1953). The NLRB may order the employer to fulfill the duty to bargain.

If the employer dominates or controls the employees' union or interferes and supports one of two competing unions, the employer is committing an unfair labor practice. Such employer support of a competing union is clearly illustrated in a situation in which two unions are competing for members in the nursing facility, as well as for recognition as the employees' bargaining organization. If the nursing facility permits one of the unions to use its facilities for its organizational activities, but denies the use of the facilities to the other union, an unfair labor practice is committed. Financial assistance to one of the competing unions also constitutes an unfair labor practice.[11]

The NLRA also places duties on labor organizations and prohibits certain employee activities that are considered unfair labor practices. Coercion of employees by the union constitutes an unfair labor practice; such activities as mass picketing, assaulting nonstrikers, and following groups of nonstrikers away from the immediate area of the facility plainly constitute coercion and will be ordered stopped by the NLRB.[12] Breach of a collective bargaining contract by the labor union is another example of an unfair labor practice.

Labor Disputes

Congress enacted the Norris–LaGuardia Act to limit the power of the federal courts to issue injunctions in cases involving or growing out of labor disputes. The act's strict standards must be met before such injunctions can be issued. Essentially, a federal court may not apply restraints in a labor dispute until after the case is heard in open court and the finding is that unlawful acts will be committed unless restrained and that substantial and irreparable injury to the complainant's property will follow. *United States v. Hutcheson*, 312 U.S. 219 (1941).

The Norris–LaGuardia Act is aimed at reducing the number of injunctions granted to restrain strikes and picketing. An additional piece of legislation designating procedures limiting strikes in health institutions is the 1974 amendment to the National Labor Relations Act.[13]

This amendment sets out special procedures for handling labor disputes that develop from collective bargaining at the termination of an existing agreement or during negotiations for an initial contract between a health institution and its employees. The procedures were designed to ensure that the needs of patients would be met during any work stoppage (strike) or labor dispute in such an institution.

The amendment provides for creating a board of inquiry if a dispute threatens to interrupt health care in a particular community.[14] The board is appointed by the director of the Federal Mediation and Conciliation Service (FMCS) within 30 days after notification of either party's intention to terminate a labor contract. The board then has 15 days in which to investigate and report its findings and recommendations in writing. Once the report is filed with the FMCS, both parties are expected to maintain the status quo for an additional 15 days.

The board's findings provide a framework for arbitrators' decisions, while recognizing both the community's need for continuous health services and the good faith intentions of labor organizations to avoid a work stoppage whenever possible and to accept arbitration when negotiations reach an impasse.

The amendment also mandates certain notice requirements by labor groups in health care institutions: (1) the institution must be given 90 days' notice before a collective bargaining agreement expires, and (2) the FMCS is entitled to 60 days' notice. Previously, only 60 days' notice to the employer and 30 days' notice to the FMCS were required. However, if the bargaining agreement is the initial contract between the parties, only 30 days' notice need be given to the FMCS.

More significantly, ten days' notice is required in advance of any strike, picketing, or other concerted refusal to work, regardless of the source of the dispute.[15] This allows the NLRB to determine the legality of a strike before it occurs and also gives health care institutions ample time to ensure the continuity of patient treatment. At the same time, any attempt to utilize this period to undermine the bargaining relationship is implicitly forbidden.

The ten-day notice may be concurrent with the final ten days of the expiration notice. Any employee violation of these provisions amounts to an unfair labor practice and may automatically result in the discharge of the employee. In addition, injunctive relief may be available from the courts if circumstances warrant.

In summary, the amendment's provisions are designed to ensure that every possible approach to a peaceful settlement is fully explored before a strike is called.[16]

Labor–Management Reporting and Disclosure Act

The Labor–Management Reporting and Disclosure Act of 1959 places controls on labor unions and the relationships between unions and their members. In addition, it requires that employers report payments and loans made to officials or other representatives of labor organizations or any promises to make such payments or loans. Expenditures made to influence or restrict the way employees exercise their rights to organize and bargain collectively are illegal unless they are disclosed by the employer. Agreements with labor relations consultants, under which such persons undertake to interfere with certain employee rights, must also be disclosed. Reports required under this law must be filed with the secretary of labor and are then made public. Both charitable and proprietary health care facilities that make such payments or enter into such agreements must file reports. Penalties for failing to make the required reports, or for making false reports, include fines up to $10,000 and imprisonment for one year.

Fair Labor Standards Act

The Fair Labor Standards Act, 29 U.S.C. Chapter 8, establishes minimum wages and maximum hours of employment. The employees of all governmental, charitable, and proprietary health care facilities are covered by this act. Employers must conform to the minimum wage and overtime pay provisions. However, bona fide executive, administrative, and professional employees are exempted from the wage and hour provisions.

The law permits employers to enter into agreements with employees, establishing a work period of 14 consecutive days as an alternative to the usual 7-day week. If the alternative period is chosen, the employer must pay the overtime rate only for hours worked in excess of 80 hours during the 14-day period. It should be noted that the alternate 14-day work period does not relieve a facility from paying overtime for hours worked in excess of 8 in any one day even if no more than 80 hours are worked during the period.

Equal Pay Act of 1963

The Equal Pay Act of 1963, 29 U.S.C. Chapter 8, is essentially an amendment to the Fair Labor Standards Act and was passed to address wage disparities based on sex. The law is applicable everywhere that the minimum wage law is applicable and is enforced by the Equal Employment Opportunity Commission (EEOC). The Equal Pay Act, simply stated, requires that employees who perform equal work receive equal pay. There are situations where wages may be unequal so long as they are based upon factors other than sex, such as in the case of a formalized seniority system or a system that objectively measures earnings by the quantity or quality of production.

The court in *Odomes v. Nucare, Inc.*, 653 F.2d 246 (6th Cir. 1981), found that the nursing facility violated the Equal Pay Act of 1963 and Title VII of the Civil Rights Act of 1964 by paying a female nurse aide less than it was paying its male orderlies for similar work. The nursing facility had argued that the orderlies performed heavy lifting chores and provided a form of security for the mostly all-female shift. ". . . uncontradicted testimony of the orderlies who testified for Mrs. Odomes was that they did little or nothing that the nurse's aides didn't do." *Id.* at 250. The security aspects of an orderly's job was at best his presence on the shift and his periodic checking of the facility's premises. The facility argued that the orderlies were involved in a training program that justified higher pay. The court considered this an "illusory postevent justification for unequal pay for equal work." *Id.* at 247.

The Supreme Court stated in *Corning Glass Works v. Brennan*, 417 U.S. 188 (1974):

> Congress' purpose in enacting the Equal Pay Act was to remedy what was perceived to be a serious and endemic problem of employment discrimination in private industry—the fact that the wage structure of many segments of American industry has been based on an ancient but outmoded belief that a man, because of his role in society, should be paid more than a woman even though his ideas are the same.

Id. at 195.

Equal Employment Opportunity

Title VII of the Civil Rights Act of 1964, as amended by the Equal Employment Opportunity Act of 1972, prohibits private employers and state and local governments from discriminating on the basis of age, race, color, religion, sex, or national origin. An exception to prohibited employment practices may be permitted when religion, sex, or national origin is a bona fide occupational qualification necessary to the operation of a particular business or enterprise. *Griggs v. Duke Power Co.*, 401 U.S. 424 (1971).

Many states have enacted protective laws with respect to the employment of females. The EEOC guidelines on sex discrimination make it clear that state laws limiting the employment of females in certain occupations are superseded by Title VII and are no defense against a charge of sex discrimination.

Racial Discrimination

Lorraine Young, a black applicant for a nurse aide position in *Buckley Nursing Home, Inc. v. Massachusetts Commission Against Discrimination*, 478 N.E.2d 1292 (Mass. App. Ct. 1985), filed a complaint against the nursing facility for alleged racial discrimination. Ms. Young had responded to a newspaper advertisement for a nurse aide position. She had filed an application on March 1, 1974, and was interviewed by the acting supervisor of nursing. The applicant called to inquire about the position on several occasions and was eventually told that the position had been filled. The advertisement ran again in the newspaper and the applicant again called in response to the advertisement. Ms. Young was told that her application was on file and that she would be called as needed. The facility hired four full-time and one part-time nurses aides for the evening shift between March 1, 1974, and July 1, 1974.

> On the upper right hand corner of Young's application, there is a handwritten notation "no openings," even though during the relevant time periods there were openings and other persons were hired for the evening shift. That notation does not appear on any other application, and none of Buckley's witnesses could identify who wrote it or when it appeared.
>
> * * *
>
> Despite testimony to the contrary, the commission found that there was discussion about Young's race and that Buckley decided not to hire her on that basis.
>
> * * *
>
> The commission thus concluded that Buckley's reason for not hiring Young (that she was not the best qualified applicant for the job) was a pretext and that she would have been hired but for her race.

Id. at 1295.

The Commission awarded Ms. Young $6,986 plus interest for lost wages and $2,000 for emotional distress. In addition to the the monetary award to Ms. Young, the nursing home had been instructed by the Commission to develop a minority recruitment program. On appeal by the facility, the trial court upheld the Commission's decision. On further appeal, the appeals court held that the evidence was sufficient to support a reasonable inference that the nursing facility's rejection of the applicant occurred after consideration of her race.

Age Discrimination in Employment Act

The Age Discrimination in Employment Act of 1967, 29 U.S.C. Chapter 14, as amended, prohibits age-based employment discrimination against individuals between 40 and 70 years of age. The purpose of this law is to promote employment of older persons on the basis of their ability without regard to their age.

Rehabilitation Act of 1973

The essential purpose of the Rehabilitation Act of 1973, 29 U.S.C. Chapter 14, is to afford protection to handicapped employees. The law is basically administered by the Department of Health and Human Services, which derives its jurisdiction from the fact that health care facilities participate in such federal programs as Medicare, Medicaid, Hill–Burton, etc. The law is therefore applied to both public and private institutions, since both participate in these programs.

Section 503 of the Act applies to government contractors whose contracts exceed $2,500 in value. Section 504, which applies to employers who are recipients of federal financial assistance, states, "No . . . qualified handicapped individual in the United States . . . shall solely by reason of his handicap, be excluded from participation in, be denied the benefits of, or be subjected to discrimination under any program as actively receiving Federal financial assistance." Section 504 applies to virtually every area of personnel administration, including recruitment, advertising, processing of applications, promotions, rates of pay, fringe benefits, job assignments, etc.

Since July 1977, all institutions receiving federal financial assistance from the Department of Health and Human Services have been required to file assurances of compliance forms. Each employer must designate an individual to coordinate compliance efforts. A grievance procedure should be in place to address employee complaints alleging violation of the regulation. All employment decisions must be made without regard to physical or mental handicaps that are not disqualifying (e.g., an employer is not obligated to employ a person with a highly contagious disease that can be easily transmitted to others).

Employers receiving federal funds are required to perform a self evaluation as to their compliance with section 504 of the Rehabilitation Act of 1973. If discriminatory practices are identified through the self-evaluation process, remedial steps are to be taken to eliminate the effects of any discrimination. Records of the evaluation are to be maintained on file for at least three years following the review for public inspection. 45 C.F.R. Sec. 4.6(c).

Bargaining Units

A major area of concern for health care institutions is the number of bargaining units allowed in any one institution. New rules and regulations issued on April 21, 1989, by the NLRB allow up to eight collective bargaining units in health care facilities as opposed to the three normally allowed prior to the regulations. The American Hospital Association (AHA) had brought an action to enjoin the NLRB from enforcing the newly promulgated regulation recognizing up to eight bargaining units. A federal district court enjoined enforcement of the rule. The NLRB and intervening unions appealed. In *American Hospital Association v. N.L.R.B.*, 899 F.2d 651 (7th Cir. 1990), the Seventh Circuit held that the rule was not arbitrary and was within the authority of the NLRB. No rule is necessary to confer the rights already conferred by statute entitling guards and professional employees to form separate bargaining units.

> In making unit determinations the Board is thus required to strike a balance among the competing interests of unions, employees (whose interests are not always identical with those of unions), employers, and the broader public. The statute can be read to suggest that the tilt should be in favor of unions and toward relatively many, rather than relatively few, units.

Id. at 654. This balancing act is not spelled out in the statute, thus requiring an NLRB decision. "The decision is particularly difficult and delicate in the health care industry because the work force of a hospital, nursing home, or rehabilitation center tends to be small and heterogeneous." *Id.* at 654–655.

On appeal, the U.S. Supreme Court, on April 23, 1991, upon unanimous decision upheld a National Labor Relations Board rule allowing hospital workers to form up to eight separate bargaining units, including those for

- physicians
- registered nurses
- other professionals
- technical employees
- clerical employees
- skilled maintenance employees
- other non-professional employees
- security guards[17]

It is anticipated that there will be increased union activity in health care facilities, thus increasing administrative costs. Management must strive to maintain open lines of communications with employees and strive to improve working conditions. An honest and open relationship with employees will go a long way towards maintaining a union-free environment.

> . . . officials at one long term care facility effectively countered an organizing attempt by educating their employees about the union and what it realistically could do for them. In March, employees of St. Anthony Home, Crown Point, IN, voted against representation by a national steelworker's union.[18]

STATE LAWS

The federal labor enactments serve as a pattern for many state labor laws that comprise the second labor regulation system touching long-term care facilities.

State labor acts vary from state to state. Therefore, it is important that each institution familiarize itself not only with federal regulations but also with state regulations affecting labor relations within the institution.

State Labor–Management Relations Act

Because the National Labor Relations Act (NLRA) excludes from coverage health care institutions operated by the state or its political subdivisions, regulation of labor–management relations in these institutions is left to state law.[19] However, most states do not have labor relations statutes. Unless the constitution in such a state guarantees the right of employees to organize and imposes the duty of collective bargaining on the employer, health care facilities do not have to bargain collectively with their employees. However, in states that do have labor relations acts, the obligation of an institution to bargain collectively with its employees is determined by the applicable statute.

State laws vary considerably in their coverage, and often employees of state and local governmental institutions are covered by separate public employee legislation. Some of these statutes cover both state and local employees, whereas others cover only state or only local employees. A number of states have statutes similar to the Norris–LaGuardia Act, restricting the granting of injunctions in labor disputes. There are anti-injunction acts in several other states that are different from this type, and decisions under them do not fall into an easily recognized pattern.

Some of the states that have labor relations acts granting employees the right to organize, join unions, and bargain collectively have specifically prohibited strikes and lockouts and have provided for compulsory arbitration whenever a collective bargaining contract cannot otherwise be executed amicably. Anti-injunction statutes would not forbid injunctions to restrain violations of these statutory provisions.

The doctrine of federal pre-emption, as applied to labor relations, displaces the states' jurisdiction to regulate an activity that is arguably an unfair labor practice within the meaning of the NLRA. Nonetheless, the U.S. Supreme Court has ruled that states can still regulate labor relations activity that also falls within the jurisdiction of the NLRB where deeply rooted local feelings and responsibility are affected. *Amalgamated Association of Street, Electric Railway & Motor Coach Employees v. Lockridge*, 403 U.S. 274 (1971).

Union Security Contracts and Right-To-Work Laws

Labor organizations frequently seek to enter union security contracts with employers. Such contracts are of two types: the closed shop contract, which provides that only members of a particular union may be hired, and the union shop contract, which makes continued employment dependent on membership in the union, although the employee need not have been a union member when applying for the job.

More than one-third of all the states have made such contracts unlawful. Statutes forbidding such agreements are generally called right-to-work laws on the theory that they protect everyone's right to work even if a person refuses to join a union. Several other state statutes or decisions purport to restrict union security contracts or specify procedures to be completed before such agreements may be made.

Wage and Hour Laws

Where state minimum wage standards are higher than federal standards, the state's standards are applicable.

Child Labor Acts

Many states prohibit the employment of minors below a certain age and restrict the employment of other minors. Child labor legislation commonly requires that working papers be secured before a child may be hired, forbids the employment of minors at night, and prohibits minors from operating certain types of dangerous machinery.

This kind of legislation rarely exempts charitable institutions, although some exceptions may be made with respect to the hours when student nurses may work.

Worker's Compensation

Worker's compensation is a program by which an employee can receive certain wage benefits due to work-related injuries. An employee who is injured while performing job-related duties is generally eligible for worker's compensation. Worker's compensation programs are administered by the states.

State legislatures have recognized that it is difficult and expensive for employees to recover from their employers and have therefore enacted worker's compensation laws.[20] Employers are required to provide worker compensation as a benefit. Worker's compensation laws give the employee a legal way to receive compensation for injuries on the job. The acts do not require the employee to prove that the injury was the result of the employer's negligence. Worker's compensation laws are based on the employer–employee relationship and not on the theory of negligence.

The scope of worker's compensation varies widely. Some states limit an employee's compensation to the amount recoverable by the worker's compensation law, and further lawsuits against the employer are barred. Other states permit employees to choose whether they accept the compensation provided by law or institute a lawsuit against the employer. Some acts go further and provide a system of insurance that may be under the supervision of state or private insurers. Recovery by an employee begins with a hearing on the claim before a board of commissioners. Following the hearing, the commissioners decide whether there was an employer–employee relationship, whether the injury is covered by the act,[21] and whether there is a connection between the employment and the injury. The commissioners then award compensation according to a predetermined schedule based on the nature of the injury. Generally, worker's compensation boards tend to be liberal in interpreting the law to provide compensation for employees.

Physical Injury

The courts have been somewhat liberal in allowing worker's compensation benefits to be paid to employees injured while on duty, even when challenged by the employer under seemingly justifiable circumstances. The employee, for example, in *Fondulac Nursing Home v. Industrial Commission*, 460 N.E.2d 751 (Ill. 1984), was found to be entitled to worker's compensation despite orders that she was not to lift patients because of a back injury. When a patient was being transferred from her wheelchair to her bed and began to fall, the nurse attempted to prevent the fall, injuring herself. The nurse acted within her scope of employment by attempting to prevent the fall—to her own detriment and her employer's best interests—by protecting the patient from injury.

Job Stress

The registered nurse in *Elwood v. SAIF*, 676 P.2d 922 (Or. Ct. App. 1984), had filed a worker's compensation claim for an occupational disease based on depression. The referee and the Workers' Compensation Board affirmed the insurer's denial of the claim and the claimant sought judicial review. The questions that needed to be answered in order to determine job stress, as in *McGarrah v. SAIF*, 296 Or. 145, 675 P.2d 159 (1983), were:

1. What were the "real" events and conditions of plaintiff's employment?
2. Were those real events and conditions capable of producing stress when viewed "objectively," even though an average worker might not have responded adversely to them?
3. Did plaintiff suffer a mental disorder?
4. Were the real stressful events and conditions the "major contributing cause" of plaintiff's mental disorder?

676 P.2d at 923.

The record established that numerous events and conditions of her employment, including her termination, were real and capable of producing stress when viewed objectively. The claimant's treating physician advised her that she was suffering from anxiety and depression and stress and advised her to seek a psychiatric evaluation. *Id.* at 924. The court held that the claimant established that her condition was compensable.

LABOR'S RIGHTS

Rights and responsibilities run concurrently. Employee rights include

- Right to organize and bargain collectively.
- Right to solicit and distribute union information during non-working hours (i.e., mealtimes and coffee breaks).
- Right to picket. Picketing is the act of patrolling, by one or more persons, of a place related to a labor dispute. It varies in purpose and form; it may be conducted by employees or non-employees and, like strikes, some picketing may be legislatively or judicially disapproved and subject to regulation.
- Right to strike. A strike may be defined as the collective quitting of work by employees as a means of inducing the employer to assent to employee demands. Employees possess the right to strike although this right is not absolute and is subject to limited exercise. The 1974 amendments to the NLRA have added new requirements with respect to strikes and picketing in an attempt to reduce the interruption of health care services. The NLRB is urged to give top priority to settling labor–management disputes resulting in the loss of health care personnel or medical services.

Employees granted the above rights have the concomitant responsibility to properly perform their work duties. A nursing home housekeeper, for example, was properly terminated following repeated oral and written reprimands concerning her improper cleaning of rooms in *Ford v. Patin*, 534 So. 2d 1003 (La. Ct. App. 1988). Her substandard performance despite repeated warnings evidenced willful and wanton disregard of her employer's interest and constituted misconduct within purview of Louisiana Rev. Stat. 23:1601(2).

MANAGEMENT RIGHTS

As with labor, management also has certain rights and responsibilities. Specific management rights are discussed below.

Right To Receive Strike Notice

Management has a right to a 10-day advance notice of a bargaining unit's intent to strike.[22]

Right To Hire Replacement Workers

Although management may not discharge employees in retaliation for union activity, concomitant with the employees' right to strike is management's right to hire replacement workers in the event of a strike. The nursing home in *Charlesgate Nursing Center v. State of Rhode Island*, 723 F. Supp. 859 (D. R.I. 1989), brought an action against the state, seeking a determination that a state statute prohibiting struck employers from utilizing the services of a third party to recruit replacement workers during a strike was unconstitutional. Employees of the nursing home went on strike June 2, 1988, and Charlesgate hired temporary replacement workers in order to provide continued services for its patients. The employees were hired through employment agencies. The actions of Charlesgate and the agencies had violated the General Laws of Rhode Island (1956) (1986 Re-enactment) Secs. 28–10–10 an 28–10–12, which read:

> 28–10–10. Recruitment prohibited—It shall be unlawful for any person, partnership, agency, firm or corporation, or officer or agent thereof, to knowingly recruit, procure, supply or refer any person who offers him or herself for employment in the place of an employee involved in a labor strike or lockout in which such person, partnership, agency, firm, or corporation is not directly interested.
>
> 28–10–12. Agency for procurement—It shall be unlawful for any person, partnership, firm or corporation, or officer or agent thereof, involved in a labor strike or lockout to contract or arrange with any other person, partnership, agency, firm or corporation to recruit, procure, supply, or refer persons who offer themselves for employment in the place of employees involved in a labor strike or lockout for employment in place of employees involved in such labor strike or lockout.

Id. at 861.

Citing these statutes, the labor unions involved in the strike notified nursing pools throughout the state that it was unlawful to provide Charlesgate with replacement workers. At the same time, the unions urged the City of Providence and the Rhode Island Attorney General to prosecute Charlesgate, at which time Charlesgate filed its suit claiming that the Rhode Island statutes were unconstitutional.

Although the strike was settled prior to any actions by the city and the Attorney General, the case was not required to be dismissed. The federal district court held that the statute was unconstitutional because it prohibited activity that Congress had intended to leave open to struck employers as a peaceful weapon of economic self-help.

Right To Restrict Union Activities to Prescribed Areas

Management has the right to reasonably restrict union organizers to certain locations in the nursing facility and to certain time periods to avoid interference with facility operations.

Right To Prohibit Union Activity during Working Hours

Management has the right to prohibit union activities during employee working hours.

Right To Prohibit Supervisors from Participating in Union Activity

Management has the right to prohibit supervisors from engaging in union organizational activity. A nursing supervisor brought a lawsuit for wrongful discharge against a nursing facility and its director of nursing. She was dismissed for her activities in attempting to form an organization to represent the nurses. The circuit court granted summary judgment for the defendants and the appeals court affirmed. On review, the Supreme Court of Wisconsin held in *Arena v. Lincoln Lutheran of Racine*, 149 Wis. 2d 35, 437 N.W.2d 538 (1989), that after the National Labor Relations Board had determined that the nurses in this case were "supervisors" rather than "employees" within the meaning of the National Labor Relations Act, federal labor law pre-empted the state court from determining whether the nurse's discharge for engaging in concerted activities was wrongful under Wisconsin law.

Nursing home personnel who are supervisors as defined in the National Labor Relations Act are treated differently than professional employees. The definition of the term supervisor found in Section 2(11) provides:

> The term "supervisor" means any individual having authority, in the interest of the employer, to hire, transfer, suspend, layoff, recall, promote, discharge, assign, reward, or discipline other employees, or responsibly to direct them, or to adjust their grievances, or effectively to recommend such action, if in connection with the foregoing the exercise of such authority is not merely a routine or clerical nature, but requires the use of independent judgment. [29 U.S.C. 152(11) (1965).]

The petitioner alleged in her complaint that she had become concerned with certain policies that included nurses' being treated in an arbitrary manner. The petitioner had held a meeting outside of Racine with the nurses to discuss their concerns and the possibility of forming an association to represent the collective interests of the nurses. The NLRA did not protect the nursing supervisor due to the fact that she was a supervisor, rather than an employee. Congress excluded supervisors from protection afforded rank-and-file employees engaged in concerted activity for their mutual benefit in order to assure management of the undivided loyalty of its supervisory personnel, by making sure that no employer would have to retain as its agent one who is obligated to a union.

Seven registered nurses at a small 72-bed nursing home were found not to function as supervisors and were, therefore, eligible for a separate bargaining unit in *N.L.R.B. v. Res-Care, Inc.*, 705 F.2d 1461 (7th Cir. 1983). While the nurses had the authority to assign nurse aides, their exercise of this authority was merely routine and did not require independent judgment. The nurses were not shown to have any authority to hire, discipline, and/or fire any of the nursing aides. Such authority, if present, would have indicated some sort of supervisory status. Allowing seven nurses to form their own collective bargaining unit, rather than merging them into a unit consisting of nurse aides and other workers, was not found to be improper nor was it an undue proliferation of bargaining units at the facility.

Certification of 17 registered nurses as an employee bargaining unit in *NLRB v. American Medical Services, Inc.*, 705 F.2d 1472 (7th Cir. 1983), was shown to be improper. The nursing home had contended that a very low ratio of supervisors to employees would occur if the NLRB's decision was upheld. Substantial evidence had been presented to the court showing that the nurses exercised substantial supervisory powers, including the authority to issue work assignments and discipline employees.

> Taft–Hartley applied some brakes, so that the balance of power between companies and unions would not shift wholly to the union side. The exclusion of supervisors is one of the breaks. If supervisors were free to join or form unions and enjoy the broad protection of the Act for concerted activity, see Sec. 7, 29 U.S.C. Sec. 157, the impact of a strike would be greatly amplified because the company would not be able to use its supervisory personnel to replace strikers. More important, the company—with or without a strike—could lose control of its work force to the unions, since the very people in the company who controlled hiring, discipline, assignments, and other dimensions of the employment relationship might be subject to control by the same union as the employees they were supposed to be controlling on the employer's behalf.

N.L.R.B. v. Res-Care, Inc., 705 F.2d at 1465.

EQUAL EMPLOYMENT OPPORTUNITY OR AFFIRMATIVE ACTION PLAN

Nursing facilities are required to comply with all applicable HHS regulations "including but not limited to those pertaining to non-discrimination on the basis of race, color, or national origin (45 C.F.R. Part 80), non-discrimination on the basis of handicap (45 C.F.R. Part 84), non-discrimination on the basis of age (45 C.F.R. Part 91), protection of human subjects of research (45 C.F.R. Part 46), and fraud and abuse (42 C.F.R. Part 455). Although these regulations are not in themselves considered requirements under this part, their violation may result in the termination or suspension of or the refusal to grant or continue payment with federal funds.[23] In order to comply with the spirit of these regulations and Executive Order 11246, nursing facilities should have an equal employment opportunity or affirmative action plan in place.

An affirmative action program would include such things as the collection and analysis of data on the race and sex of all applicants for employment and a statement in the personnel policy and procedure manuals and employee handbooks that would read, for example, "Nursing Facility, Inc., is an equal opportunity/affirmative action employer and does not discriminate on the basis of race, color, religion, sex, national origin, age, handicap, or veteran status."

RESIDENT RIGHTS DURING LABOR DISPUTES

Just as labor and management have a variety of rights and responsibilities, the same is true for residents. For example, residents' rights take precedence over employee and management rights when a patient's right to privacy or well-being is in jeopardy due to labor disputes.

INJUNCTION

An injunction is an order by a court directing that a certain act be done or not done. Persons who fail to comply with court orders are said to be in "contempt of court." The earliest uses of injunctions in labor relations was by employers to stop strikes or picketing by employees. Today, the general rule limits the availability of injunctive relief to halt work stoppages. The federal government and many states have enacted anti-injunction acts. These acts restrict the power of the courts to limit injunctions in labor disputes by setting strictly defined standards that must be met before injunctions can be granted to restrain activities such as strikes and picketing.

ADMINISTERING A COLLECTIVE BARGAINING AGREEMENT

Once a collective bargaining agreement has been negotiated "in good faith," it should be administered with care and good faith as well.

The first line supervisors are responsible for administering the agreement at the grass roots level. They should familiarize themselves with the provisions of the agreement. Formal orientation programs can be provided by an institution's human resources department. Special emphasis should be placed on the use of corrective discipline, as provided under the contract, and on how to respond to grievances. The institution's management through its human relations department maintains the ultimate responsibility in the facility for the fair and effective administration of its union contract(s).

Maintaining propitious records of all grievances, grievance meetings, and grievance resolutions is the responsibility of supervisors and management alike. Regardless of whether a grievance is meritorious and settled by management, or whether it is spurious and therefore denied, clear and complete records should be maintained. An ability to document resolutions of particular problems, as well as management's approach to grievances, is especially important if arbitration is required to settle a grievance.

Employers and unions often provide for arbitration because the procedure is generally quicker and less expensive than it would be if court adjudication were required, and because labor arbitrators have greater expertise in labor affairs than do most judges.

Arbitration procedures are set in motion when the union files a demand for arbitration either with the employer or with the arbitration agency named in the contract. The arbitration hearing is a relatively informal proceeding at which management frequently chooses to be represented by counsel. The arbitrator's decision is binding on both parties.

The arbitrator's decision can be upset by showing any of the following:

1. The arbitrator has clearly exceeded his authority under the collective bargaining agreement.
2. The decision is the product of fraud or duress.
3. The arbitrator has been guilty of impropriety.
4. The award violates the law or requires a violation of the law.

OCCUPATIONAL SAFETY AND HEALTH ACT

Congress enacted the Occupational Safety and Health Act of 1970, 29 U.S.C. Sec. 651, to establish administrative machinery for the development and enforcement of standards for occupational health and safety.[24] The legislation was enacted based on Congressional findings that personal injuries and illnesses arising out of work situations impose a substantial burden upon and are substantial hindrances to interstate commerce in terms of lost production, wage loss, medical expenses, and disability compensation payments. The Congress declared that its purpose and policy was to assure, so far as possible, every working man and woman in the nation safe and healthful working conditions and to preserve our human resources by

1. encouraging employers and employees in their efforts to reduce the number of occupational safety and health hazards at their places of employment, and stimulating employers and employees to institute new and to perfect existing programs for providing safe and healthful working conditions
2. providing that employers and employees have separate but dependent responsibilities and rights with respect to achieving safe and healthful working conditions
3. authorizing the Secretary of Labor to set mandatory occupational safety and health standards applicable to businesses affecting interstate commerce, and creating an Occupational and Health Review Commission for carrying out adjudicatory functions under the Act

4. building upon advances already made through employer and employee initiative for providing safe and healthful working conditions
5. providing for research in the field of occupational safety and health, including the psychological factors involved, and developing innovative methods, techniques, and approaches for dealing with occupational safety and health problems
6. exploring ways to discover latent diseases, establishing causal connections between diseases and work in environmental conditions, and conducting other research relating to health problems, in recognition of the fact that occupational health standards present problems often different from those involved in occupational safety
7. providing medical criteria that will assure, insofar as practicable, that no employee will suffer diminished health, functional capacity, or life expectancy as a result of his or her work experience
8. providing for training programs to increase the number and competence of personnel engaged in the field of occupational safety and health
9. providing for the development and promulgation of occupational safety and health standards
10. providing an effective enforcement program that includes a prohibition against giving advance notice of any inspection and sanctions for any individual violating this prohibition
11. encouraging the states to assume the fullest responsibility for the administration and enforcement of their occupational safety and health laws by providing grants to the states to assist in identifying their needs and responsibilities in the area of occupational safety and health, developing plans in accordance with the provisions of this Act, improving the administration and enforcement of state occupational safety and health laws, and conducting experimental and demonstration projects in connection therewith
12. providing for appropriate reporting procedures with respect to occupational safety and health that procedures will help achieve the objectives of this Act and accurately describe the nature of the occupational safety and health problem
13. encouraging joint labor–management efforts to reduce injuries and disease arising out of employment.[25]

The employer must comply with the occupational and health standards under the Act and employees must follow the rules, regulations, and orders issued under the Act that are applicable to their actions and conduct on the job. The duties of employers and employees under the act are as follows:

(a) Each employer—

(1) shall furnish to each of his employees employment and a place of employment which is free from recognized hazards that are causing or are likely to cause death or serious physical harm to his employees;

(2) shall comply with occupational safety and health standards promulgated under this Act.

(b) Each employee shall comply with occupational safety and health standards and all rules, regulations, and orders pursuant to this Act which are applicable to his own actions and conduct.[26]

The OSHA Survey

The Occupational Safety and Health Administration (OSHA) is responsible for administering the Act, issuing standards, and conducting on-site inspections to ensure compliance with the Act. OSHA develops and promulgates occupational safety and health standards for the workplace. It develops and issues regulations, conducts investigations and inspections to determine the status of compliance, and issues citations and proposes penalties for noncompliance.

In recent developments, OSHA inspectors have called for stiffer penalties for health and safety violations in order to deter violations. "OSHA inspectors surveyed by Congress' General Accounting Office said further criminal enforcement authority was needed to enforce this nation's workplace health and safety standards."[27]

State Regulation

Employees or their representatives have the right to file their complaints with an OSHA office and request a survey when they believe that conditions in the workplace are unsafe or unhealthful. If a violation of the Act is found at the time of a survey, the employer receives a citation stating a time frame within which a violation must be corrected.

The states also have statutes charging employers with the duty to furnish employees with a safe working environment. The city and county in which a health care facility is located may also prescribe rules regarding the health and safety of employees. Many communities have enacted sanitary and health codes that require certain facilities or standards.

Legal Liability

From a liability point of view, an employer can be held legally liable for damages suffered by employees through exposure to dangerous conditions that are in violation of OSHA standards. Proof of an employee's exposure to noncompliant conditions is generally necessary in order to find an employer liable.

NOTES

1. 29 U.S.C. §151 *et seq.*
2. *Id.*
3. NLRA Amendments of 1974, Pub. L. No. 93–360.
4. NATIONAL LABOR RELATIONS BOARD, LEGISLATIVE HISTORY OF THE LABOR–MANAGEMENT RELATIONS ACT OF 1947, at 303, 359 (1949). There exists almost no debate regarding this exclusion, although Senator Tydings of Maryland did justify this approach on the rationale that nonprofit hospitals were charitable institutions subject to local governmental regulations and, at least in 1947, were in dire financial straits. *Id.* at 1464–65.
5. *Id.* §2 (14).
6. *Id.* §9.
7. *Id.*
8. *Id.* §9(b)(1) & (b)(3).
9. *Id.* §8.
10. *Id.* §8, 9.
11. *Id.* §8(a)(1) & (a)(3).
12. *Id.* §8(b)(7); Landrum–Griffin Amendments of 1959, Pub. L. No. 86–257 (1959).
13. *Id.* §8(g).
14. *Id.*
15. *Id.* §8(d).
16. SUBCOMMITTEE ON LABOR OF THE SENATE COMMITTEE ON LABOR AND PUBLIC WELFARE, 93d Cong., 2d Sess., LEGISLATIVE HISTORY OF THE COVERAGE OF NON-PROFIT HOSPITALS UNDER THE NATIONAL LABOR RELATIONS ACT OF 1974, at 412–14 (1974).
17. *Supreme Court Upholds NLRB Bargaining-Unit Rule*, 27(17) AHA News, April 29, 1991, at 1.
18. *Despite NLRB Ruling, Hospitals Can Counter Unions: Experts*, 27(21) AHA News, May 27, 1991, at 4.
19. NLRA, *supra* note 5, §2(3); 29 U.S.C. §152(3), Pub. L. No. 93–360 (1974).
20. REPORT OF THE NATIONAL COMMISSION ON STATE WORKMEN'S COMPENSATION LAWS (1972). The statute that authorized the study and subsequent report was the Occupational Safety and Health Act of 1970.
21. This refers to the particular state statute in effect at the time of the injury.
22. 29 U.S.C. §158(g).
23. 42 C.F.R. §483.75 (1989).
24. 29 U.S.C. §651 *et seq.*
25. Pub. L. No. 91–596, Dec. 29, 1970, §2, 84 Stat. 1590; *see also* 29 U.S.C.A. §651 (1990).
26. Pub. L. No. 91–596, Dec. 29, 1970, §5, 84 Stat. 1593; 29 U.S.C.A. §654 (1990).
27. *OSHA's Inspectors Call for Stiffer Penalties for Violations*, XXI (1) THE NATION'S HEALTH, January, 1991, at 7.

Chapter 18

Employment, Discipline, and Discharge

According to a study for the Bureau of National Affairs, more than 25,000 wrongful discharge cases are pending in state and federal courts.[1] "The study estimates that wrongful discharge cases more than doubled between 1982 and 1987."[2] For the health care executive, an unexpected termination may mean a significant setback in career progression, financial hardship, and loss of self-esteem. For the institution and its community, a termination means a lack of stability in the management structure and possible disruption and realignment of services provided. There is a growing consensus that the current high turnover rates are unhealthy and provide a disservice to an industry already suffering from cost constraints and other pressures.[3]

In 1989, the American College of Healthcare Executives published Phase I results of its CEO turnover study. The report showed that overall turnover had increased from 16.9 percent in 1981–82 to 24.2 percent in 1986–87, and there was every indication that rates would be a major concern in the near future. Although not all turnover reflects termination, there is evidence that a large proportion of CEOs leave involuntarily.[4]

Fairly balancing the rights of the employee and the needs of the organization is an extremely complex objective. This chapter provides some direction in this balancing act.

EMPLOYMENT-AT-WILL

The common law "employment-at-will" doctrine provides that employment is at the will of either the employer or the employee and that employment may be terminated by the employer or the employee at any time for any or no reason, unless there is a contract in place that specifies the terms and duration of employment. Historically, termination of employees for any reason was widely accepted. However, contemporary thinking does not support this concept.

> In recent years the rule that employment for an indefinite term is terminable by the employer whenever and for whatever cause he chooses without incurring liability has been the subject of considerable scholarly debate, and judicial and legislative modification. Consequently, there has been a growing trend toward a restricted application of the at-will employment rule whereby the right of an employer to discharge an at-will employee without cause is limited by either public policy considerations or an implied covenant of good faith and fair dealing.

44 A.L.R. 4th 1136. In *Sides v. Duke Hospital*, 328 S.E.2d 818 (N.C. Ct. App. 1985), the Court of Appeals of North Carolina found it to be an

> . . . obvious and indisputable fact that in a civilized state where reciprocal legal rights and duties abound the words "at will" can never mean "without limit or qualification," as so much of the discussion and the briefs of the defendants imply; for in such a state the rights of each person are necessarily and inherently limited by the rights of others and the interests of the public. An at will prerogative without limits could be suffered only in an anarchy, and there not for long—it certainly cannot be suffered in a society such as ours without weakening the bond of counter balancing rights and obligations that holds such societies together.
>
> * * *
>
> If we are to have law, those who so act against the public interest must be held accountable for the harm inflicted thereby; to accord them civil immunity would incongruously reward their lawlessness at the unjust expense of their innocent victims.

The concept of the employment-at-will doctrine is embroiled in a combination of legislative enactments and judicial decisions. Some states have a tendency to be more employer oriented, such as New York, while others, like California, emerge as being much more forward thinking and in harmony with the constitutional rights of the employee. A study of 120 wrongful discharge cases in California between 1980 and 1986, conducted by the Rand Corporation, revealed that plaintiffs won 67.5 percent of the time and were awarded an average of $646,855.[5]

> The employment at will common law doctrine is not truly applicable in today's society and many courts have recognized this fact. In the last century, the common law developed in a laissez-faire climate that encouraged industrial growth and improved the right of an employer to control his own business, including the right to fire without cause an employee at will . . . The twentieth century has witnessed significant changes in socioeconomic values that have led to reassessment of the common law

> rule. Businesses have evolved from small and medium size firms to gigantic corporations in which ownership is separate from management. Formerly there was a clear delineation between employers, who frequently were owners of their own businesses, and employees. The employer in the old sense has been replaced by a superior in the corporate hierarchy who is himself an employee.

Pierce v. Ortho Pharmaceutical Corp., 417 A.2d 505, 509 (N.J. 1980).

As discussed below, exceptions to the employment at-will doctrine involve contractual relationships, public policy issues, defamation, fairness, and retaliatory discharge. Besides public policy issues in general, it would seem that the doctrine has little applicability in today's modern society.

Contractual Relationships

Express Agreement

An employer's right to terminate an employee can be limited by express agreement with the employee or through a collective bargaining agreement to which the employee is a beneficiary. No such agreement was found to exist in *O'Connor v. Eastman Kodak Co.*, 492 N.Y.S.2d 9 (N.Y. 1985), where the court held that an employer had a right to terminate an employee at will at any time and for any reason or no reason. The plaintiff did not rely on any specific representation made to him during the course of his employment interviews, nor did he rely on any documentation in the employee handbook, which would have limited the defendant's common law right to discharge at will. The employee had relied on a popular perception of Kodak as a womb-to-tomb employer.

The employment-at-will doctrine provides employees with few employment rights. Employers who experience favorable court decisions in wrongful discharge claims are often the losers due to the bad press and the negative effects a discharge has on employee morale. "Wrongful discharge claims are difficult, time consuming and expensive lawsuits to defend and, when they reach the jury, employers are losing about 75% of the time."[6]

In another case, the employee manual was found not to contain an express limitation on the employer's right to terminate an employee at will. The discharged employee in *Rock v. Sear-Brown Associates, P.C.*, 524 N.Y.S.2d 935 (N.Y. App. Div. 1988), had brought an action against his employer for wrongful discharge. The court dismissed the complaint, and the employee appealed. The appellate court held that an employee could not state a claim for wrongful discharge.

Implied Contracts

The rights of employees have been expanding through judicial decisions in the various states. Court decisions have been based on verbal promises, historical practices of the employer, and documents such as employee handbooks and administrative policy and procedure manuals that describe employee rights. The following are a few of the many cases that involve published personnel policies and procedures.

An employee brought suit against his employer for wrongful termination in *Weiner v. McGraw-Hill*, 57 N.Y.2d 458, 443 N.E.2d 441, 457 N.Y.S.2d 193 (1982). The court held that although the plaintiff was not engaged by the defendant for a fixed term of employment, he pleaded a good cause of action for breach of contract. The plaintiff was allegedly discharged without the "just and sufficient cause" or the rehabilitative efforts specified in the defendants' handbook and allegedly promised at the time the plaintiff accepted employment. Furthermore, on several occasions when the plaintiff had recommended that certain of his subordinates be dismissed, he was allegedly instructed to proceed in strict compliance with the handbook and policy manuals. The employment application that the plaintiff had signed stated that his employment would be subject to the provisions of McGraw–Hill's "handbook on personnel policies and procedures."

An employee handbook or other policy statement may modify an at-will employment contract. The provisions of an employee handbook were held binding in *Duldulao v. St. Mary of Nazareth Hospital Center*, 505 N.E.2d 314 (Ill. 1985). The Supreme Court of Illinois held that: (1) a presumption that an employee hired for an indefinite term was an employee at will could be rebutted by evidence that the parties contracted to the contrary; (2) language in the employee handbook to the effect that a non-probationary employee could be discharged after written notice was sufficient to modify the at-will nature of the plaintiff's employment; and (3) the plaintiff qualified as a "non-probationary employee," for purpose of the language in the handbook.

A nurse's aide was awarded $20,000 in *Watson v. Idaho Falls Consolidated Hospitals, Inc.*, 720 P.2d 632 (Idaho 1986), for damages when the hospital, as employer, violated the provisions of its employee handbook in the manner in which it terminated her employment. Evidence that the employee was making $1,000 a month at the time of her discharge and was not able to find suitable employment following her discharge supported the award of $20,000 in her favor for wrongful discharge. Although the nurse's aide had no formal written contract, the employee handbook and the hospital policies and procedures manual constituted a contract in view of evidence to the effect that these documents had been intended to be enforced and complied with by both employees and management. Employees read and relied on the handbook as creating terms of an employment contract and were required to sign for the handbook in order to establish receipt of a revised handbook explaining hospital policy, discipline, counseling, and termination. A policy and procedure manual placed on each floor of the hospital also outlined termination procedures.

The nurse in *Churchill v. Waters*, 731 F. Supp. 311 (C.D. Ill. 1990), brought a civil rights action against the hospital and hospital officials following her discharge. The federal district court held for the defendants on motion for summary judgment, finding that the hospital employee handbook did not give the nurse a protected property interest in continued employment. "Absent proof that the handbook contained clear promises which indicated the intent to bind the parties, no contract was created." *Id.* at 321–22. The handbook contained a disclaimer expressly disavowing any attempt to be bound by it and stated that its contents were not to be considered conditions of employment. The handbook was "presented as a matter of information only and the language contained herein [was] not intended to constitute a contract between McDonough District Hospital and . . . the employee." *Id.* at 315–16.

"Employment guidelines and manuals are very helpful in obtaining employee good will and maintaining good employee relations. They can also be excellent tools in maintaining a union-free environment. Therefore, the use, drafting, and implementation of an employment manual should be taken seriously. When drafting such manuals, employers should keep in mind the legal consequences of each provision and take care to avoid restrictive or tightly worded language. An employee handbook can both be written in accordance with the stated guidelines and help to maintain good employee communication and effective employee relations."[7]

Public Policy Issues

The public policy exception to the employment-at-will doctrine provides that employees may not be terminated for reasons that are contrary to public policy.

Public policy originates with legislative enactments that prohibit, for example, the discharge of employees on the basis of handicap, age, race, color, religion, sex, national origin, pregnancy, filing of safety violation complaints with various agencies (e.g., the Occupational Safety and Health Administration), or union membership. Any attempt to limit, segregate, or classify employees in any way that would tend to deprive any individual of employment opportunities on these bases is contrary to public policy.

Public policy can also arise as a result of judicial decisions that address those issues not covered by statutes, rules, and regulations. "[I]t can be said that public policy concerns what is right and just and what affects the citizens of the state collectively. It is to be found in the state's constitution and statutes and, when they are silent, in its judicial decisions." *Palmateer v. International Harvester Co.*, 421 N.E.2d 876, 878 (Ill. 1981).

> Public policy favors the exposure of crime, and the cooperation of citizens possessing knowledge thereof is essential to effective implementation of that policy. Persons acting in good faith who have probable cause to believe crimes have been committed should not be deterred from reporting them by the fear of unfounded suits by those accused.

Joiner v. Benton Community Bank, 411 N.E.2d 229, 231 (Ill. 1980).

The Supreme Court of New Jersey held in *Pierce v. Ortho Pharmaceutical Corp.*, 417 A.2d 505 (N.J. 1980) that an employee at will has a cause of action for "wrongful discharge" when the discharge is contrary to public policy; however, unless an employee identifies a specific expression of public policy, he or she may be discharged with or without cause. Dr. Pierce in this case had continuously opposed the investigation being conducted on a particular drug at Ortho and eventually resigned because of reassignment to another position that she considered a demotion. She later filed a complaint for alleged wrongful discharge. Ortho moved for a summary judgment on the basis that Pierce resigned from her position. "The trial judge denied the motion on that ground because he found that there was a fact question whether Ortho induced Dr. Pierce's resignation." *Id.* at 508. The court found that Dr. Pierce did not have a cause of action for wrongful discharge. Judge Pashman, in dissenting to the majority ruling, stated

> . . . the majority has prevented the plaintiff from proving at trial that her discharge was based on a refusal to engage in a clear violation of statutory policy or one of several codes of professional ethics. It also rejects plaintiff's contractual allegations without any examination of their possible factual basis, let alone an examination that is properly "indulgent." While I generally agree with the legal principles expressed in the majority's decision, I cannot accept its grudging and inconsistent application of them. Plaintiff has been denied the benefit of the rule which she has sought to vindicate her professional conscience. Since I would permit her that benefit, I respectfully dissent.

Id. at 521.

The court in *Brown v. Physicians Mutual Insurance Co.*, 679 S.W.2d 836 (Ky. Ct. App. 1984), held that a complaint alleging that discharge of an employee by her employer after she attempted to report procedural irregularities was contrary to public policy was sufficient to state a cause of action for wrongful discharge. Employees of insurance companies are required to report violations of the Insurance Code to the Insurance Department.

Whistleblowing

Whistleblowing has been defined as an act of someone "who, believing that the public interest overrides the interest of the organization he serves, publicly 'blows the whistle' if the organization is involved in corrupt, illegal, fraudulent, or harmful activity."[8]

> . . . according to the public policy exception, an employer may not rely on the at-will doctrine as a basis for escaping liability for discharging an employee because of the doing of, or the refusing to do, such an act. Moreover, statutes in several jurisdictions protect an employee from an employer's retaliation for engaging in certain types of protected activities, such as whistleblowing.

99 A.L.R. Fed. 775.

Age

According to the United States Supreme Court in *Texas Department of Community Affairs v. Burdine*, 450 U.S. 248, 253 (1981),a prima facie case of age discrimination requires that evidence sufficient to support a finding for the complaintant must establish all of the following:

1. The complaintant is in a protected age group.
2. The complaintant is qualified for his or her job.
3. The complaintant was discharged.
4. The discharge occurred in circumstances that give rise to the inference of age discrimination.

A prima facie case of age discrimination was not established in *Pena v. Brattleboro Retreat*, 702 F.2d 322 (2nd Cir. 1983), where a 63-year-old female administrator of a psychiatric nursing facility alleged that she was dismissed as administrator so that a younger administrator could take over her position. The evidence established that the younger assistant administrator, a woman in her early thirties, had been hired at the suggestion of the administrator so that she could eventually take over the position of administrator upon the administrator's retirement. A federal district court found in favor of the administrator upon jury verdict, and an appeal was taken. The Second Circuit held that the former administrator had failed to prove either explicit or constructive discharge. A constructive discharge occurs when the employer, rather than acting directly, "deliberately makes an employee's working conditions so intolerable that the employee is forced into an involuntary resignation." *Younger v. Southwestern Savings and Loan Assn.*, 509 F.2d 140 144 (5th Cir. 1975).

> The Retreat's treatment of Mrs. Pena cannot even remotely be described as intolerable. Mrs. Pena was simply asked to train her successor for a year and a half, rather than the six months she herself envisioned. This was no more than a change in job responsibilities based on a reasonable business decision on the part of the Retreat . . . . Mrs. Pena was faced with no loss of pay or change in title.

Pena, 702 F.2d *supra*, at 325. The Retreat claimed that Mrs. Pena resigned on her own because of her inability to adjust to the Retreat's business decisions. The Age Discrimination in Employment Act does not protect employees who resign in protest against business decisions. *Id.* at 326.

Color

The Civil Service Commission was found to have acted improperly in suspending a black LPN as a result of a physical altercation with a white co-worker in *Theodore v. Department of Health & Human Services*, 515 So. 2d 454 (La. Ct. App. 1987). The white nurse had been accidentally struck by a crib being pushed by the black nurse. Evidence at trial supported the black nurse's contentions that she had apologized for the accident. The white nurse struck the first blow and spoke inflammatory slurs. The black nurse's reaction had been defensive. The facts revealed no grounds for suspension or disciplinary action against the black nurse.

The Bethany Methodist Corporation's medical and skilled nursing care facility had terminated a black certified nursing assistant because of its determination that she had abused a patient on four separate occasions in *Billups v. Methodist Hospital of Chicago*, 922 F.2d 1300 (7th Cir. 1991). The appellate court upheld a lower court order entering a summary judgment in favor of the defendant. "Billups did not offer any of the traditional forms of indirect evidence in attempting to prove racial discrimination, such as statistics or evidence of comparable situations." *Id.* at 1304–1305. "There is no evidence in the record suggesting that Bethany terminates black employees more frequently for physically abusing a patient, while retaining non-black employees." *Id.* at 1305.

Sex

Title VII of the Civil Rights Act of 1964 "requires the elimination of artificial, arbitrary, and unnecessary barriers to employment that operate invidiously to discriminate on the basis of race . . . ." *Griggs v. Duke Power Company*, 401 U.S. 424 (1971). In *Jones v. Hinds General Hospital*, 666 F. Supp. 933 (D. Miss. 1987), a prima facie case of sex discrimination was established by evidence showing that a hospital laid off female nursing assistants while retaining male orderlies who performed the necessary functions. The court held that Title VII of the Civil Rights Act was not violated by the hospital's use of gender as a basis for laying off its employees. Gender was a bona fide occupational qualification for orderlies since a substantial number of male patients objected to the performance of catheterizations and surgical prepping by female assistants.

Pregnancy Discrimination Act

The x-ray technician in *Hayes v. Shelby Memorial Hospital*, 726 F.2d 1543 (11th Cir. 1984), brought an employment discrimination action against the hospital. The technician was fired by the hospital when it learned that she was pregnant. The federal district court found that the hospital had violated the Pregnancy Discrimination Act. In affirming the lower court's decision, the appellate court held that the hospital failed to consider less discriminatory alternatives to firing the technician.

Americans with Disabilities Act

Findings of the United States Congress demonstrate that there are some 43,000,000 Americans that have one or more physical or mental disabilities. The number of disabled Americans is increasing as the population grows older. Society has tended to isolate and segregate individuals with disabilities, and despite some improvements discrimination against individuals with disabilities continues to be a serious and pervasive social problem. Discrimination continues in such crucial areas as employment, housing, public accommodations, education, transportation, health services, etc. Unlike individuals who have experienced discrimination on the basis of race, color, sex, national origin, religion, or age, those who have been disabled have had no legal recourse to redress such discrimination. Individuals with disabilities continually encounter various forms of discrimination, including outright intentional exclusion; the discriminatory effects of architectural, transportation, and communication barriers; the failure to make modifications to existing facilities and practices; exclusionary qualification standards and criteria; segregation; and relegation to lesser services, programs, activities, benefits, jobs, or other opportunities. Census data, national polls, and other studies have documented that people with disabilities, as a group, occupy an inferior status in society. The nation's proper goals regarding individuals with disabilities are to assure equality of opportunity, full participation, independent living, and economic self-sufficiency for such individuals.[9] It is the purpose of the Americans With Disabilities Act to:

1. provide a clear and comprehensive national mandate for the elimination of discrimination against individuals with disabilities
2. provide clear, strong, consistent, enforceable standards addressing discrimination against individuals with disabilities
3. ensure that the federal government plays a central role in enforcing the standards established in the Act on behalf of individuals with disabilities
4. invoke the sweep of congressional authority, including the power to enforce the fourteenth amendment and to regulate commerce, in order to address the major areas of discrimination faced day-to-day by people with disabilities[10]

The general rule of discrimination under Title I of the Act provides that

> No covered entity shall discriminate against a qualified individual with a disability because of the disability of such individual in regard to job application procedures, the hiring, advancement, or discharge of employees, employee compensation, job training, and other terms, conditions, and privileges of employment.[11]

A defense to a charge of discrimination under the Act would require a showing that the screening out of a specific disability was job-related and consistent with business necessity, and that performance cannot be accomplished by "reasonable" accommodation.[12]

Reporting of Patient Abuse

An employer may not discharge an employee for fulfilling societal obligations or in those instances where the employer acts with a socially undesirable motive.[13] A tort claim for wrongful discharge was stated in *McQuary v. Air Convalescent Home, Inc.*, 684 P.2d 21 (Or. Ct. App. 1984), by allegations that the plaintiff was wrongfully discharged from her position at the nursing facility as In-Service Director of Nurses Training and Education in retaliation for threatening to report to state authorities instances of alleged patient mistreatment. Such mistreatment purportedly involved violation of a patient's rights under the Nursing Home Patient's Bill of Rights. In order to prevail, the discharged employee was not required to prove that patient abuse had actually occurred, but only that she acted in good faith.

> This conclusion is consistent with established Oregon law. Statutes which protect employees against retaliation do not require that the alleged violation which the employee claims be ultimately proved. See, e.g., ORS 652.355 (protects an employee who merely consults an attorney or agency about a wage claim); ORS 654.062(5) (protects any employee who makes a complaint under the Oregon Safe Employment Act); ORS 659.030(1)(f) (prohibits discrimination against an employee who filed a civil rights complaint); ORS 633.120(3) (prohibits discrimination against an employee for filing an unfair labor practices complaint). We have, in fact, upheld awards for retaliation despite holding that the original complaint did not show discrimination.
>
> * * *
>
> Similar considerations of public policy lead to our conclusion that an employee who reports a violation of a nursing home patient's statutory rights in good faith should be protected from discharge for that action.

Id. at 24.

This case, which had been dismissed in the lower court, was reversed and remanded for trial.

Interference with Employment Opportunities

Liability for discrimination is not limited strictly to employer–employee relationships, but can be applied in situations in which discriminatory practices can affect the ability of a non-employee to obtain a job with a third party. This occurred in *Pardazi v. Cullman Medical Center*, 838 F.2d 1155 (11th Cir. 1988), where the court held that the physician stated a claim for relief under Title VII of the Civil Rights Act of 1964, based on the allegation that the hospital's denial of staff privileges interfered with his employment relationship with a third party. Dr. Pardazi, an Iran-educated medical practitioner, had entered into an employment contract with an Alabama corporation that required Dr. Pardazi to become a staff member of the defendant hospital. Dr. Pardazi argued that the hospital's discriminatory practices in denying his appointment denied him the right of an attorney at rehearing, extended his observation period from four months to one year (a deviation from the medical staff bylaws), and interfered with his employment opportunities. The lower court's summary judgment for the hospital was reversed and the case remanded.

Defamation Actions

Employers across the country are facing a new kind of potential liability with every employee they hire—a defamation action if the relationship doesn't work out. Observers say an increasing number of defamation claims are being brought by current and former workers, apparently because of a greater awareness by those employees—and a growing recognition by the courts—of new protections available to them.[14] According to the Bureau of National Affairs study of wrongful discharge cases between 1982 and 1987, "plaintiffs recovered damages in 78.9% of all defamation claims filed against former employers."[15]

Defamation actions are being attached to—or are taking the place of—wrongful discharge suits. "[P]laintiffs must overcome an employer's qualified privilege and show malice in order to recover."[16]

Dismissal was properly ordered for claims of wrongful termination and defamation in *Eli v. Griggs County Hospital and Nursing Home*, 385 N.W.2d 99 (N.D. 1986), where a nurse's aide was terminated on the basis of an incident in the hospital dining room. In the presence of patients and visitors she cursed her supervisor and complained that personnel were working short-staffed. Given the nature of her employment and the high standard of care that persons reasonably expected from a nursing care facility, such behavior justified her termination on a charge of reported breach of patient-specific and facility-specific information. No defamation resulted from the entry of such charges in the aide's personnel file, since the record established that the charges were true.

The nurse's aide in *Watson v. Idaho Falls Consolidated Hospitals, Inc.*, 720 P.2d 632 (Idaho 1986) claimed that the head nurse intentionally interfered with her employment relationship with the hospital, that both the head nurse and the hospital had intentionally inflicted emotional distress, and that accusations prior to discharge constituted slander. The defendants made a motion for summary judgment, which was granted in part as to the nurse's aide's claim for slander. Although the nurse's aide did not appeal the issue of slander, it seems clear that actions for defamation will appear in an ever-increasing number of cases.

Retaliatory Discharge

There is a tendency for those in power to abuse that power through threats, abuse, intimidation, and retaliatory discharge, all of which are cause for legal action. Employees who become the targets of a vindictive supervisor often have difficulty in proving a bad faith motive. In an effort to reduce the probability of wrongful discharge, some states, such as Connecticut,[17] Maine,[18] Montana,[19] and Michigan,[20] have enacted legislation that protects employees from terminations found to be arbitrary and capricious. The Montana Supreme Court upheld state legislation that protects workers against arbitrary discharge, while at the same time limiting the damages they can win.[21]

"Employees have . . . brought claims alleging abusive discharge in violation of public policy. This type of action is usually found to sound in tort, and thus in certain circumstances punitive damages have been awarded."[22] The burden of proof for establishing some hidden motive for discharge from employment rests on discharged employees.

> The National Labor Relations Act and other labor legislation illustrate the governmental policy of preventing employers from using the right of discharge as a means of oppression.
>
> * * *
>
> Consistent with this policy, many states have recognized the need to protect employees who are not parties to a collective bargaining agreement or other contract from abusive practices by the employer.
>
> * * *
>
> Recently those states have recognized a common law cause of action for employees at will who were discharged for reasons that were in some way "wrongful." The courts in those jurisdictions have taken various approaches: some recognizing the action in tort, some in contract.

Pierce v. Ortho Pharmaceutical Corp., 417 A.2d., at 509.

The court in *Khanna v. Microdata Corp.*, 215 Cal. Rptr. 860 (Ct. App. 1985), held that substantial evidence supported a finding that the employer fired the employee in bad faith retaliation for bringing a lawsuit against the employer, thus violating an implied covenant of good faith and fair dealing. Under the traditional common law rule, codified in California Labor Code Section 2922, an employment contract of indefinite duration is in general terminable at the will of either party. Over the past several decades, however, judicial authorities in California and throughout the United States have established the rule that, under both common law and the statute, an employer does not enjoy an absolute or totally unfettered right to discharge even an at-will employee . . . ." 215 Cal. Rptr. at 865. A cause of action was stated for the employer's breach of an implied-in-fact covenant to terminate only for good cause.

In *Shores v. Senior Manor Nursing Center*, 518 N.E.2d 471 (Ill. App. Ct. 1988), a formerly employed nurse's assistant brought an action against the nursing facility on the basis of retaliatory discharge. The circuit court dismissed the complaint for failure to state a cause of action and the decision was appealed. The appellate court held that the allegation of the former nursing facility employee that she was discharged in retaliation for reporting to the nursing home administrator that the charge nurse was improperly performing her functions as a nurse, which allegedly violated the Nursing Home Care Reform Act, stated a cause of action for retaliatory discharge. The circuit court was reversed and the case remanded for further proceedings.

The former director of nursing administration brought an action against the hospital and others for breach of contract, violation of civil rights, and interference with contractual relations in *Hobson v. McClean Hospital Corp.*, 402 Mass. 413, 522 N.E.2d 975 (1988). The Supreme Judicial Court of Massachusetts held (1) the complaint stated a cause of action for breach of an employment contract and interference with the employment contract, (2) the complaint stated a cause of action for discharge in violation of public policy, but (3) the complaint did not state a cause of action under the Civil Rights Act. The director of nursing administration alleged that the hospital bylaws for professional staff conferred privileges on employees and that the hospital terminated her without good cause (". . . wrongfully terminated employee in retaliation for her enforcement of State municipal laws and regulations." *Id.* at 976. There were no counselings and no warnings.

Fairness—The Ultimate Test

"Is it fair?" is the ultimate question that a supervisor must ask when considering a termination. In general, "bad faith" and "inexplicable terminations," are subject to the scrutiny of the courts. Some courts and legislative enactments have overturned the view that employers have total discretion to terminate workers who are not otherwise protected by collective bargaining agreements or civil services regulations. Montana legislation grants every employee the right to sue the employer for wrongful discharge. The mere fact that an employment contract is terminable at will does not give the employer an absolute right to terminate it in all cases. The court in *Cleary v. American Airlines, Inc.*, 199 Cal. Rptr. 722 (1980), held that the longevity of the employee's services, together with the express policy of the employer, operated as a form of estoppel, precluding any discharge of the employee by the employer without good cause, and, thus, the employee stated a cause of action for wrongful discharge.

There is an implied covenant of good faith and fair dealing in every contract that neither party will do anything that will injure the right of the other to receive benefits from the agreement.

The employee in *Pugh v. See's Candies, Inc.*, 116 Cal. App. 3d 311, 171 Cal. Rptr. 917 (1981), was found to have demonstrated a prima facie case of wrongful termination in violation of an implied promise that the employer would not act arbitrarily in dealing with the employee. The employer's right to terminate an employee is not absolute. It is limited by fundamental principles of public policy and by expressed or implied terms of agreement between the employer and the employee.

Procedural issues are as important as issues of discrimination. The Supreme Court of Michigan in *Renny v. Port Huron Hospital*, 398 N.W.2d 327 (Mich. 1986), found, as did the jury, that the employee's discharge hearing was not final and binding because it did not comport with elementary "fairness." The court found that there was sufficient evidence for the jury to find that the employee had not been discharged for just cause. The existence of a just-cause contract is a question of fact for the jury where the employer establishes written policies and procedures and does not expressly retain the right to terminate an employee at will. The fact that the hospital followed the grievance procedure with the plaintiff is evidence that a just-cause contract existed on which the plaintiff relied.

The employee handbook provided for a grievance board as a fair way to resolve work-related complaints and problems. This was not a mandatory procedure to which the hospital's employees had to submit. The employee was not bound by the grievance board determination that her discharge was proper, in that evidence supported a finding that she was not given adequate notice of who the witnesses against her would be. She was not permitted to be present when the witnesses testified, and she was not given the right to present certain evidence.

There was sufficient evidence for the jury to conclude that the plaintiff had in fact suffered damages in the amount of $100,000. Evidence presented indicated that her subsequent professional employment did not equal her earnings prior to discharge and that she had experienced increased expenses due to the loss of her health insurance as well as other financial losses that she suffered as a result of her discharge.

An employee, especially a supervisor, who believes he or she has been unfairly discharged will be most likely to seek access to the following information in defense of his or her claim:

- minutes of any meetings
- written reports, typed or handwritten
- personnel file
- tapes
- letters, cards, and handwritten notes written on the employee's behalf from the public
- personnel handbook
- personnel and departmental policies and procedures books
- oral testimony from fellow employees and supervisors

Employers must carefully and fairly document any disciplinary proceedings that might be subject to discovery by a disgruntled employee. Failure to do so could place a board or a supervisor at an uncomfortable disadvantage should a complaint reach the courts.

Unemployment Compensation

Fair dealing in termination should also include fair dealing with the terminated employee who files for unemployment benefits. The nursing facility in *Euclid Manor Nursing Home v. Board of Review*, 501 N.E.2d 635 (Ohio Ct. App. 1985), appealed from a court decision affirming an order of the Bureau of Employment Services granting unemployment benefits to the claimant. The claimant had only worked for the home four weeks prior to being terminated. She had knowingly been hired for a supervisory position even though she was a recent graduate with one year of experience in a non-supervisory position. The appeals court held that the nursing home's termination of the claimant was without "just cause," so that termination did not preclude claimant from receiving benefits.

In another case, *Mankato Lutheran Home v. Miller*, 358 N.W.2d 96 (Minn. Ct. App. 1984), a nursing assistant was found not to be disqualified from receiving unemployment benefits because of a single episode of profanity directed toward her supervisor while she was ill, frustrated and, in part, provoked by actions of her supervisor. The nursing assistant had no prior record of misconduct in five years of employment; however, her illness and frustration at having to work, after she had repeatedly indicated that she was not feeling well, increased over the course of several hours until she exploded emotionally. She had asked her supervisor, Ms. Darkow, if she could go home but was refused because of the probability of being unable to replace her in the middle of a shift.

> At about 5:30 A.M. Darkow entered a patient's room where Miller was helping a resident get dressed. When she asked how Miller was feeling, Miller became upset and said, "What the hell do you care, you don't think I'm sick anyway. I could drop over dead and still have to do these . . . (Bleep) people." Darkow retorted that Miller should not have come to work if she was so sick, and Miller yelled back "I never had this . . . (Bleep) pain until I came to this . . . (Bleep) hole.

Id. at 98. Although the assistant's outburst was directed toward her supervisor, one of two residents in the room who heard the incident was upset by it. *Id.* The episode did not represent a disregard for the employer's interests or of the nursing assistant's duties and responsibilities.

Fair dealing does not always imply that every discharged employee should be entitled to unemployment benefits. For example, in *Forbis v. Wesleyan Nursing Home, Inc.*, 325 S.E. 2d 651 (1985), unemployment compensation was denied because of an employee's discharge resulting from theft of a patient's clock. The theft constituted willful and wanton disregard for the nursing home's interests. The Employment Security Commission upon its investigation made the following findings of fact:

> 2. The claimant was discharged . . . for theft [of] patient property.
> 3. . . . [A] patient accused the claimant of taking the patient's clock.
> 4. Upon being confronted with the patient's accusation, the claimant produced the missing clock from her pocket and admitted taking it.

Id. at 652.

In another case, a nursing assistant was properly denied unemployment benefits as a result of being terminated for poor work attendance, even though her most recent absence had been excused. The employee's record indicated that the center had demonstrated great tolerance in allowing the employee to continue employment for as long as it did. *Love v. Heritage House Convalescent Center*, 463 N.E.2d 478 (Ind. Ct. App. 1983).

Voluntary termination because of a change in working conditions will not necessarily make an employee eligible for unemployment benefits. In *Montclair Nursing Home v. Wills*, 371 N.W.2d 121 (Neb. 1985), a licensed practical nurse was found not to be eligible for unemployment benefits when she resigned following reassignment to a night shift. Voluntary termination because of a change in working hours was not considered sufficient good cause to grant unemployment benefits, absent an "improper" purpose or motive in the change in the employee's work hours.

TERMINATION

A decision to terminate an employee should be carefully reviewed by a member of management familiar with the issues of wrongful discharge. Oral counseling, written counseling, written counseling with suspension, and written counseling with termination are the textbook responses to disciplinary action and discharge. Textbook theories are fine in a black and white world, but few people live in such a world. The following listing presents some alternatives to the undesirable task of terminating employees.

- Use inter- and intra-departmental transfers when indicated. Transfers are generally more effective in larger corporations such as multi-site health care systems where relocation is geographically possible.
- Substitute suspension for termination when possible. Do not have the courts do it for you.
- Provide an opportunity for early retirement.
- Consider a re-deployment of personnel, a hiring freeze, a reduction of overtime, etc., before personnel cutbacks are made due to financial difficulties.

The employer's right to terminate an employee is not absolute. It is limited by fundamental principles of public policy and by express or implied terms of agreement between the employer and the employee.

> Formulating a standard for substantive fairness in employee dismissal law requires accommodating a number of different interests already afforded legal recognition. The legal interest of employees to be protected against certain types of unfair and injurious action . . . are at the core of any employee dismissal proposal. Arrayed against these interests are employer and societal interests in effective management of organizations, which require that employees not be shielded from the consequences of their poor performance or misconduct, and that supervisors

> not be deterred from exercising their managerial responsibilities by the inconvenience of litigating employees' claims.[23]

Whatever form of discipline is utilized, it should be designed to produce a more effective and productive employee. Prior to termination of an employee, the employer should review the following questions:

1. Was the termination
   - a violation of any policy or procedure outlined in an administrative manual, the employee handbook, the personnel department's policies and procedures, or any other health care facility policies and procedures or regulations?
   - arbitrary and capricious?
   - discriminatory on the basis of age, disability, race, creed, color, religion, gender, national origin, or marital status?
   - a violation of any contract—oral or written?
   - a violation of any public policy—federal, state, or local?
   - consistent with the reasons for discharge?
   - discriminatory against the employee for filing a lawsuit?
   - fixed prior to any appeal actions that might be available to the employee? If an appeal was granted, was the employee given an opportunity to be represented by counsel?
2. Was there
   - retaliatory action because of a refusal to perform an illegal act or a questioning of a management practice?
   - defamation of character?
   - a conspiracy?
   - a personal vendetta?
   - threat or intimidation?
   - unlawful activity?
   - an attempt to bribe?
   - a denial of constitutional rights to freedom of speech?
   - an interference with an employee's rights as secured by the laws or Constitution of the United States?

Employment Disclaimers

A disclaimer is the denial of a right that is imputed to a person or that is alleged to belong to him or her. Although a disclaimer is often a successful defense for employers in wrongful discharge cases, it should not be considered a license to discharge at will and at the whim of the supervisor in an arbitrary and capricious manner.

Employers can help prevent successful lawsuits for wrongful discharge that are based on the premise that an employee handbook or departmental policy and procedure manual is an implied contract by incorporating disclaimers in published manuals, such as that described in *Battaglia v. Sisters of Charity Hospital*, 508 N.Y.S.2d 802 (N.Y. App. Div. 1986), where a personnel manual could not be interpreted to limit the hospital's power to terminate an at-will employee. Language in the manual indicated that the personnel manual was not a contract; that it could be modified, amended, or supplemented; and that the hospital retained the right to make all necessary management decisions for the delivery of patient care services and the selection, direction, compensation, and retention of employees.

Disclaimers must be clear to the employee. The court in *Harvet v. Unity Medical Center, Inc.*, 428 N.W.2d 574 (Minn. Ct. App. 1988), held in a wrongful discharge suit that the hospital's employee handbook was sufficiently definite to form an employment contract.

> Unity's handbook contained detailed provisions on conduct and procedures for discipline. As the trial court observed, "there can be no question that [respondent's] handbook provisions are sufficiently definite to form a contract." The handbook represents much more than Unity's general statement of policy. Moreover, the terms of the handbook were sufficiently definite to allow a fact finder to determine whether there had been a breach.
>
> * * *
>
> Respondent contends the handbook contained the following reservations on the part of the employer indicating it was not being offered as a contract: "Exceptions to any personnel policy or procedure may be permitted on a documented form showing of good and sufficient cause."
>
> * * *
>
> In the present case the trial court correctly found, "the clause does not clearly tell employees that the handbook is not part of an employment contract."

Id. at 577.

The employer's disclaimers were considered clear in *Simonson v. Meader Distribution Company*, 413 N.W.2d 146 (Minn. Ct. App. 1987), where an employee filed a breach of contract suit alleging a dismissal was outside company-adopted disciplinary guidelines. The court held that the company could and did reserve the discretion to discipline employees outside adopted guidelines. The policy manual contained the following three specific reservations of management discretion:

> Management reserves the right to make any changes at any time by adding to, deleting, or changing any existing policy.

> The rules set out below are as complete as we can reasonably make them. However, they are not necessarily all-inclusive, because circumstances that we have not anticipated may arise. Some currently unanticipated circumstances may warrant the application of discipline, including discharge.
>
> Management may vary from the above policies if, in its opinion, the circumstances require.

Id. at 147.

Health care facilities can be successful when confronted with wrongful discharge suits based on breach of contract by placing similar language in their personnel manuals.

Termination for Cause Clause

A termination for cause only clause in an employment contract is binding. An employment contract in *Eales v. Tanana*, 663 P.2d 958 (Alaska 1983), that provided that an employee hired up to retirement age could be terminated only for cause was upheld by the court.

Violation of Published Policies

Unemployment compensation was proper denied a nursing assistant for breach of a no-smoking rule in *Selan v. Commonwealth Unemployment Compensation Board of Review*, 415 A.2d 139 (Pa. Commw. Ct. 1980). The nursing facility's personnel handbook clearly provided that smoking was allowed only in specified areas.

> Smoking can be very offensive. It also creates a health and fire problem.
>
> You must refrain from smoking in offices, resident areas, elevators, corridors, or any area where it might be hazardous. In fact, you should not smoke in the public view. All "no smoking signs" must be observed. Your Department Director will inform you of the areas in which you are permitted to smoke. Smoking is permitted during break times and at meal times in these designated smoking areas.
>
> Smoking is permitted in vehicles only if residents are not present.
>
> Use ashtrays to keep The Home clean and to prevent fires. Special care must be exercised when oxygen or other inflammable gases may be present.

Id. at 140.

The nursing home assistant admitted that she was smoking but argued that she did not break the facility's smoking rules. The court disagreed. Evidence was sufficient to show that the employee knowingly violated Methodist Home's rule by smoking in a patient's bathroom. "Deliberate violation of a reasonable employer rule, without due cause, constitutes willful misconduct warranting disqualification for unemployment compensation. 43 P.S. Sec. 802(e)." *Id.* at 139.

Termination Because of Financial Necessity

No breach of employment contract occurred in *Wilde v. Houlton Regional Hospital*, 537 A.2d 1137 (Me. 1987), when, because of financial difficulties and over-staffing, a hospital terminated the employment of two nurses, a ward clerk, and a dietary supervisor. Even if the employees were correct in contending that their indefinite contracts of employment had been modified by virtue of a "dismissal for cause" provision in the employee's handbook and by management's oral assurances that they were permanent, full time employees whose jobs were secure so long as they performed satisfactorily, the employees' discharge for financial or other legitimate business reasons did not offend the employment contracts as thus modified. A private employer had an essential business prerogative to adjust its work force as market forces and business necessity required, and the layoffs in question violated no compelling public policy.

> [T]he appellants have failed to set forth specific facts showing that they were discharged for any reasons other than financial difficulties and overstaffing. The record does not suggest, for example, that financial difficulties were a pretext for discharges that were actually motivated by Houlton Regional's bad faith or retaliatory purpose.

Id. at 1138.

Termination Because of Hostile Attitude

A county nursing facility employee's discharge was warranted in *Langford v. Lane*, 921 F.2d 677 (6th Cir. Tenn. 1991), where the employee refused, in front of other employees and patients, to discuss with the administrator her hostile attitude toward management. The employee's refusal to speak with the administrator directly threatened the administrator's authority and constituted insubordination, which was sufficient independent justification for the employee's discharge. The employee's refusal was not constitutionally protected speech.

The chief x-ray technician in *Paros v. Hoemako Hospital*, 681 P.2d 918 (Ariz. Ct. App. 1984), was dismissed because of a chronic argumentative and hostile attitude inconsistent with the performance of supervisory duties. The trial court entered a summary judgment in favor of the hospital and the administrator. On appeal, the appeals court held that the discharge was properly based on good cause and precluded recovery for breach of contract and wrongful discharge.

Termination Because of Misconduct

A nurse's aide in *Daniels v. Hillcrest Homes, Inc.*, 594 S.W.2d 64 (Ark. Ct. App. 1980), was terminated for the following alleged reasons: (1) the aide was uncooperative with other aides; (2) she did not report to work as scheduled; (3) she was abusive to residents; and (4) her boyfriend had on occasions interfered with her job by coming to her place of work. *Id.* at 65. The Arkansas Unemployment Compensation Board of Review determined, by the evidence presented (three unsworn handwritten statements), that the nurse's aide was not terminated because of misconduct and that she was eligible for unemployment benefits. The circuit court reversed the Board's determination and an appeal was taken. The Court of Appeals of Arkansas held that the Board's decision granting unemployment benefits was supported by substantial evidence.

> Credibility of witnesses and the weight to be accorded the testimony are matters to be resolved by the Administrative Agency. The trial judge could reverse if the findings of the Board of review were arbitrary, capricious, unreasonable and without substantial evidence to support them or in fraud or corruption. Moreover, a reviewing court may not substitute its findings for those of the Administrative Agency even though the court might reach a different conclusion if it had made the original determination upon the same evidence considered by the Agency. Even if the evidence is undisputed, the drawing of inferences is for the Agency, not the courts.

Id. at 65, 66. It is important for nursing facilities to recognize from this case the importance of well documented employee counselings and disciplinary actions.

Termination for Improper Billing Practices

The hospital in *Jagust v. Brookhaven Memorial Association, Inc.*, 541 N.Y.S.2d 41 (N.Y. App. Div. 1989), was found to have properly dismissed a staff physician from his administrative position as director of the hospital's family practice residency program without a hearing. The hospital learned that the physician had engaged in improper billing practices by submitting bills for services that he never rendered. The physician was an employee at will as far as his administrative position was concerned. Neither the hospital's administrative procedure manual nor the employee handbook stated that the employee was subject to discharge for cause. Procedural protection was provided in the medical staff bylaws; however, the bylaws pertained to medical staff privileges and not administrative positions.

Termination Because of Theft

A nurse's discharge in *Waara v. Mesabi Regional Medical Center*, 415 N.W.2d 362 (Minn. Ct. App. 1987), involved misconduct so gross as to deny unemployment compensation where it was based on charges that she had stolen supplies of Demerol for her own use and that she had falsified patient records to conceal such thefts.

Termination Because of Poor Work Performance

A nurse's aide had been terminated from the county infirmary for misconduct in that, among other things, she failed to timely report bumping and injuring a resident's leg, failed to properly feed a resident as ordered by the resident's physician, and on another occasion fed a resident food that burned the resident's mouth. Upon review in *Yerry v. Ulster County*, 512 N.Y.2d 592 (N.Y. Ct. App. Div. 1987), the court held that eyewitness testimony and believable hearsay was sufficient to sustain the findings of the hearings officer who recommended her termination.

> As to the imposition of discipline, when petitioner's serious performance deficiencies are considered in light of her experience and the grave responsibility her work demanded in caring for helpless and dependent patients, we find that the penalty imposed was not disproportionate to the offenses. She showed an insensitivity and a lack of ability that made her unsuitable for the work and constituted a danger to the well-being of the infirmary's elderly residents.

Id. at 593.

Unemployment compensation was properly denied to a nurse's aide in *Starks v. Director of the Division of Employment Sec.*, 462 N.E.2d 1360 (Mass. 1984), who had been discharged for leaving a resident unattended and unrestrained on a commode and for using the property (medicated cream) of another resident, both of which are violations of the employer's policies. The court held that the examiner's findings of fact were adequate to support a conclusion that the claimant was discharged solely for misconduct in willful disregard of the employer's interest. *Id.* at 1360. The examiner had found that the employee had been adequately trained and was capable of accomplishing her work and that she had already been warned that her job was in jeopardy. *Id.* at 1361.

No cognizable claim was stated in *Hinson v. Cameron*, 742 P.2d 549 (Okla. 1987), by a nurse's aide whose at-will employment was terminated by a hospital on the basis of a supervisor's charge that the aide failed to administer an enema to a patient. The nurse's aide had not been ordered to perform an illegal act, and thus the tort of wrongful discharge could not be made out. In this case, the hospital's employee manual could not be read as conferring tenured employment or job security. The Supreme Court of Oklahoma held that although the employee manual listed examples of some grounds for termination it was not an exclusive listing of all grounds for termination. Even though there might be an implied covenant of good faith and fair dealing in every at-will employment relationship, that covenant does not operate to forbid employment severance except for good cause.

Termination and Damages

An employee who is wrongly discharged may maintain a cause of action in contract or tort or both. In a tort action for wrongful discharge, the court can award punitive damages. This remedy is not available under the law of contract.

> Recent headlines highlight that the damages awarded in employment related litigation may not be limited to back pay, fringe benefits and other forms of compensatory relief. In June 1988, a federal jury in the Eastern District of Kentucky awarded a total of $3 million in punitive damages to two former executives of Ashl and Oil, Inc. who prevailed in a wrongful termination suit. . . . The plaintiffs alleged that they were dismissed for opposing and then failing to cover up illegal payments made to foreign government representatives. The jury assessed punitive damages against the corporation, its chairman, former chairman and a senior vice president.[24]

A California Supreme Court decision that prohibits plaintiffs from seeking punitive and emotional distress damages from former employers in wrongful dismissal cases applies retroactively to thousands of cases pending in that state's courts. In *Newman v. Emerson Radio Corp.*, 772 P.2d 1059 (Cal. 1989), the court, by a 4–3 vote, decided that its December 29 decision in *Foley v. Interactive Data Corp.*, 765 P.2d 373, 47 Cal. Rptr. 3d 211 (1988), applies to all wrongful dismissal cases pending as of January 30. The Supreme Court of California held in *Foley* that a wrongful discharge claim asserting a breach of an implied covenant of good faith and fair dealing may give rise to contract, but not tort, damages. As a result of this ruling, punitive damages will not ordinarily be available to successful wrongful discharge plaintiffs.

The Montana Supreme Court held that a Montana statute that limits the damages recoverable in wrongful discharge suits to four years' wages and benefits does not violate the state constitution. *Meech v. Hillhaven West, Inc.*, 776 P.2d 488 (Mont. 1989). According to the court, the state constitution's guarantee of "full legal redress" affords the plaintiff, a former nursing home administrator, only a right to judicial access to obtain remedies, not a fundamental right to full redress. The statute abolishes common law causes of action for discharge and creates a statutory action. It is the first of its kind in the nation. Punitive damages are available only upon clear and convincing evidence that the employer acted with actual malice or committed actual fraud.

EMPLOYMENT PRACTICES

Health care facilities can improve the quality of personnel in their institutions by implementing more effective screening practices. Since it is unlikely that an applicant will reveal any criminal convictions on his or her application, thorough background checks on prospective employees is mandatory. Many states recognize liability for negligent hiring when an employer knew or should have known that an employee posed a foreseeable risk of harm or danger to others.[25] Texas mandates background checks on individuals applying for nursing home positions.[26] Because employment laws do vary from state to state, it is important that background investigations be conducted within operative state law.

It is possible for employers to reduce their exposure to liability for wrongful discharge by developing appropriate guidelines. The best way for the human resources manager to prevent negligent-hiring litigation for the employer is to become familiar with the risks and avoid hiring workers who are likely to become problem employees.

- Take appropriate precautions to prevent the hiring of those who might be a hazard to others.
- Develop clear policies and procedures on hiring, disciplining, and terminating employees.
- Review each applicant's background and past work behavior.
- Become familiar with any state laws that might be applicable when hiring an individual with a past criminal record.
- Develop an application that realistically determines an applicant's qualifications prior to hiring.
- Develop a two-tiered interview system for screening applicants. (The interviews should be conducted first by an appropriately trained member of the personnel department and then by the department head of the service to which the applicant is applying.)
- Solicit references with applicant's permission utilizing a release form, and follow up with a telephone call for further information.
- Clearly define personnel policies and procedures in the form of a personnel handbook and present a job description to each new employee. Signed documentation should be maintained in the employee's personnel folder indicating that the employee received, read, and understood the nursing facility's employee handbook and job description.
- Develop constructive performance evaluations that reinforce good behavior and provide instruction in those areas needing improvement. The performance evaluation should include a written statement regarding the employee's performance.
- Develop a progressive disciplinary action policy.
- Provide in-service education programs for supervisors on such subjects as employee interviews, evaluations, and discipline. (Various colleges, universities, and consultants provide in-service education programs for employers.)

- Be mindful of the importance of developing appropriate employment contract language, as well as administrative manuals and employee handbooks.

Employers must clearly communicate to prospective employees that their employment is at the will of the employer and can be terminated at any time. During the course of employment, handbooks and personnel manuals must provide a fair and unambiguous standard for employee discipline and termination.

NOTES

1. M. Geyelin, *Fired Managers Winning More Lawsuits*, The Wall Street Journal, September 7, 1989, at B1.

2. *Id.* at B1.

3. *The Governing Board's Quest for "Supermanager,"* 5 HEALTHCARE EXECUTIVE, September/October 1990, at 19.

4. *Id.* at 18.

5. M. Geyelin, *supra* note 1, at B1.

6. OFFICE OF GENERAL COUNSEL OF AMERICAN HOSPITAL ASSOCIATION, THE WRONGFUL DISCHARGE OF EMPLOYEES IN THE HEALTH CARE INDUSTRY 1 (Legal Memorandum No. 10) (1987).

7. P.I. WEINER, S.H. BOMPEY, & M.G. BRITTAIN, JR., WRONGFUL DISCHARGE CLAIMS, N.Y.C.: Practicing Law Institute 98 (1986).

8. WHISTLEBLOWING: THE REPORT OF THE CONFERENCE OF PROFESSIONAL RESPONSIBILITY 6 (R. Nader, P. Petkas, & K. Blackwell, eds., 1972). *See also* 99 A.L.R. Fed. 778.

9. Act of July 26, 1990, Pub. L. No. 101–336, 1990 U.S. CODE CONG. & ADMIN. NEWS (104 Stat.) 327–329.

10. *Id.* at 329.

11. *Id.* at 331–332.

12. *Id.* at 333–334.

13. *Delaney v. Taco Time Intl.*, 681 P.2d 114 (Or. 1984), involved an employer found liable by the Supreme Court of Oregon for the wrongful discharge of an at-will employee who was discharged for fulfilling a societal obligation in that he refused to sign a false and arguably tortious statement that cast aspersions on the work habits and moral behavior of a former employee.

14. *Employers Face Upsurge in Suits Over Defamation*, Nat'l L. J., May 4, 1987, at 1.

15. M. Geyelin, *supra* note 1, at B1.

16. *Id.* at B1.

17. CONN. GEN. STAT. ANN., §31–51m(a) (West 1987).

18. ME. REV. STAT. ANN. tit. 26, §§831–840 (Cum. Supp. 1987).

19. MONT. CODE. ANN. § 39–2–901 (1987).

20. MICH. COMP. LAWS ANN. §§15.361–.369 (West 1981).

21. M. Geyelin, *supra* note 1, at B1.

22. Furfaro & Josephson, *Punitive Damages in Employment Cases*, N.Y.L.J., Apr. 7, 1989, at 4.

23. H.H. PERRITT, EMPLOYEE DISMISSAL LAW AND PRACTICE 354 (1984).

24. *Id.* at 3.

25. J. Green, *Programs Help Uncover Skeletons in Job Applicants Closets*, 25(19) AHA News, May 14, 1990, at 6.

26. *Id.*

Chapter 19

Medical Malpractice—The Crisis—The Solution?

The medical malpractice crisis continues to be a major dilemma for the health care industry. Although there have been many approaches to resolving the crisis, there appears to be no one magic formula. The solution will require a variety of efforts, including tort reform.

The Robert Wood Johnson Foundation in 1985 viewed medical malpractice as an issue that potentially threatened the accessibility, affordability, and quality of health care. As a result of this concern, it funded 19 research and demonstration grants for approximately $4.5 million over a two-year period. Findings from a variety of projects indicate that

- The tort and insurance liability systems, as they are now structured, provide neither an efficient nor an equitable means of compensation for injured parties against medical negligence.
- Current systems of risk management and professional regulation, in general, do a poor job of identifying and correcting negligent behavior.
- There is considerable potential to prevent injuries through the development of new, more formal professional standards and through the identification and correction of incident-prone situations and settings. There is also potential, albeit more limited, to reduce the frequency of maloccurrence by better addressing the problem of negligence-prone physicians.
- Several alternatives to the existing insurance/tort system may hold promise for more efficient and equitable compensation of injured claimants and for more effective injury prevention.[1]

The Pepper Commission, in its report on "Access to Health Care and Long-Term Care for All Americans," recommended that:

> The Prospective Payment Commission and the Physician Payment Review Commission will be directed to convene experts, providers,

> lawyers, consumers to study and conduct demonstration projects related to medical malpractice reform in order to make recommendations to Congress on actions to be taken on the federal level. The appropriate committees of jurisdiction in Congress should also hold hearings on the malpractice issue, and the access legislation should incorporate professional liability reform.[2]

The traditional negligence-based system for adverse medical outcomes has seriously broken down. Compensation as a deterrent to malpractice has failed to hold the number of claims to a reasonable level. Expensive jury awards and malpractice insurance premiums continue to have a negative impact on the nation's health care system, bringing it ever closer to a day of reckoning with financial disaster.

Although many states have made some progress in tort reform, a more aggressive approach on a national basis is necessary. "Tinkering with the nation's medical-malpractice system apparently has helped to stabilize premiums. But health care and legal experts contend that the system will require a complete overhaul before it can function fairly for either patients or physicians."[3] There are efforts under way to generate malpractice reform on a national basis. Early in 1990, President Bush directed the Domestic Council to recommend federal reforms of the medical-malpractice system.[4]

The tort system, as it is presently designed, fosters the practice of defensive medicine. A Harvard Medical Practice Study team found that

> [P]hysicians are three times more likely to believe they will be sued in a given year than actually are. Physicians who believe themselves at greater risk of being sued order more tests and procedures ("defensive medicine"). They also tend to reduce the scope of their practices, performing fewer risky procedures and treating fewer high-risk patients.[5]

Those physicians who wish to practice and survive have accepted the concept of practicing "defensive medicine." Defensive medicine is believed to be one of the most harmful effects produced by the threat of malpractice litigation. Defensive medicine is practiced to forestall potential litigation and provide an advantageous legal defense should a lawsuit be instituted. Medical records are becoming more defensive and will become even more so with closer scrutiny by insurance carriers. Because of the risk and potential for liability in most diagnostic and therapeutic procedures, physicians are practicing defensive medicine.

The fear of malpractice litigation precipitates an ineffective use of scarce health care resources. Defensive medicine often results in either under-treatment, by avoiding high-risk tests and procedures, or over-treatment, such as the excessive utilization of diagnostic tests.

Because the federal government is a major payer of health care benefits, greater attention will be given to the costly effects of defensive medicine and the need for tort reform.

> Many of those involved in medical malpractice legal reforms say that it's easy to see why the players on the federal level have taken such an interest. "The government is paying for close to 50 percent of the nation's health care bill among Medicare, Medicaid, CHAMPUS, Veteran's Administration, and federal employee benefit health programs," says a staff member of Sen. Orrin G. Hatch (R-UT). The President and members of Congress are concerned that defensive medicine—in addition to other malpractice defense costs—is contributing to the high cost of health care.[6]

It has been estimated that defensive medicine cost the health care industry $19.3 billion in 1988.[7]

In order for tort reform to be successful, it will probably be necessary for the federal government to tie financial incentives to such reform. The Bush Administration, in a May 15, 1991 proposal, sponsored at the request of the White House by Senator Orrin Hatch, would give the states until 1995 "to adopt recommended liability reforms or lose access to a federally sponsored pool of funds that would pay malpractice awards."[8] Specific reforms would include: (1) placing caps on non-medical payments (e.g., limiting malpractice awards for pain and suffering to $250,000); (2) settling disputes outside the courtroom through mediation and arbitration; (3) barring double recovery of damages; (4) eliminating of joint and several liability; (5) providing for structured awards; and (6) establishing guidelines for clinical practice.[9]

The emotions regarding the President's plan run high. There are some who strongly believe that the President's plan for tort reform is misguided. Richard Carlson in a Newsday editorial comments:

> Besides being wrong and ineffective in so many ways, the Bush bill is dangerous because it seeks to remove one of the few lights on what is a very private and dimly lit world: that of medical practice in the United States.
>
> * * *
>
> Let patients sue for millions, let them be awarded millions, until people say, "Wait, this makes no sense, there is something corrupt and unhealthy here."
>
> Then perhaps the creaking cottage industry of American medicine will be dismantled and constructed anew in an atmosphere of service, communication and trust, beneficial to care-user and care-giver alike.[10]

MEDIATION AND ARBITRATION

Mediation is the process whereby a third party, the mediator, attempts to mediate a settlement between the parties of a complaint. The mediator cannot force a settlement.

Arbitration is the process by which parties to a dispute voluntarily agree to submit their differences to the judgment of an impartial mediation panel for resolution. It is used as a means to evaluate, screen, and resolve medical malpractice disputes before they reach the courts. Arbitration can be accomplished by mutual consent of the parties or statutory provisions. A decision made at arbitration may or may not be binding, depending on prior agreement between the parties or statutory requirements.

Among the many factors contributing to the malpractice crisis is the high cost of litigation. Trial by jury is lengthy and expensive. If case disputes can be handled out of court, the process and expense of a lawsuit can be greatly reduced. Arbitration is one means for simplifying and expediting the settlement of claims.

Medical malpractice arbitration panels can facilitate professional malpractice actions. A 1975 Alabama law provides that after a health care provider has rendered services to a patient out of which a claim has arisen, the parties may agree to settle the dispute by arbitration. Such agreement is binding and irrevocable.[11] A 1988 Florida statute provides that upon completion of presuit investigation, with preliminary reasonable grounds for a medical negligence claim intact, the parties may elect to have damages determined by an arbitration panel. Arbitration is undertaken with the understanding that damages shall be limited as specified in the arbitration statute.[12] Michigan law provides that the health care provider may not revoke the agreement after its execution.[13]

On the federal level, Senator Pete V. Domenici (Republican—New Mexico) introduced a bill that would require mandatory arbitration. The bill would allow states or private agencies to resolve disputes.[14]

PRETRIAL SCREENING PANEL

Pretrial screening panels are designed to evaluate the merits of medical injury claims in order to encourage the settlement of claims outside the courtroom. "Panels render an opinion on provider liability and, in some cases, on damages. In most states, the panel's decision on the merit of the claim is admissible in court."[15] Unlike binding arbitration, the decision of a screening panel is not binding and is imposed as a condition precedent to trial, whereas arbitration is conducted in lieu of a trial. Mandatory screenings of alleged negligence cases are useful in discouraging frivolous lawsuits from proceeding to trial.

In 1986, Maine passed a number of liability-reform measures, which included pretrial screening of medical-malpractice lawsuits. The Maine statute provides that medical injury claims must be submitted to a screening and mediation panel, unless all parties agree to bypass a panel hearing. Any panel findings that are unanimous and unfavorable to either the defendant or claimant are admissible as evidence at any subsequent trial.[16] The law appears to have helped to reduce the number of "frivolous" suits.[17]

The Supreme Court of Alaska held in *Keyes v. Humana Hospital Alaska, Inc.*, 750 P.2d 343 (Alaska 1988), that a statute creating mandatory pretrial review of medical malpractice claims by an expert advisory panel did not impermissibly infringe on the plaintiff's constitutional right to a trial by jury. The statute was a reasonable legislative response to the medical malpractice insurance crisis. The constitutionality of a Virginia statute in *Speet v. Bacaj*, 377 S.E.2d 397 (Va. 1989), provided that admission of a medical review panel's opinion into evidence did not infringe upon the plaintiff's right to a trial by jury as guaranteed by the Virginia Constitution.

COLLATERAL SOURCE RULE

The collateral source rule is a common law principle that prohibits a court or jury from taking into account when setting an award the fact that part, or even all, of the plaintiff's damages have already been covered by other sources of payment (e.g., health insurance, disability, and compensation). Several states have modified the collateral source rule so that evidence regarding other sources of payment to the plaintiff may be introduced for purposes of reducing the amount of the ultimate award to the plaintiff. The jury would then be permitted to assign the evidence such weight as it chooses. The award could be reduced to the extent the plaintiff received compensation from other sources.

Imposition of the collateral source rule can often result in recoveries to plaintiffs far in excess of their economic loss. Such excessive payments contribute significantly to the high cost of malpractice insurance and the high cost of medicine to the public. Where evidence regarding collateral sources of payment can be introduced in order to mitigate the damages payable to a plaintiff, excessive recoveries may be discouraged.

A Tennessee statute provided that

> In a malpractice action in which liability is admitted or established, the damages awarded may include (in addition to other elements of damages authorized by law) actual economic losses suffered by the claimant by reason of the personal injury, including but not limited to cost of reasonable and necessary medical care, rehabilitation services, and custodial care, loss of services and loss of earned income, but only to the extent that such costs are not paid or payable and such losses are not replaced, or indemnified in whole or in part, by insurance provided by an employer, either governmental or private, by social security benefits, service benefit programs, unemployment benefits, or any other source except the assets of the claimants or of the members of the claimants' immediate family and insurance purchased in whole or in part, privately and individually.[18]

The malpractice litigants in *Baker v. Vanderbilt University,* 616 F. Supp. 330 (D. Tenn. 1985), sought a court order declaring the provisions of the Tennessee statute abrogating the collateral source rule in medical malpractice cases to be unconstitutional. The district court held that the Tennessee statute did not deny the litigants equal protection as compared with victims of other torts.

CONTINGENCY FEE LIMITATIONS

A contingency fee is payment for services rendered by an attorney predicated on the favorable outcome of a case. Payment is based on a pre-established percentage of the total award. Some states set this percentage by statute or court rule. Under a contingency agreement, if there is no award to the plaintiff, the attorney receives no payment for services rendered.

Physicians argue that the contingency fee arrangement serves to encourage frivolous prosecution and an inordinate number of lawsuits. Lawyers reason that if they or their clients must bear the initial cost of a lawsuit, only those with obvious merit will be brought forward. The contingency fee structure also allows those unable to bear the cost of litigation to initiate a suit for damages.

Limiting contingency fees on a sliding scale basis, with the percentage decreasing as the award to the plaintiff increases, and/or providing for a lesser fee if a claim is settled without going to trial seems to have some merit. A Connecticut law provides that in any contingency fee arrangement, the fee shall not exceed: (1) 33 1/3 percent of the first $300,000; (2) 25 percent of the next $300,000; (3) 20 percent of the next $300,000; (4) 15 percent of the next $300,000; and (5) 10 percent of any amount which exceeds $1,200,000.[19] A Maine law provides for: (1) 33 1/3 percent of the first $100,000 recovered; (2) 25 percent of the next $100,000 recovered; and (3) 20 percent of any amount recovered over one million dollars.[20]

Some states provide for a maximum percentage of the amount recovered by the plaintiff. Florida, for example, provides that attorney fees may not exceed 15 percent where the claimant has agreed to binding arbitration. Where a defendant has refused a claimant's offer to arbitrate, claimant's attorney fees may not exceed 25 percent.[21] Michigan provides a maximum allowable fee of 33 1/3 percent,[22] while Oklahoma allows 50 percent of the net amount of a judgment.[23]

A third approach to limiting contingency fees occurs in those states where regulations provide for court review of attorney fees. Hawaii, for example, provides that in all tort actions in which a judgment is entered by a court of competent jurisdiction, attorney fees for both the plaintiff and the defendant shall be limited to a reasonable amount as approved by the court.[24] In New Hampshire, at the time of settlement or judgment of any action, all counsel of record are required to submit a complete review of all fees received for services for said action. All fees for actions resulting in settlement or judgment of $200,000 or more are subject to approval by the court.[25]

PRECALENDAR CONFERENCE

Precalendar conferences should be encouraged in order to settle disputes between the parties to a lawsuit. Trial proceedings are costly and should be avoided when a less costly course of action such as a precalendar conference is feasible.

DISCOVERY PROCEEDINGS

Discovery is a very costly aspect of pretrial proceedings. Adjudication of malpractice cases can be expedited by limiting the time allotted for such proceedings.

EXPERT WITNESSES

The qualifications of expert witnesses should be disclosed prior to trial. Only qualified experts should be permitted to present expert testimony in court.

STATUTES OF LIMITATIONS

Statutes of limitations should begin to run when an injury is discovered and the physician–patient relationship has ended. The time frame within which a lawsuit must be initiated must be reasonable.

FRIVOLOUS CLAIMS

Health providers, in some instances, are filing countersuits after being named in what they believe to be malicious, libelous, slanderous, frivolous, and non-meritorious medical malpractice suits. Remedies for such actions vary from one jurisdiction to the next. In order for a physician to prevail in a suit against a plaintiff or plaintiff's attorney, the physician must show that the suit was frivolous, that the motivation of the plaintiff was not to recover for a legitimate injury, and that the physician has suffered damages as a result of the suit. The plaintiff's attorney has a legal and ethical responsibility to make sure that any suits filed are backed by sufficient and reasonable facts.

There have been arguments that defendants should be allowed to recover court costs and damage awards from both the plaintiff(s) and their attorneys for frivolous claims and counterclaims. The courts have thus far not looked favorably on countersuits for frivolous and unscrupulous negligence actions. Some state legislatures have taken limited action in this area. An Arkansas statute, for example, provides that in any civil action in which the court finds that there was a complete absence of a judicial issue of either law or fact raised by the losing party or his attorney, the court shall award, with certain stipulations, an attorney fee in an amount not to exceed $5,000 or 10 percent of the amount in controversy, whichever is less, to the prevailing party.[26]

In *Berlin v. Nathan*, 64 Ill. App. 3d 940, 381 N.E.2d 1367 (1978), a radiologist, a surgeon, and a hospital were sued for alleged malpractice by a patient who sought $250,000 because the defendants did not properly diagnose a fracture of her little finger. The radiologist missed the break, but he claimed that it was not evident on the x-ray taken at the hospital and that there was no error on his part. Furthermore, the finger was placed in a splint just as if it had been broken, so the treatment was correct regardless of the diagnosis. The radiologist countersued, so that the malpractice suit and countersuit were tried together. When the jury was selected, the patient withdrew the malpractice suit, but the radiologist persisted with his case. The jury awarded the radiologist $2,000 as compensation and $6,000 in punitive damages, presumably convinced that the patient and her attorneys acted improperly in bringing the lawsuit and that the lawyers were negligent in their investigation of the patient's case before filing suit.

When the case was taken to an appellate court, the decision of the lower court was reversed on the grounds that the physician had failed to plead special damages and (because the countersuit had been filed prematurely) had failed to plead a favorable result in the original suit. The appellate court went on to say that a showing of special damages is essential in a case of this type in order that the public's right to free access to the court system not be impeded by the threat of counter-litigation. The court reasoned that persons who feel they have legitimate claims should not be dissuaded from using the court system solely because of the fear of liability in the event their claim is unsuccessful.

The appellate court holding in the Berlin case represents the majority judicial view across the country regarding countersuits. Courts generally do not find in favor of the countersuing party because they fear that persons who would otherwise bring such suits will be discouraged simply because of a concern over the possibility of a countersuit.

JOINT AND SEVERAL LIABILITY

The doctrine of joint and several liability provides that a person causing an injury concurrently with another person can be held liable for the entire judgment awarded by a court. It is proposed by some that each defendant in a multi-defendant action should be limited to payment for the percentage of fault ascribed to him or her. Some states have taken action to modify the doctrine. A 1986 Wyoming statute, for example, provides that each defendant to a lawsuit is only liable for that proportion of the total dollar amount of damages according to the percentage of the amount of fault attributed to him.[27] A Minnesota statute provides that a defendant whose fault is 15 percent or less may be jointly liable for a percentage of the whole award not greater than four times his percentage of fault.[28]

MALPRACTICE CAPS

Various states are attempting to stem the tide of rising malpractice costs by passing laws that impose restrictions on limiting the total dollar damages allowable in malpractice actions. The White House is preparing a package designed to encourage states to cap non-economic damages at $250,000 and incentives for states to adopt measures designed to rein in the malpractice litigation process. The proposal would give compensation to states that adopt recommendations that include structured payments of damages and programs to settle malpractice cases out of court.[29]

Guidelines should be established that juries can follow in setting punitive damage awards. Attorneys for the American Hospital Association, in an amicus curiae brief filed December 21, 1990 with the Oklahoma Supreme Court, argued that juries should receive guidance from the courts to assure that the punitive damages they assess are rational and fair. A jury's award of $10 million in punitive damages against Tulsa-based Hillcrest Medical Center was appealed to a higher court.[30]

Many states have enacted laws that limit malpractice awards. A Kansas statute, for example, provides that in any personal injury action the total amount recoverable by each party from all defendants for non-economic losses shall not exceed $250,000.[31] Maryland allows for up to $350,000 for non-economic damages.[32]

While there have been challenges to such enactments, it would appear that limitations on malpractice recoveries are not unconstitutional. The Supreme Court of Idaho in *Jones v. State Board of Medicine*, 97 Idaho 859, 555 P.2d 399 (1976), held that the state's limitation on malpractice recoveries ($150,000) need not necessarily be unconstitutional. The court held that there was no inherent right to an unlimited amount of damages and that the state had a legitimate interest in controlling excessive medical costs caused by large malpractice recoveries, and thus the statute could be held constitutional.

A Virginia statute that places a cap of $750,000 on damages recoverable in a malpractice action was found not to violate the Seventh Amendment separation of powers principles or the Fourteenth Amendment due process or equal protection clauses. *Boyd v. Bulala*, 877 F.2D 1191 (4th Cir. 1989), *reversing* 56 U.S.L.W. 2285.

It is unlikely that setting a cap on awards for pain and suffering will do very much to reduce the costs of malpractice insurance. "Placing limits on malpractice awards is no solution to the lack of coordinated planning that reflects this country's approach to health care. Capping awards would do nothing to help patients."[33] A study examining the impact of Indiana's 1975 tort-reform laws on injured patients revealed that claimants are treated "quite generously," despite a seemingly strict system that caps damages at $750,000 and mandates pre-trial screenings. The average claim in Indiana is about $430,000 compared with $290,000 in Michigan and $303,000 in Ohio.[34] The malpractice reforms in Indiana, which set upper limits on damage rewards and a mandatory review of malpractice claims by a physician panel, did not deter people from filing malpractice claims.[35]

NO-FAULT SYSTEM

A no-fault system compensates injured parties for economic losses regardless of fault. It is intended to compensate more claimants with smaller awards. As a result of a major study commissioned by the state of New York, the Commissioner of Health "proposed a no-fault system that would compensate victims of medical injury whether or not they can prove medical negligence."[36]

A no-fault system of compensation has its drawbacks. The deterrence factor in the present tort system would be absent in a no-fault system. The system's lower administrative costs can be an incentive to file lawsuits, and, therefore, not produce the desired outcome of reducing the incidence of malpractice claims. Estimates from a 1975 California study indicated that a no-fault system would cost California approximately $800 million annually. The tort system was only costing $250 million at the time.[37]

PEER REVIEW ORGANIZATIONS

Public Law No. 92–603 of the Social Security Amendments of 1972 and Public Law No. 94–182 of the Social Security Act of 1975 created a nationwide review agency known as Professional Standard Review Organizations (PSROs) under Title XI of the Social Security Act. Their purpose is to assure that medical care provided to patients is of high quality and reflects the most appropriate and efficient utilization of institutional health care services.

PSRO norms, standards, and criteria were to be utilized as guidelines of acceptable medical care to measure the standard of care rendered to beneficiaries of Medicare, Medicaid, and maternal and child health programs. PSROs compiled and studied physician profiles of care to determine whether services rendered in a given area were consistent with the standards of learning and skill of the average reputable physician, either nationwide or in communities similar to those under examination.

In 1982 Congress repealed the PSRO program, replacing it with the Peer Review Improvement Act (Title XI, §143, Part B). Under this act, peer review organizations (PROs) perform functions similar to those of the PSROs. Hospitals must have agreements with PROs as a condition of receiving Medicare payments under the prospective payment system (PPS), as required by the Deficit Reduction Act of 1984 (Pub. L. No. 98–369). PROs can deny reimbursement for substandard care. They can also recommend that a practitioner be suspended from the Medicare and Medicaid programs, as well as be fined for a pattern of poor performance.

Peer review documents are generally protected from discovery so long as they are maintained in compliance with a formalized quality assurance program. The U.S. Supreme Court in *Patrick v. Burget*, 486 U.S. 94 (1988), by an 8–0 vote reversed the decision of the Ninth Circuit Court of Appeals, which had held that the peer review process was exempt from antitrust scrutiny under the so-called state action doctrine.

> Because we conclude that no state actor in Oregon actively supervises hospital peer-review decisions, we hold that the state action doctrine does not protect the peer-review activities challenged in this case from application of the federal antitrust laws. In so holding we are not unmindful of the policy argument that respondents and their amici have advanced for reaching the opposite conclusion. They contend that effective peer review is essential to the provision of quality medical care and that any threat of antitrust liability will prevent physicians from participating openly and actively in peer-review proceedings. This argument, however, essentially challenges the wisdom of applying the antitrust laws to the sphere of medical care, and as such is properly directed to the legislative branch. To the extent that Congress has declined to exempt medical peer review from the reach of the antitrust laws, peer review is immune from antitrust scrutiny only if the state effectively has made this conduct its own. The State of Oregon has not done so.

Id. at 1665–1666. Compliance with the Health Care Quality Improvement Act is the only way health care facilities and their medical staffs can hope to protect credentialing and peer review activities from antitrust liability. The Supreme Court endorsed the Act in the *Patrick* opinion, holding that the Home Care Quality Improvement Act "which was enacted well after the events at issue in this case and is not retroactive, essentially immunizes peer review action from liability if the action was taken in the reasonable belief that [it] was in the furtherance of quality health care." *Id.* at 1665.

A physician who resigned following evaluation of his suspected alcohol, drug, or emotional problem filed a complaint against the hospital and the assistant administrator on the theories of slander, coercion, intentional infliction of emotional distress, and intentional interference with his employment contract as medical director of the hospital's department of perinatology. Alcohol had been detected on the physician's breath while he was performing certain medical procedures. Interviews were conducted by a chemical dependency specialist with members of the hospital's staff who had contact with the plaintiff. According to the witnesses, the plaintiff was subject to mood swings, became abrupt and tactless with patients, boasted of becoming intoxicated, and would occasionally leave work and return "wired." The plaintiff had been described as bizarre and paranoid. In conducting the interviews with the hospital staff, the witnesses believed that something was wrong with the plaintiff, but they were reluctant to speak because of their fondness for him.

Acting on the advice of the chemical dependency specialist, the vice president of medical staff affairs for the hospital formed a committee that met for the purpose of confronting the physician regarding the alleged behavior problem. The physician reluctantly agreed to an evaluation by a physician experienced in treating impaired physicians. The plaintiff was evaluated later that day at a nearby hospital. The record is silent as to the results of that evaluation, except to indicate that the plaintiff did not require hospitalization. The circuit court dismissed the complaint, and the physician appealed. On appeal, the appellate court held that the Hospital Licensing Act provided the defendants with absolute immunity from liability for the hospital peer review committee's investigation of the physician's conduct. *Cardwell v. Rockford Memorial Hospital Association*, 183 Ill. App. 3d 1072, 132 Ill. Dec. 516, 539 N.E.2d 1322 (1989).

PROFESSIONAL MISCONDUCT

State boards of medical misconduct have been established in several states. New York has a panel within the state department of health to deal with issues of medical misconduct. The panel is appointed by the commissioner of health. Committees are appointed from among the members to investigate each complaint of professional misconduct received, regardless of the source.

Professional misconduct generally includes

- obtaining a license fraudulently
- practicing a profession fraudulently, beyond its authorized scope, with gross incompetence on a particular occasion, or with negligence or incompetence on more than one occasion
- practicing a profession while the ability to practice is impaired by alcohol, drugs, physical disability, or mental disability
- refusing to provide professional service to a person because of such person's race, creed, color, or national origin
- permitting, aiding, or abetting an unlicensed person to perform activities requiring a license
- being convicted of committing an act constituting a crime

The penalties that may be imposed on a licensee found guilty of professional misconduct include

- suspension of the license to practice
- revocation of the license to practice
- limitation on registration or issuance of any further licenses
- imposition of a fine

In New York, the board of regents may stay such penalties and place the licensee on probation, or it may restore a license that has been revoked. New York State Education Law, Section 6509.

The chief executive officer, the chief of the medical staff, and the department chairpersons of every institution established pursuant to Article 2803–e, as amended, of the New York State Public Health Law shall, and any other person may, report to the board without malice any information that reasonably appears to show that a physician is guilty of professional misconduct. Section 2803–e of the law provides that hospitals must report within 60 days the termination or curtailment of privileges of physicians for alleged malpractice, incompetence, misconduct, or alleged mental or physical impairment; resignation or withdrawal of association or privileges from a facility to avoid disciplinary action; and the facility's receipt of information that indicates that a professional licensee has been convicted of a crime.

The physician in *Gunduy v. Commissioner of Education*, 460 N.Y.S.2d 664 (N.Y. App. Div. 1983), appealed the commissioner of education's decision to revoke his license for being convicted under federal law on seven counts of an indictment. The physician was involved in the possession and distribution of large amounts of amphetamines and furnished false information in required reports and records. The court confirmed the commissioner's decision and noted that professionals have considerable responsibility not to abuse the trust that licensure places on them by violating the laws controlling dangerous drugs.

REGULATION OF INSURANCE PRACTICES

Many believe that the regulation of insurance practices is necessary to prevent windfall profits. Both the medical profession and the legal profession believe that insurance carriers have raised premiums disproportionately to their losses and that, despite their claims of substantial losses, they have reaped substantial profits.

STRUCTURED AWARDS

Structured awards are set up for the periodic payment of judgments by establishing a reversible trust fund for specified parts of awards due patients. The purpose of a structured award is to provide compensation during a patient's lifetime. It would eliminate an unwarranted windfall to the patient's beneficiaries in the event of death. Some states have sought to deal with award limitations by mandating so-called structured recoveries where recoveries exceed a certain dollar amount. Arizona, for example, provides for mandatory periodic payment of future economic damages where there has been an effective election by a party.

Structured recoveries provide that money awarded to the plaintiff be placed in a trust fund and invested appropriately so that those funds will be available to the plaintiff over a long period of time. The rationale behind such legislation is that an immediate award of a large sum of money is not necessary in order for a plaintiff to be well taken care of after suffering injuries at the hands of the defendant. The prudent investment of a smaller amount of money can produce a recovery commensurate with the needs and the rights of the plaintiff. This, in turn, requires a smaller cash outlay by the defendant or the defendant's insurance company, thereby holding down the costs of malpractice insurance and the ultimate cost of medical care to the consumer.

CONCLUSION

Although the medical malpractice crisis has historically centered around the inability of many physicians to obtain malpractice insurance at reasonable rates, it is unlikely that tort reform alone will solve the problems associated with medical injuries and the resulting lawsuits.

The ever-increasing proliferation of regulations by policymakers, which have been designed to control costs and improve the quality of care, has alienated health care providers and added fuel to the practice of defensive medicine.

Physicians, who are on the front lines, have often been excluded from the decision-making processes that threaten their autonomy and financial security. A concerted effort must be made to include them in policy development and implementation. The present system of punishment for all because of the inadequacies of the few has proven to be costly and far from productive. The key to improving quality and controlling costs is cooperation not alienation. Policymakers have failed in this arena and must return to a common sense approach in policy development by including those who are on the front lines of medicine.

Greater efforts must be made to reduce the risks leading to injury. This is best accomplished at the bedside; after all is said and done, an ounce of prevention is better than a pound of cure.

NOTES

1. The Robert Wood Johnson Foundation, *The Medical Malpractice Program: Overview*, ABRIDGE, Spring 1991, at 1.

2. U.S. BIPARTISAN COMMISSION ON COMPREHENSIVE CARE, ACCESS TO HEALTH CARE AND LONG-TERM CARE FOR ALL AMERICANS 3 (March 2, 1990).

3. *Tinkering on Tort Reform Not Enough to Solve Problem: Experts*, 27(11) AHA News, March 18, 1991, at 1.

4. *Experts Debate Reforming Medical-Malpractice System*, 26(41) AHA News, October 15, 1990, at 2.

5. The Robert Wood Johnson Foundation, *Malpractice Research Points Toward Reform*, III(4) ADVANCES, Winter 1990, at 11.

6. *Tort Reform Legislation: Can It Help Hospitals*, HOSPITALS, May 20, 1990, at 29.

7. *Malpractice on Agenda*, XXI(3) NATION'S HEALTH, March 1991, at 5.

8. *White House Pro Incentives in Malpractice Reform*, 27(20) AHA News, May 20, 1991, at 1.

9. *Id.*

10. R. Carlson, *Bush's Malpractice Plan: Cap It!*, 51(289) Newsday, June 19, 1991, at 49.

11. ALA. CODE §6–5–485 (1975).

12. FLA. STAT. §§766.207–.212 (1988).

13. MICH. COMP. LAWS §§600.5040–.5065 (1975).

14. *Malpractice Plan Calls for Mandatory Arbitration*, 27(23) AHA News, June 10, 1991, at 2.

15. The Robert Wood Johnson Foundation, *Legal Reform*, ABRIDGE, Princeton, Spring 1991, at 3.

16. ME. REV. STAT. ANN. tit. 24, §§2851–2859 (1986).

17. *Maine: Malpractice Reform*, 26(37) AHA News, September 17, 1990, at 7.

18. TENN. CODE. ANN. §29–26–119 (1975).

19. CONN. GEN. STAT. §52–251c (1986).
20. ME. REV. STAT. ANN. tit. 24, §2961 (1986).
21. FLA. STAT. §§766.207, 766.209 (1988).
22. MICH. CT. R. 8.121(B).
23. OKLA. STAT. tit. 5, §7 (1953).
24. HAW. REV. STAT. §607–15.5 (1986).
25. N.H. REV. STAT. ANN. §508:4–e (1986).
26. ARK. STAT. ANN. §16–22–309 (1987).
27. WYO. STAT. §1–1–109 (1986).
28. MINN. STAT. §604.02 (1988).
29. *Bush to Offer Malpractice Cap Bill*, Newsday, March 20, 1991, at 4.
30. *Briefs*, 26(50) AHA News, December 24, 1990, at 1.
31. KAN. STAT. ANN. §60–19a02 (1988).
32. MD. CTS. & JUD. PROC. CODE ANN. §11–108 (1986).
33. R. Carlson, *supra* note 10, at 89.
34. *Experts Debate Reforming Medical Malpractice System*, *supra* note 4, at 2.
35. The Robert Wood Johnson Foundation, *supra* note 5, at 11.
36. Zinman, *Study Finds Hospitals 'Harm' Some*, 50(177) Newsday, March 1, 1990, at 17.
37. The Robert Wood Johnson Foundation, *Insurance Reform*, ABRIDGE, Spring 1991, at 4.

Chapter 20

Miscellaneous Topics

The topics reviewed in this chapter have far-reaching health care and economic implications for the entire health care industry. Although a vast amount of information is available in print on each topic surveyed, every effort has been made to provide the reader with current information on the scope of the subject reviewed as well as a variety of the complicated issues involved.

QUALITY ASSURANCE

Quality assurance, risk management, and utilization review have traditionally been treated as separate departments. However, the needs of each department often revolve around utilization of the same information sources, thus making a case for combining the three departments. This reduces duplication of administrative costs, such as staffing, records keeping, etc.

Quality assurance (QA) programs in nursing facilities involve more than ensuring that food is hot and beds are clean. QA is concerned with the total care of every resident in the facility and is directed toward assuring that desirable and appropriate outcomes are achieved. The Omnibus Budget Reconciliation Act of 1987 (OBRA 87) requires that a facility must maintain a quality assessment and assurance committee. OBRA regulations provide that

> (1) Effective October 1, 1990, a facility must maintain a quality assessment and assurance committee consisting of—
> (i) The director of nursing services;
> (ii) A physician designated by the facility; and
> (iii) At least 3 other members of the facility's staff.
> (2) The quality assessment and assurance committee—
> (i) Meets at least quarterly to identify issues with respect to which quality assessment and assurance activities are necessary; and

(ii) Develops and implements appropriate plans of action to correct identified quality deficiencies.[1]

The Pepper Commission, in its report on "Access to Health Care and Long-Term Care for All Americans," indicated the importance and need for organized QA programs in nursing facilities. The Pepper Commission report recommended that the federal government develop and implement a comprehensive national system of quality assurance that would include

- The development of national practice guidelines and standards of care, already begun by the newly created Agency for Health Care Policy and Research. Physicians and physician organizations should be widely utilized in developing and reviewing practice guidelines and parameters.
- The development and implementation of a uniform data system that covers all health care encounters, regardless of payment source setting. These data would provide a common foundation for all payers' quality assessment activities and for examining the effectiveness of medical care and identifying health policy and research concerns.
- The development and testing of new, more effective methods of quality assurance and assessment.
- The development and oversight of local review organizations that have skills in data integration and analysis, quality assessment, and quality assurance.[2]

The Joint Commission on Accreditation of Health Care Organizations recommends a ten-step process to monitor and evaluate quality of care in the long-term care facility. This monitoring and evaluation process is designed to assist health care facilities to focus on quality of care issues. The monitoring portion of the process addresses establishing patterns or trends in care while the evaluation portion of the process is designed to explore the presence or absence of an opportunity to improve quality of care. The ten steps are

1. Assign responsibility for monitoring and evaluation activities;
2. Delineate the scope of care provided by the organization;
3. Identify the most important aspects of care provided by the organization;
4. Identify indicators (and appropriate clinical criteria) for monitoring the important aspects of care;
5. Establish thresholds (levels, patterns, trends) for the indicators that will trigger evaluation of the care;
6. Monitor the important aspects of care by collecting and organizing the data for each indicator;
7. Evaluate care when thresholds are reached to identify opportunities to improve care or problems;
8. Take actions to improve care or correct identified problems;

9. Assess the effectiveness of the actions and document the improvement in care; and
10. Communicate the results of the monitoring and evaluation process to relevant individuals, departments, or services and to the organization-wide quality assurance program.[3]

"Long-Term Care Standards Manual," Joint Commission of Accreditation of Health Care Organizations, Chicago, 1990, at 3–7.

State regulations address quality of care issues. New York, for example, provides:

> *415.12 Quality of Care.* Each resident shall receive and the facility shall provide the necessary care and services to attain or maintain the highest practicable physical, mental and comprehensive assessment and plan of care subject to the resident's right of self-determination.
>
> * * *
>
> *415.27 Quality Assessment and Assurance.* The facility shall establish and maintain a coordinated quality assessment and assurance program which integrates the review activities of all nursing home programs and services to enhance the quality of life and resident care and treatment.
> (a) Facility-wide quality assurance. Quality assurance shall be the responsibility of all staff, at every level, at all times. Supervisory personnel alone cannot ensure quality of care and services. Such quality must be a part of each individual's approach to his or her daily responsibilities.[4]

To distinguish between quality of care and quality of life issues we can look to the dietary department in a nursing facility. From the quality of care perspective one would consider food in terms of adequate nutritional value and proper selection of diet for a particular resident. In contrast, quality of life issues are those that recognize the importance of food in our lives. Cookouts, theme parties, and special meals on religious and other holidays acknowledge that meal times are as important to residents for socializing as they are for eating.[5]

Key to a successful QA program is the assignment of responsibility for coordinating QA activities to an appropriate individual, preferably one who has demonstrated the ability and interest in developing, implementing, and monitoring a quality program. In the early developmental stages or revamping of an existing QA program, it might be helpful to employ a consultant with expertise in QA activities.

Quality Assurance Committees

A quality assurance committee has responsibility for reviewing services rendered in the nursing facility with a goal of improving care. The committee should include representation from the governing board, administration, and medical staff.

The committee should periodically review the credentials, physical and mental capacity, and competency of health professionals employed or associated with the nursing facility. Other functions of the committee include

- instituting continuing education programs for health professionals in their areas of responsibility
- instituting general education programs that include patient safety, fire prevention, etc.
- promptly resolving resident complaints
- coordinating malpractice prevention programs that identify and assist in preventing negligent acts
- verifying credentials prior to granting privileges

Medicare and Medicaid

The Medicare/Medicaid Programs include a quality assurance focal point to carry out the quality assurance provisions of the Medicare and Medicaid programs, the development and implementation of health and safety standards for providers of care in federal health programs, and the implementation of End Stage Renal Disease Program and the Professional Standards Review provisions.[6]

Disclosure of Information

OBRA regulations provide that a state or the Secretary of Health and Human Services may not require the disclosure of the records of a "quality assessment and assurance committee," except for making a determination regarding a facility's compliance with the requirement for maintaining the committee.[7]

Misuse of the peer review process can result in legal action. Peer review documents are exempt from discovery so long as the statutory protected materials are used for legitimate purposes. The ophthalmologist in *Summit Health Ltd. v. Pinhas*, Ill. S. Ct. 61 (1990), *affirming* 894 F.2d 1024, claimed that a hospital and its medical staff misused the peer review process by initiating proceedings against him, conspiring to exclude him from the Los Angeles ophthalmological services market because he refused to follow unnecessary costly procedures used at Midway Hospital Medical Center. The United States Supreme Court held that there was a sufficient connection with interstate commerce to support federal jurisdiction under Section 1 of the Sherman Act. Even though the effect of conspiring to exclude one individual from practicing in a particular market may be minimal, the potential for further abuse cannot be discounted. "When the competitive significance of respondent's exclusion from the market is measured, not by a particularized evaluation of his practice, but by a general evaluation of the restraint's impact on other participants in that market, the restraint is covered by the Act."

Performance Standards

Regulators who set performance standards to achieve desired outcomes in a resident's care must recognize that there may be a variety of ways to meet the desired outcome. Regulations often focus on negative outcomes and punishment of those health care professionals who have failed to meet set standards. This system of enforcement encourages the practice of defensive medicine, often resulting in over- or under-treatment. To be effective, a quality assurance program must not merely identify performance problems and develop complex procedures designed to prevent future problems; it must also educate, educate, and re-educate.

RISK MANAGEMENT

Risk management is the identification of potential accidents with an emphasis on claims prevention. A risk management program is designed to reduce and prevent injuries to patients, employees, visitors, and other third parties. Its aim is to reduce the number of negligence claims and subsequent financial losses from malpractice suits.

Increasing insurance costs and general financial constraints are putting pressure on nursing facilities to take part in the prevention of medically related injuries. In risk management, a team effort is necessary to improve the quality of care and eliminate or minimize the number of incidents that become potential lawsuits.

> In response to the growing realization that the malpractice problem may become much more directly relevant for them in the near future, many nursing home administrators, governing boards, and medical and nursing directors are exploring, albeit cautiously, the advisability of instituting legal risk-management systems within their facilities.[8]

In a survey of nursing home risk management programs by Marshall B. Kapp, professor in the department of community health, and Ronald J. Markert, Professor in the department of medicine at Wright State University in Dayton, Ohio, administrators were asked about their perception of the effectiveness of risk management programs.

> When queried whether they believed that their risk management system had helped to improve the quality of care, 86 percent (65 of 76) of the facilities in this category answered in the affirmative. Ninety percent (68 of 76) of respondents opined that the existence of a risk management system improved their ability to administer the facility. Fifty-eight percent (44 of 76) of the administrators felt that their risk management program helped to prevent or reduce the severity of lawsuits against the facility.

* * *

> Most notably, 90 percent (68 of 76) of administrators answered that development of a formal risk management system within their facility had been worth the expense and effort involved and that they would recommend a risk management system to their colleagues.[9]

Board of Directors

The board of a nursing facility must concern itself with reviewing the competence of the medical staff. Standards of performance also must be set, in order to evaluate medical care. Standards also must be set to measure the quality of all equipment utilized by the facility and a preventive maintenance program must be established to correct deficiencies. Public expectations place a broad responsibility on health care facilities to ensure safe care regardless of who renders it. The nursing facility board's ultimate responsibility for adequate patient care mandates its involvement in the risk management process.

Administration

There must be cooperation among all levels of personnel. Members of the medical staff must be encouraged to voice their concerns and present their problems. The administrator should review resident care status reports. An administrative representative should be present at all medical staff meetings. Incident reports should be reviewed by an administrative representative. An on-going effort must be made on the part of management to provide an educational program in risk management to board members, physicians, and employees.

Medical Staff

The medical staff must establish and enforce professional performance standards. The conduct of each physician must then be evaluated against these established standards. Appropriate committees of the medical staff should support the risk management process.

Risk Management Committee

A risk management committee with representation from the medical staff and appropriate department heads should be either established or combined with the activities of a safety committee. The committee chairperson should be trained in medical audits and the risk management process. The risk manager should be responsible for the development and coordination of strategic prevention programs. This committee serves to monitor all potential hazards. Information from all nursing facility committees (i.e., pharmacy, transfusion, infections, safety, utilization, tissue, medical records, and credentials) regarding potential liability hazards should be funneled into this committee for review, evaluation, and appropriate action. The facility's attorney should be readily available for legal guidance.

Elements of a Risk Management Program

Valuable components of a risk management program include

- preparation of incident reports
- evaluation of the frequency and severity of incident exposure
- definition of the cause of each incident
- formulation and implementation of corrective actions to reduce risk and exposure to liability
- training and education of staff to assist in reducing the number of incidents
- continuing attention of a safety committee
- use of a suggestion box
- a public relations program (Employees should be trained in completing timely incident reports that clearly document the facts and that are utilized not to cover up unfortunate incidents, but to train personnel and identify problems.)
- prompt investigation and care following accidental injury to a patient

Incident Reports

It should be noted that incident reports are discoverable and subject to subpoena. Therefore, consideration should be given to referring questionable incident reports (e.g., incidents that might result in a negligence suit) to the facility's attorney for legal advice. This may help prevent discovery on the basis of attorney–client privilege. Incident reports should not be placed in a resident's medical record.

UTILIZATION REVIEW

Medicare

As a condition for participation in the federal Medicare program, skilled nursing facilities are required to have a utilization review program.

> The skilled nursing facility carries out utilization review of the services provided in the facility at least to in-patients who are entitled to benefits

> under the program(s). Utilization review has as its overall objectives both the maintenance of high quality patient care and assurance of appropriate and efficient utilization of facility services. There are two elements to utilization review: medical care evaluation studies that identify and examine patterns of care provided in the facility, and review of extended duration cases which is concerned with efficiency, appropriateness, and cost effectiveness of care.[10]

Medicare is very specific in its requirements of the skilled nursing services for which it pays. It requires that the services be

1. ordered by a physician
2. so inherently complex that the service must be provided by and under the supervision of technical or professional health personnel
3. required on a daily basis
4. furnished for a condition that arose as a result of a recent hospitalization[11]

Medicaid

Under OBRA requirements all three of the existing Medicaid utilization control mechanisms will no longer be required of nursing facilities (NFs), effective October 1, 1990. Section 412(e)(1) of OBRA 87 abolishes the requirements for physician certification and recertification, section 4212(d)(2) removes the requirement for professional review and inspections of care, and section 4211(h)(3) removes the requirement for utilization control by the facility's utilization review committee.[12] This has been replaced by a standardized system of resident assessment and care planning (section 415.11).

ACQUIRED IMMUNODEFICIENCY SYNDROME

The acquired immunodeficiency syndrome (AIDS) is generally accepted as a syndrome—a collection of specific, life-threatening, opportunistic infections and manifestations that are the result of an underlying immune deficiency. It is caused by a virus called human immunodeficiency virus (HIV) and is the most severe form of the HIV infection. AIDS is a fatal disease that destroys the body's capacity to ward off bacteria and viruses that would ordinarily be fought off by a properly functioning immune system. Although there is no effective long-term treatment of the disease, there are indications that proper management of the disease can improve the quality of life and delay progression of the disease.

AIDS is spread by direct contact with infected blood or body fluids, such as vaginal secretions, semen, and breast milk. At the present time there is no evidence that the virus can be transmitted through food, water, or casual body contact. The HIV virus does not survive well outside the body. Although there is presently no cure for AIDS, early diagnosis and treatment with new medications can help HIV-infected persons remain healthy for longer periods of time. High-risk groups include homosexual males, intravenous drug users, Haitian immigrants, and those who require transfusions of blood and blood products, such as hemophiliacs.

The first case of AIDS appeared in the literature in 1981.[13] Since that time numerous reports have followed, describing patients with unusual immune defects, later identified as being caused by the AIDS virus. Since identification of the first AIDS case in 1981, more than 120,000 cases have been reported to the Centers for Disease Control (CDC) through January 1990.[14] (See Figure 20-1 below).

To date, about 54 percent of all reported cases have resulted in death. An estimated 1.5 million Americans are afflicted with the virus that causes AIDS, with a large percentage of them expected to develop the full symptoms of the disease.[15] The Centers for Disease Control recently reported that the AIDS epidemic has killed 100,777 people since it was first recognized almost 10 years ago. It has been estimated that another 165,000 to 215,000 patients may die within the next three years. Of the deaths that have occurred so far, 31,196 were reported in 1990 alone.[16] It is projected that cumulatively about 270,000 Americans will have contracted AIDS by 1991, with 179,000 deaths from the disease.[17] (See Figure 20-1.) The costs associated with treating persons with AIDS are certain to rise. It has been estimated that life and health insurance claims related to the AIDS syndrome totaled one billion dollars in 1989.[18] As with other parts of the world, HIV infection is appearing with increasing frequency in the non-IV drug-using, heterosexual population. In addition, it is no longer confined to major urban areas.[19]

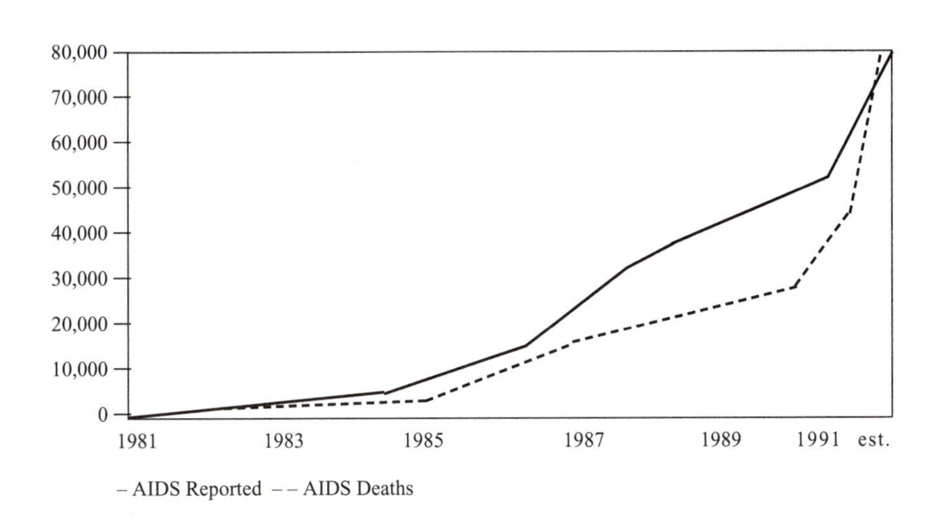

Figure 20-1 AIDS Reported Compared to Deaths 1981–91

AIDS and Health Care Workers

The number of AIDS cases cared for in health care facilities is on the rise, as are the costs associated with treatment.[20] A national breakdown by profession of reported AIDS cases among health care workers since the early 1980s revealed the following:[21]

Nurses	1,358
Health Aides	1,101
Technicians	941
Therapists	319
Dentists & Hygienists	171
Paramedics	116
Surgeons	47
Others	1,680
Total	**6,436**

Source: Centers for Disease Control, 3/31/91.

"An estimated 50,000 health workers are thought to be infected with HIV; nearly all are believed to be still working."[22] The American Medical Association and the American Dental Association, in a somewhat unpopular fashion, are recommending that physicians and dentists inform their patients if they are carrying the AIDS virus.

> All doctors and dentists who have the AIDS virus should either inform their patients they are infected or cease practicing surgery, other forms of invasive medicine and most dentistry, the American Medical Association and American Dental Association said yesterday in a controversial reversal of their previous positions.[23]

An AIDS notification bill in Illinois, if approved by the governor, would require notifying more than 67,000 patients that they may be at risk of being infected with the AIDS virus. The patients were exposed when they underwent invasive procedures performed by 204 health care workers who tested positive for the virus.[24]

The ever-increasing likelihood that health care workers will come into contact with persons carrying the HIV virus demands the development of and compliance with approved safety procedures. This is especially important for those who come into contact with blood and body fluids of HIV-infected persons.

> The federal Centers for Disease Control is following over 1,000 health care workers who have experienced blood-to-blood or blood-to-mucous membrane exposure to the body fluids of AIDS patients; many of these workers have had needlestick injuries while treating AIDS patients. To

date, about 25 health care workers who experienced punctures or other exposures to blood have become infected. These cases demonstrate the need for health care workers to strictly follow safety guidelines to prevent direct exposure to blood and body fluids in the care of patients.[25]

AIDS Emergency Act

Because the incidence of the HIV virus affects various localities of the United States disproportionately, the Senate and House of Representatives enacted the Ryan White Comprehensive AIDS Resources Emergency Act of 1990. The purpose of the Act is to

> provide emergency assistance to localities that are disproportionately affected by the Human Immunodeficiency Virus epidemic and to make financial assistance available to States and other public or private nonprofit entities to provide for the development, organization, coordination and operation of more effective and cost efficient systems for the delivery of essential services to individuals and families with the HIV disease.[26]

Under the HIV Care Grants section of the Act, a state may use grant funds

> (1) to establish and operate HIV care consortia within areas most affected by HIV disease that shall be designated to provide a comprehensive continuum of care to individuals and families with HIV disease . . .
> (2) to provide home- and community-based care services for individuals with HIV disease . . .
> (3) to provide assistance to assure the continuity of health insurance coverage for individuals with HIV disease . . .
> (4) to provide treatments, that have been determined to prolong life or prevent serious deterioration of health to individuals with HIV disease . . . .[27]

Mandatory Testing and Confidentiality

Both health care workers and patients claim mandatory HIV testing violates their Fourth Amendment right to privacy. The dilemma is how to balance these rights against the rights of the public in general to be protected from a deadly disease. The American Medical Association at its June 23–27, 1991 meeting in Chicago "rejected mandatory testing of health care workers, but adopted a resolution supporting voluntary HIV testing."[28]

State laws have been developed that protect the confidentiality of HIV-related information. In addition, some states have developed informational brochures and consent, release, and partner notification forms. The unauthorized disclosure of confidential HIV-related information can subject an individual to civil and/or criminal penalties.[29]

A formidable and troublesome ethical question continues to go unanswered—should a physician suffering from AIDS notify his or her patients that he or she has tested positive for the AIDS virus? Guidelines drafted by the CDC call on health care workers who perform "exposure-prone" procedures to voluntarily undergo tests to determine whether or not they are infected. The guidelines also recommend that patients be informed.[30]

Any new AIDS-related regulations must address the rights and responsibilities of both patients and health care workers. Although this will require a delicate balancing act, it must not be handled as a back burner issue by legislators.

Medical Records

Health care institutions must be sure to adopt appropriate and effective policies and procedures for protecting the rights of patients with AIDS. As with mental health records, a higher degree of confidentiality is generally expected of the treating institution due to the negative impact on persons who have contracted AIDS.

Discrimination

Discrimination against persons who have contracted the AIDS virus is often found to be in violation of their constitutional rights. The sufferings and hardships of those who have contracted the disease extend to family as well as "best friends." The infringements of those afflicted with AIDS include discrimination in access to health care, education, employment, housing, insurance benefits, and military service. Those who believe that they have been discriminated against can contact their state's human rights commission.

Access to Health Care

The American Civil Liberties Union in New York City charged in a recent report that nursing homes discriminate against AIDS patients. "The report is based on a study of 13,000 AIDS discrimination incidents that occurred between 1983 and 1988. The report shows that 'public accommodations'—including nursing homes—accounted for 16 percent of the incidents."[31] A Long Island man stricken with AIDS spent the final three years of his life searching for a nursing home. He died in Nassau County Medical Center after he had been rejected by 22 different homes. The Health Systems Agency, along with the efforts of some state and local officials, were able to "persuade nursing homes in Nassau and Suffolk counties to open their doors to people with AIDS."[32]

There is a growing need for nursing home care for AIDS patients, particularly for those who are homeless or have no family support system. An AIDS survey conducted by mail in Oregon revealed that 79 percent of those hospitals responding had adequate resources to care for AIDS patients, 26 percent of skilled nursing facilities, and 69 percent of home health agencies.[33] In response to the need for nursing home care, some health departments (e.g., New York) are encouraging the development of specialized HIV/AIDS nursing homes that will combine medical services and drug treatment for AIDS patients who have become infected through drug abuse.[34]

Employment

AIDS-related employment issues involve a two-sided coin, with employment discrimination on one side and the refusal of employees to care for AIDS patients on the flip side. The growing consensus of case law indicates that employment-related discrimination is unlawful.

Employees who have contracted the AIDS virus and whose symptoms warrant should be placed in positions that are non-threatening to the health and safety of patients and employees. In severe cases, it may be necessary to place the employee on a medical leave of absence.

Situations may arise from time to time where employees may refuse to treat AIDS patients. There are two basic approaches that can be taken in dealing with such problems. The most beneficial course of action for the employee and the institution would be to embark upon a thorough program of educating the staff. The alternative and less desirable response to the problem may require that disciplinary steps be initiated against the employee. Such action could be justified on the basis that the health care facility has a right to manage its work force by assigning staff in a responsible manner to carry out its mission of caring for the sick.

In the final analysis, there are numerous competing issues (e.g., humanitarian, legal, moral, ethical, and religious) pertaining to the rights of patients and caregivers who have contracted the AIDS virus, as well as those who have not, and employers. As the search for answers continues, the debates and controversies will be heated. Hopefully, solutions will be forthcoming which will meet the needs of those who have been infected with the AIDS virus, and those who are involved with providing health care to them.

Reporting Requirements

Because of the social stigma associated with AIDS, there is a worldwide tendency to under report the incidence of the disease. This is particularly true in developing countries, where the problem is compounded by the lack of efficient reporting systems. For example, in Africa, for every person with AIDS, between 50 and 100 more are estimated to be infected with the HIV virus. Most cases are not reported, and some governments are unwilling to admit to the problem. Few African countries possess the medical resources to deal with this disease epidemic. Whole sectors of African economies face ruin. The social stigma is not endemic to African countries. In the United States, health information is merely more readily available due to sophisticated reporting systems.[35]

> AIDS is now a reportable communicable disease in every state. . . . Physicians and hospitals must report every case of AIDS—with the patient's name—to government public health authorities. New York State does not require reports of ARC or of positive blood test for HIV antibodies, but some states do. . . . Cases reported to local health authorities are also reported to the federal Centers for Disease Control (CDC), with the patients' names encoded by a system known as Soundex. CDC records come under the general confidentiality protections of the federal Privacy Act of 1974. However, the statute permits disclosures to other federal agencies, under certain circumstances.[36]

Occupational Safety and Health Act

The Occupational Safety and Health Act (OSHA) requires that health care facilities implement strict procedures to protect employees against the AIDS virus. OSHA requires strict adherence to guidelines developed by the Centers for Disease Control in Atlanta. Complaints investigated by OSHA can result in the issuance of fines for failure to comply with regulatory requirements.

Education for the Nursing Facility

> . . . if SNFs are to be the future resources for care for persons with AIDS, the responses of the CNEs in these facilities suggest that a concerted effort is needed to market the idea to their sponsors; the fears they expressed point to the need for further community education and involvement.[37]

A wide variety of AIDS-related educational materials are available on the market. One of the most important sources of AIDS information is the Centers for Disease Control in Atlanta, Georgia. Every effort must be made to sensitize the staff, residents, and families for the AIDS admission. The process of staff education in preparing to care for residents with AIDS is extremely important and must include a training program on prevention and transmission in the work setting. Educational requirements specified by the Occupational Safety and Health Administration for health care employees includes epidemiology, modes of transmission, preventive practices, and universal precautions.

CERTIFICATE OF NEED

The National Health Planning and Resources Development Act of 1974, Public Law No. 93–641, sought to encourage state review of all plans calling for the construction, expansion, or renovation of health facilities or services by conditioning receipt of certain federal funds on the establishment of an approved state "Certificate of Need" (CON) program. Most states responded to this law by instituting state CON programs that complied with federal standards. Although the federal law is now history, CON programs remain in effect in many states. According to a survey by the American Hospital Association, CON programs remain in effect in some form in 39 states and the District of Columbia. The CON process has been eliminated in eleven states.[38] Many states continue to maintain control over Medicaid expenditures for nursing home care by controlling the number of beds through the CON process.

CON requirements have been criticized by health care providers because they require review of those expenditures "by or on behalf of a health care facility," but may allow groups of physicians or independent laboratories to make large expenditures for equipment or services without triggering the state review mechanism.

Disapprovals of CONs often occur because they do not comply with state health plans that are designed to prevent overbedding in predefined geographic areas. Some CON applicants have attempted to seek revisions in state health plans in order to obtain approval of their project. *Nursing Home of Dothan, Inc. v. Alabama State Health Planning and Development Agency*, 542 So. 2d 935 (Ala. Civ. App. 1989), was one such case. The nursing home had filed a CON application with the State Health Planning Agency (SHPA) to construct a 110 bed nursing home. SHPA informed Dothan that the State Health Plan failed to indicate a need for additional beds and advised Dothan to seek an amendment to the State Health Plan before proceeding with the CON process. The defendant filed the proposed amendment with the State Health Coordinating Council, which approved the defendant's request for additional beds. The amendment, which required the governor's approval, was rejected by him. Upon appeal of the circuit court's finding for SHPA, denying Dothan's proposed amendment to the state health plan and subsequent denial of the CON application, the appeals court held that the governor properly disapproved the requested amendment.

Disapproval of a CON application can also be based on the financial feasibility of the project. A CON proposal to construct a long-term care nursing facility with 65 percent Medicaid beds was found to have been properly denied in *National Health Corporation v. South Carolina Department of Health and Environmental Control*, 380 S.E.2d 841 (S.C. Ct. App. 1989). The Department of Health and Environmental Control's decision was considered proper, reasonable, and consistent with applicable laws and regulations. The unsuccessful applicant had failed to establish its project's financial feasibility due to the unavailability of Medicaid funding. Discrepancies also existed between its budgets and its cost reports.

> The record contains clear evidence that Medicaid funds would not be available for the NHC beds. The Board also found that inconsistencies in four budgets submitted by NHC and the discrepancies between those budgets and the cost reports submitted by NHC to State Health and

> Human Services Finance Commission raised serious questions regarding the financial feasibility of the NHC project.

Id. at 845. The agency's competitor had demonstrated the financial feasibility of its project and was, therefore, granted a CON.

There can be disagreement among justices within the same court as to whether or not an applicant has established the criteria for need within a specific geographic area. The record in *Heritage of Yankton, Inc. v. South Dakota Department of Health*, 432 N.W.2d 68 (S.D. 1988), was found to have supported denial of a CON application for additional beds based on the argument that there was no need for additional beds in the service area. The Department of Health was found not to have acted arbitrarily and capriciously in denying the application. It provided valid reasons for rejecting new information submitted at a rehearing. The Department of Health rejected an argument that a bed shortage in the county demonstrated a need for more beds.

> The Department argues it has never considered county boundaries in determining bed need, and that the population of the facility's service area is the proper area for consideration. In view of its policy to maintain high occupancy rates in all facilities, the Department also rejected Heritage's claim that the Department's formula forces the elderly to be separated from their families and home communities.

Id. at 71.

Justice Henderson stated in a dissenting opinion

> This health care facility submitted three items of new evidence which had not been previously considered. This consisted of population projections for the area and an in-and-out migration data with information pertaining to the existence of alternative services. The Department, summarily, expressed that it refused to consider this new evidence. Instead of opening its mind and then opening the door of reconsideration with relevant evidence, the Department of Health chose to be unyielding with its grip on the single formula and methodology it employed. If this health facility's evidence had been reconsidered, an open mind would see that there was an extensive need for beds existing in the city of Yankton and Yankton county.
>
> * * *
>
> I cannot in good conscience, join the majority opinion which prevents elderly citizens from having a bed, with medical care and treatment, administered compassionately, in a community where their children and grandchildren reside. I would elevate reality over a single methodology and accordingly dissent.

> "[T]herefore never send to know for whom the bell tolls; it tolls for thee." John Donne (1573-1631), *Devotions upon Emergent Occasions*, Meditation XVII. My mind drifts to Ernest Hemingway. And a clod of dirt. Chipped away at the shores of Europe by the sea. "If a clod be washed away by the sea, Europe is the less. . . ." *Supra.* All from whence Hemingway's great novel was born. And, yes, not a person is turned away from a bed of repose, in his older years, but South Dakota is lesser—in spirit. A refrain also comes to my mind: "And crown thy good, with Brotherhood, from sea to shining sea."

Id. at 76, 77.

NOTES

1. 42 C.F.R. §403.75 (1989).

2. U.S. Bipartisan Commission on Comprehensive Care, Access to Health Care and Long-Term Care for All Americans 3 (March 2, 1990).

3. Joint Commission of Accreditation of Health Care Organizations, Long Term Care Standards Manual 3–7 (1990).

4. N.Y. Comp. Codes R. & Regs. tit. 10, §415 (1990).

5. S. B. Goldsmith, Choosing a Nursing Home 2 (1990).

6. *Id.* at 308.

7. Key Medicare and Medicaid Legislation: 1990, OBRA 1990, Special Member Briefing, Chicago: American Hospital Association, January 1991, at 161.

8. M.B. Kapp & R.J. Markert, *Legal Risk-Management Programs in Nursing Homes: Who Has Them and Do They Work*, 35(4) Hospital and Health Services Management 604 (1990).

9. *Id.* at 607.

10. 42 C.F.R. §405.1137 (1989).

11. Goldsmith, *supra* note 5, at 80–82.

12. 55 Fed. Reg. 10,952 (1990).

13. A. Cantwell, Jr., M.D., AIDS: The Mystery and the Solutions, Los Angeles (1986), at 54.

14. New York State Department of Health, Albany, 100 Questions and Answers, AIDS 6 (May 1990).

15. *Id.* at 7.

16. *A Possible 215,000 AIDS Deaths in Next 3 Years*, XXI(2) The Nation's Health, February, 1991, at 1.

17. Brown, *AIDS Discrimination in the Workplace: The Legal Dilemma*, Case and Comment, Nov.-Dec. 1989, at 1.

18. *AIDS Insurance Claims Totaled $1 Billion in 1989*, 26(45) AHA News, November 12, 1990, at 2.

19. R.B. Roberts, *Introduction*, Changing Issues in the Management of HIV Infection, Symposium 2 (September, 1990).

20. *Public Hospitals Squeezed by AIDS Patients' Costs*, XXX(1) The Nation's Health, January 1991, at 4.

21. *LI Dentist Was HIV-Positive*, 51(314) Newsday, July 14, 1991, at 40.

22. L. Garrett, *Doctors with Aids Asked to Inform Patients or Quit*, 51(137) Newsday, January 18, 1981, at 13.

23. *Id.*

24. *AIDS-Notification Bill Passes*, 27(30) AHA News, July 29, 1991, at 7.

25. N.Y. STATE DEPARTMENT OF HEALTH, *supra* note 14, at 6.

26. Pub. L. No. 101–381, August 18, 1990, 1990 U.S. CODE CONG. & ADMIN. NEWS (104 Stat.) 576.

27. *Id.* at 586.

28. *AMA Rejects Mandatory Testing of Health Care Workers*, XXI(8) THE NATION'S HEALTH, August 1991, at 5.

29. N.Y. STATE DEPARTMENT OF HEALTH, *supra* note 14, at 17.

30. *CDC's HIV-Testing Guidelines Get Mixed Reviews*, 27(29) AHA News, July 22, 1991, at 1.

31. *Long-Term Care*, 64 HOSPITALS, November 20, 1990, at 20.

32. *The High Cost of the State's "Little Cuts,"* 51(209) Newsday, March 31, 1991, at 7.

33. C.M. White & M.C. Berger, *Response of Hospitals, Skilled Nursing Facilities, and Home Health Agencies in Oregon to Aids: Reports of Nursing Executives*, 81(4) AMERICAN JOURNAL OF PUBLIC HEALTH, April 1991, at 495.

34. N.Y. STATE DEPARTMENT OF HEALTH, *supra* note 14, at 11.

35. *Incalculable Cost of AIDS*, ECONOMIST (U.K.), Mar. 12, 1988, at 44.

36. LAMBDA LEGAL DEFENSE AND EDUCATION FUND, INC., LIVING WITH AIDS at 7 (1987).

37. RESPONSE OF HOSPITALS, SKILLED NURSING FACILITIES, AND HOME HEALTH AGENCIES IN OREGON TO AIDS: REPORTS OF NURSING EXECUTIVES, at 496.

38. *U.S. Wrap-Up*, 27(28) AHA News, July 15, 1991, at 7.

Appendix A

Glossary

Abandonment The unilateral severance by the physician of the professional relationship between himself or herself and the patient without reasonable notice at a time when the patient still needs continuing attention.

Abortion The premature termination of pregnancy at a time when the fetus is incapable of sustaining life independent of the mother.

Activities program A planned schedule of recreational, social, and other purposeful activity for nursing home patients/residents, designed to make their life more meaningful, to stimulate and support their desire to use their physical and mental capabilities to the fullest extent, to enable them to maintain a sense of usefulness and self-respect, but not specifically designed to correct or remedy any disability.

Administration on Aging (AoA) The Administration on Aging, an agency of the U.S. Department of Health and Human Services, is devoted exclusively to the concerns and potential of older people. The AoA develops federal programs and coordinates community services. For information write: Office of Management and Policy, 330 Independence Avenue, S.W., Washington, DC 20201, or call (202) 245–0641.

Administrative agency A government body charged with administering or implementing particular legislation.

Admissibility (of evidence) Refers to the issue of whether a court, applying the rules of evidence, is bound to receive or permit introduction of a particular piece of proof.

Adult day care centers Places where senior citizens receive care one to five days a week. The care is generally provided on a full or half day basis and can involve meals, transportation, social activities (e.g., shopping and entertainment), and a variety of therapies (e.g., art and music).

Adult homes Facilities that provide a home for elderly persons who are basically healthy and able to care for themselves. They provide some sense of security and are an alternative to living alone. These facilities attempt to provide a home-like atmosphere.

Affidavit A voluntary statement of facts, or a voluntary declaration in writing of facts, that a person swears to be true before an official authorized to administer an oath.

Agency The relationship in which one person acts for or represents another with the latter's authority, for example, insurance agent and insurance company.

Allegation A statement that a person expects to be able to prove.

American Association of Homes for the Aging (AAHA) A national organization of more than 3,700 not-for-profit nursing homes, continuing care retirement communities, senior housing facilities, and community service organizations serving more than 600,000 older Americans each year. The AAHA provides services that include representation and advocacy before Congress and federal agencies on major issues, continuing education, public relations programs, publications, enhancement of financial strength through group purchasing, and long-term care insurance programs. For information write: Suite 500, 901 E Street, N.W., Washington, DC 20004–2837, or call (202) 783–2242.

American Association of Retired Persons (AARP) The nation's leading organization for people age 50 and over. It serves their needs and interests through legislative advocacy, research, informative programs, and community services provided by a network of local chapters and experienced volunteers throughout the country. The AARP offers members a wide range of special membership benefits, including the magazine *Modern Maturity* and a monthly bulletin. For information write: 1909 K Street, N.W., Washington, DC 20049, or call (202) 872-4700.

American Bar Association, Commission on the Legal Problems of the Elderly A program of the American Bar Association that analyzes and responds to the legal needs of older people in the United States. For information write: Second Floor, South Lobby, 1800 M Street, N.W., Washington, DC 20036, or call (202) 331–2297.

Appellant The party who appeals the decision of a lower court to a court of higher jurisdiction.

Appellee The party against whom an appeal to a higher court is taken.

Area Agency on Aging Local agencies designated by the governor of each state that are concerned with all matters that relate to the needs of the elderly in the community. A variety of services funded by the Older Americans Act are available through the Area Agency on Aging, such as information and referral, transportation, home delivered meals, homemaker/home health aides, and other supportive services.

Assault An intentional act that is designed to make the victim fearful and produces reasonable apprehension of harm.

Assignment The transfer of rights, responsibilities, or property from one party to another.

Attainder A legislative act that is directed against a specified person finding him or her guilty of some offense and imposing a penalty upon him or her.

Attestation The act of witnessing a document in writing.

Audiology The comprehensive diagnostic auditory assessment of an individual's hearing loss, rehabilitation services, and hearing aide orientation, instruction, advisement and consultation.

Autonomy The right of an individual to make his or her own independent decisions.

Battery The intentional touching of one person by another without the consent of the person being touched.

Best evidence rule A legal doctrine requiring that primary evidence of a fact (such as an original document) be introduced, or that an acceptable explanation be given before a copy can be introduced or testimony given concerning the fact.

Bona fide In good faith; openly, honestly, or innocently; without knowledge or intent of fraud.

Borrowed servant doctrine Refers to a situation where an employee is temporarily under the control of someone other than his or her primary employer. The traditional example is that of a nurse employed by a hospital who is "borrowed" and under the control of the attending surgeon during a procedure in the operating room. The temporary employer of the borrowed servant can be held responsible for the negligent acts of the borrowed servant under the doctrine of respondeat superior.

Caregiver One who provides care to a resident/patient.

Case citation A means of describing where the court's opinion in a particular case can be located. It identifies the parties in the case, the text in which the case can be found, the court writing the opinion, and the year in which the case was decided. For example, the citation "*Bouvia v. Superior Court (Glenchur)*, 225 Cal. Rptr. 297 (Cal. Ct. App. 1986)" is described as follows:

- *Bouvia v. Superior Court (Glenchur)*—Identifies the basic parties involved in the lawsuit.
- 225 Cal. Rptr. 297—Identifies the case as being reported in volume 225 of the California Reporter at page 297.
- Cal. Ct. App. 1986—Identifies the case as being in the California Court of Appeals in 1986.

Case law The aggregate of reported cases on a particular legal subject as formed by the decisions of those cases.

Certiorari A writ that commands a lower court to certify proceedings for review by a higher court. This is the common method of obtaining review by the United States Supreme Court.

Charitable immunity A legal doctrine that developed out of the English court system and held charitable institutions blameless for their negligent acts.

Civil law The body of law that describes the private rights and responsibilities of individuals. It is that part of law that does not deal with crimes. It involves actions filed by one individual against another (e.g., actions in tort and contract).

Clinical privileges Upon qualification, the diagnostic and therapeutic procedures an institution allows a physician to perform on a specified patient population. Qualification includes a review of a physician's credentials, such as medical school diploma, state licensure, residency training, etc.

Closed shop contract A labor–management agreement that provides that only members of a particular union may be hired.

Common law The body of principles that has evolved and continues to evolve and expand from court decisions. Many of the legal principles and rules applied by courts in the United States had their origins in English common law.

Complaint In a negligence action, the first pleading that is filed by the plaintiff's attorney. It is the first statement of a case by the plaintiff against the defendant and states a cause of action, notifying the defendant as to the basis for the suit.

Concurring opinion See Opinion of the court.

Confidentiality See Privileged communication.

Congressional Record The document in which the proceedings of Congress are published. It is the first record of debate officially reported, printed, and published directly by the federal government. Publication of the record began March 4, 1873.

Consent Simply stated, a voluntary act by which one person agrees to allow someone else to do something.

Coroner's jury A special jury called by the coroner to determine whether evidence concerning the cause of death indicates that death was brought about by criminal means.

Counterclaim A defendant's claim in opposition to a claim of the plaintiff.

Crime An act against society in violation of the law. Crimes are prosecuted by and in the name of the state.

Criminal law The division of the law dealing with crime and punishment. It involves a legal action filed by a state or by the United States against a particular individual or individuals.

Criminal negligence The reckless disregard for the safety of others. It is the willful indifference to an injury that could follow an act.

Day care A service in which a person receives care during the day only and does not remain overnight in the facility.

Decedent A deceased person.

Decubitus ulcer A lesion or cavity on the skin often caused by lying in one position for a prolonged period of time.

Defamation The injury of a person's reputation or character caused by the false statements of another made to a third person. Defamation includes both libel and slander.

Defendant In a criminal case, the person accused of committing a crime. In a civil suit, the party against whom the suit is brought, demanding that he or she pay the other party legal relief.

Dementia Severe impairment of mental function and global cognitive abilities of long duration in an alert individual.

Demurrer A formal objection by one of the parties to a lawsuit that the evidence presented by the other party is insufficient to sustain an issue or case.

Deposition A sworn statement of fact, made out of court, that may be admitted into evidence if it is impossible for a witness to attend a trial in person.

Diagnostic related groups (DRG) A prospective payment system for hospital care based on patient diagnosis.

Directed verdict When a trial judge decides either that the evidence and/or law is clearly in favor of one party or that the plaintiff has failed to establish a case and that it is pointless for the trial to proceed further, the judge may direct the jury to return a verdict for the appropriate party. The conclusion of the judge must be so clear and obvious that reasonable minds could not arrive at a different conclusion.

Discharge summary That part of a medical record that summarizes a patient's initial complaints, course of treatment, final diagnosis and suggestions for follow-up care.

Discovery To ascertain that which was previously unknown through a pretrial investigation; it includes testimony and documents that may be under the exclusive control of the other party. Discovery facilitates out-of-court settlements.

Dissenting opinion See Opinion of the court.

Do-not-resuscitate (DNR) A directive of a physician to withhold cardiopulmonary resuscitation in the event a patient experiences cardiac or respiratory arrest.

Durable power of attorney A legal instrument enabling an individual to act on another's behalf. In the health care setting, it includes the authority to make medical decisions for another.

Emergency A sudden unexpected occurrence or event causing a threat to life or health. The legal responsibilities of those involved in an emergency situation are measured according to the occurrence.

Employee One who works for another in return for pay.

Employer A person or firm that selects employees, pays their salaries or wages, retains the power to dismiss them, and can control their conduct during working hours.

Euthanasia An act conducted for the purpose of causing the merciful death of a person who is suffering from an incurable condition.

Evidence Proof of a fact, which is legally presented in a manner prescribed by law, at trial.

Expert witness A person who has special training, experience, skill, and knowledge in a relevant area and who is allowed to offer an opinion as testimony in court.

Facility In the context of this text, a "facility" is in most instances referring to a "nursing facility," unless within the context of its usage it is referring to all forms of health care institutions, so as to include acute care hospitals.

Federal Council on Aging (FCoA) Created in 1973, the functional successor to the earlier and smaller Advisory Council on Older Americans (authorized by the Older Americans Act of 1965). The functions of the FCoA include the continuing review and evaluation of federal policies and programs, serving as a spokesperson, and providing public forums for discussing and publicizing the needs of older Americans. For information write: 330 Independence Avenue, S.W., Washington, DC 20201 or call (202) 619–2451.

Federal question A legal question involving the United States Constitution or a statute enacted by Congress.

Felony A serious crime usually punishable by imprisonment for a period of longer than one year or by death.

Gerontological Society of America A professional organization that promotes the scientific study of aging in the biological and social sciences. For information write: Suite 350, 1275 K St., N.W., Washington, DC 20005–4006 or call (202) 842–1275.

Gerontology The study of the process of aging.

Good Samaritan laws Laws designed to protect those who stop to render aid in an emergency. These laws generally provide immunity for specified persons from any civil suit arising out of care rendered at the scene of an emergency, provided that the one rendering assistance has not done so in a grossly negligent manner.

Governing board The official body of an institution vested with the legal responsibility for its operation.

Government facility A facility operated under federal, state, or local government auspices.

Grand jury A jury called to determine whether there is sufficient evidence that a crime has been committed to justify bringing a case to trial. It is not the jury before which the case is tried to determine guilt or innocence.

Grand larceny The theft of property valued at more than a specified amount (usually $50), thus constituting a felony instead of a misdemeanor.

Guardian A person appointed by a court to protect the interests of and make decisions for a person who is incapable of making his or her own decisions.

Habeas corpus The writ to challenge the legality of imprisonment or detention.

Health According to the World Health Organization, "[a] state of complete physical, mental, and social well-being and not merely the absence of disease or infirmity."

Health Care Financing Administration (HCFA) The federal agency that coordinates the federal government's participation in the Medicare and Medicaid programs. For information write: 200 Independence Avenue, S.W., Washington, DC or call (202) 245–6145.

Health care proxy A document that delegates the authority to make one's own health care decisions to another adult, known as the health care agent, when one has become incapacitated or is unable to make his or her own decisions.

Hearsay rule A rule of evidence that restricts the admissibility of evidence that is not the personal knowledge of the witness. Hearsay evidence is admissible only under strict rules.

Holographic will A will handwritten by the testator.

Home health agency Any public agency or private organization, or a subdivision of such an agency or organization, whether operated for profit or not, that provides home health services. Home health care involves an array of services provided to patients in their homes or foster homes because of acute illness, exacerbation of chronic illness, and disability. Such services are therapeutic and/or preventive.

Home health aide A person who has completed a basic training program in personal care services to provide selected aspects of resident/patient care under nursing supervision, and other professional supervision when required by the type of care provided, to patients receiving home health agency services.

Hospice A long-term care facility for terminally ill persons. It is provided in a setting more economical than that provided in a hospital or nursing home. Hospice care is generally sought after a decision has been made to discontinue aggressive efforts to prolong life. A hospice program includes such characteristics as support services by trained individuals, family involvement, and control of pain and discomfort.

Hydration The intravenous addition of fluids to the circulatory system.

Impeachment A legislative proceeding designed to remove an executive or judicial officer from office because of misconduct.

In loco parentis A legal doctrine that permits the courts to assign a person to stand in the place of parents and possess their legal rights, duties, and responsibilities toward a child.

Incompetent An individual determined by a court to be incapable of making rational decisions on his or her own behalf.

Independent contractor One who agrees to undertake work without being under the direct control or direction of the employer.

Indictment A formal written accusation, found and presented by a grand jury, charging a person therein named with criminal conduct.

Informed consent A legal concept that provides that a patient/resident has a right to know the potential risks and benefits of a proposed procedure.

Injunction A court order either requiring one to do a certain act or prohibiting one from doing a certain act.

Interrogatories A list of questions sent from one party in a lawsuit to the other party to be answered under oath.

Judge An officer who guides court proceedings to ensure impartiality and enforces the rules of evidence. The trial judge determines the applicable law and states it to the jury. The appellate judge hears appeals and renders decisions concerning the correctness of the actions of the trial judge, the law of the case, and the sufficiency of the evidence.

Jurisdiction The right of a court to administer justice by hearing and deciding controversies.

Jurisprudence The philosophy or science of law on which a particular legal system is built.

Jury A certain number of persons selected and sworn to hear the evidence and determine the facts in a case.

Larceny The taking of another person's property without consent with the intent to permanently deprive the owner of its use and ownership.

Liability As it relates to damages, an obligation one has incurred or might incur through a negligent act.

Liability insurance A contract to have someone else pay for any liability or loss thereby in return for the payment of premiums.

Libel A false or malicious writing that is intended to defame or dishonor another person and is published so that someone other than the one defamed will observe it.

License A permit from the state allowing certain acts to be performed, usually for a specific period of time.

Life care community A self-sufficient residential community that provides residential, social, medical, and nursing services to its members.

Litigation A trial in court to determine legal issues, rights, and duties between the parties to the litigation.

Living will A document in which an individual expresses in advance his or her wishes regarding the application of life sustaining treatment in the event he or she is incapable of doing so at some future time.

Long-term care The provision of a variety of services (e.g., personal, medical, and social) to individuals who are unable to care for themselves. Such services are generally required by the elderly, as a result of diminishing health, or by others who might be disabled from some illness or other disability. Long-term care facilities utilized for providing services and programs include nursing facilities, adult day care centers, and home health agencies.

Malfeasance The execution of an unlawful or improper act.

Malpractice Professional misconduct, improper discharge of professional duties, or failure to meet the standard of care of a professional that resulted in harm to another. The negligence or carelessness of a professional person, such as a nurse, pharmacist, physician, accountant, etc.

Mandamus An action brought in a court of competent jurisdiction to compel a lower court or administrative agency to perform or not to perform a specific act.

Mayhem The crime of intentionally disfiguring or dismembering another.

Medicaid The medical assistance provided in Title XIX of the Social Security Act. Medicaid is a state administered program for the medically indigent.

Medical staff All physicians and dentists appointed by the governing authority and responsible to such authority for the adequacy and quality of the medical care rendered to the residents/patients in a facility.

Medicare The medical assistance provided in Title XVIII of the Social Security Act. Medicare is a health insurance program administered by the Social Security Administration for persons aged 65 years and over and for disabled persons who are eligible for benefits. Medicare Part A benefits provide coverage for inpatient hospital care, skilled nursing facility care, home health care, and hospice care. Medicare Part B benefits provide coverage for physician services, outpatient hospital services, diagnostic tests, various therapies, durable medical equipment, medical supplies, and prosthetic devices.

Misdemeanor An unlawful act of a less serious nature than a felony, usually punishable by a jail sentence for a term of less than one year and/or a fine.

Misfeasance The improper performance of an act.

National Council on the Aging (NCA) A nonprofit membership organization for professionals and volunteers that serves as a national resource for information, technical assistance, training, and research relating to the field of aging. For information write: West Wing 100, 600 Maryland Avenue, S.W., Washington, DC 20024 or call (202) 479–1200.

National Institute on Aging (NIA) The NIA is the principal federal agency for conducting and supporting biomedical, social, and behavioral research related to the aging process as well as the diseases and special problems of older persons. For information write: Public Information Office, Federal Building, Room 6C12, 9000 Rockville Pike, Bethesda, MD 20892 or call (301) 496–1752.

National Foundation for Long-Term Health Care A private nonprofit organization that works on behalf of professionals who provide long-term care to older persons and the chronically ill. For information write: Suite 402, 1200 15th Street, N.W., Washington, DC 20005 or call (202) 659–3148.

National Geriatrics Society A nonprofit educational scientific organization that works to advance the quality of care provided to older, chronically ill, disabled, or convalescent patients. For information write: 212 West Wisconsin Avenue, Milwaukee, WI 53203.

Negligence The omission or commission of an act that a reasonably prudent person would or would not do under given circumstances. It is a form of heedlessness or carelessness that constitutes a departure from the standard of care generally imposed on members of society.

Next of kin Those persons who by the law of descent would be adjudged the closest blood relatives of the decedent.

Non compos mentis "Not of sound mind"; suffering from some form of mental defect.

Nonfeasance The failure to act, when there is a duty to act, as a reasonably prudent person would in similar circumstances.

Notary public A public official who administers oaths and certifies the validity of documents.

Nuncupative will An oral statement intended as a last will made in anticipation of death.

Nursing assistant/aide An unlicensed worker employed and trained to assist licensed and/or registered nursing personnel in the personal care needs of patients/residents.

Nursing facility See Nursing home below.

Nursing home A facility with three or more beds that provides nursing care or personal care to adults, such as help with bathing, correspondence, walking, eating, using the toilet, or dressing, and/or supervision over such activities as money management, ambulation, and shopping. A nursing facility may be either free standing or a distinct unit of a larger facility.

Occupational therapy The art and science of evaluation and treatment of physical and psychological dysfunctions through the use of such activities as creative, manual, industrial, educational, recreational, social, and self-help activities to enable the patient/resident to achieve his or her optimal level of self-care and productivity.

Older Americans Act An act that established a National Network on Aging, which is comprised of the U.S. Administration on Aging, State and Area Agencies on Aging, tribal organizations, and service providers. Through this network older persons in each community have access to supportive and nutrition services. The type of services available in each community varies based on the needs of the people and resources of a given area.

Ombudsman A person who is designated to speak and act on behalf of a patient/resident, especially in regard to his or her daily needs.

Opinion of the court In an appellate court decision, the reasons for the decision. One judge writes the opinion for the majority of the court. Judges who agree with the result, but for different reasons, may write concurring opinions explaining their reasons. Judges who disagree with the majority may write dissenting opinions.

Ordinance A law passed by a municipal legislative body.

Palliative care Care that is intended to keep a person comfortable, but not intended to prolong life.

Peer review organization (PRO) An organization that has a contract with the Health Care Financing Administration (HCFA) to review, under Part B of Title XI of the Social Security Act, the health care services or items furnished or proposed to be furnished to Medicare beneficiaries.

Perjury The willful act of giving false testimony under oath.

Petit (petty) larceny The theft of property valued below a set monetary amount. This offense is usually classified as a misdemeanor.

Physical therapy The art and science of preventing and treating neuro-muscular or musculo-skeletal disabilities through evaluation of an individual's disability and rehabilitation potential; utilization of such physical agents as heat, cold, electricity, water, light; and neuromuscular procedures that, through their physiological effect, improve or maintain the patient's optimum functional level.

Plaintiff The party who brings a civil suit seeking damages or other legal relief.

Police power The power of the state to protect the health, safety, morals, and general welfare of the people.

Preadmission screening Assessment of the appropriateness of nursing facility placement prior to admission.

Privileged communication A statement made to an attorney, physician, spouse, or anyone else in a position of trust. Because of the confidential nature of such information, the law protects it from being revealed even in court. The term is applied in two distinct situations. First, the communications between certain persons, such as physician and patient, cannot be divulged without consent of the patient. Second, in some situations the law provides an exemption from liability for disclosing information where there is a higher duty to speak, such as statutory reporting requirements.

Probate The judicial proceeding that determines the existence and validity of a will.

Probate court A court with jurisdiction over wills. Its powers range from deciding the validity of a will to distributing property.

Prognosis An informed judgment regarding the likely course and probable outcome of a disease.

Proprietary nursing facility A nursing facility operated under private commercial ownership.

Proximate In immediate relation with something else. In negligence cases, the careless act must be the proximate cause of injury.

Real evidence Evidence furnished by tangible things, such as weapons, bullets, and equipment.

Rebuttal The giving of evidence to contradict the effect of evidence introduced by the opposing party.

Registered nurse One who is qualified for the title of R.N. by meeting the educational and licensure requirements of the state in which he or she is licensed.

Regulatory agency An arm of the government that enforces legislation regulating an act or activity in a particular area—for example, the federal Food and Drug Administration.

Rehabilitation therapy services Therapy services that include, but are not limited to, occupational therapy, physical therapy, speech pathology, or audiology.

Release A statement signed by one person relinquishing a right or claim against another.

Remand The referral of a case by an appeals court back to the original court, out of which it came, for the purpose of having some action taken there.

Res gestae "The thing done"; all of the surrounding events that become part of an incident. If statements are made as part of the incident, they are admissible in court as res gestae in spite of the hearsay rule.

Res ipsa loquitur "The thing speaks for itself"; a doctrine of law applicable to cases where the defendant had exclusive control of the thing that caused the harm and where the harm ordinarily could not have occurred without negligent conduct.

Res judicata That which has been acted on or decided by the courts.

Resident, nursing home An individual who has been admitted to and resides in a nursing home and who is entitled to receive care, treatment, and services.

Resource utilization group A prospective payment system of reimbursement for nursing facility care under Medicaid based on the characteristics and care needs of a facility's residents.

Respite care A program of informal support for family members who are in need of relief from their own care-giving responsibilities. It can, for example, be given in the caregiver's home or a nursing facility.

Respondeat superior "Let the master answer"; an aphorism meaning that the employer is responsible for the legal consequences of the acts of the servant or employee who is acting within the scope of his or her employment.

Restraint Restraints can be either "physical" or "chemical." A physical restraint involves a device (e.g., safety belts, safety bars, geriatric chairs and bedrails) that restricts or limits voluntary movement and that cannot be removed by the resident.

Slander A false oral statement, made in the presence of a third person, that injures the character or reputation of another.

Social Security Administration (SSA) The SSA is the federal agency responsible for the social security retirement, survivors and disability insurance and supplemental security income programs. For information write: Office of Public Inquiries, 402 Security Boulevard, Baltimore, MD 21235 or call (301) 594–1234.

Speech pathology The nonmedical evaluation, diagnosis, and treatment of human language, voice, and speech disorders and their etiologies.

Standard of care A description of the conduct that is expected of an individual in a given situation. It is a measure against which a defendant's conduct is compared.

Stare decisis "Let the decision stand"; the legal doctrine that prescribes adherence to those precedents set forth in cases that have been decided.

Statute of limitations A legal limit on the time allowed for filing suit in civil matters, usually measured from the time of the wrong or from the time when a reasonable person would have discovered the wrong.

Statutory law Law that is prescribed by legislative enactments.

Stipulation An agreement, usually in writing, by attorneys on opposite sides of an issue as to any matter pertaining to the proceedings. A stipulation is not binding unless agreed upon by the parties involved in the issue.

Subpoena ad testificandum A court order requiring one to appear in court to give testimony.

Subpoena duces tecum A court order that commands a person to come to court and to produce whatever documents are named in the order.

Subrogation The substitution of one person for another in reference to a lawful claim or right.

Suit A court proceeding where one person seeks damages or other legal remedies from another.

Summary judgment Generally, an immediate decision by a judge, without jury deliberation.

Summons A court order directed to the sheriff or other appropriate official to notify the defendant in a civil suit that a suit has been filed and when and where to appear.

Surrogate decision maker An individual who has been designated to make decisions on behalf of an individual determined incapable of making his or her own decisions.

Tertiary care Highly specialized care generally provided in a major medical center, often a teaching hospital.

Testimony An oral statement of a witness given under oath at a trial.

Tort A civil wrong committed by one individual against another. Torts may be classified as either intentional or unintentional. If a tort is classified as a criminal wrong (e.g., assault, battery, and false imprisonment), the wrongdoer could be held liable in a criminal action as well as a civil action.

Tort-feasor A person who commits a tort.

Trial court The court in which evidence is presented to a judge or jury for decision.

Union shop contract A labor–management agreement making continued employment contingent on joining the union.

Venue The geographic district in which an action is or may be brought.

Verdict The formal declaration of a jury's findings of fact, signed by the jury foreman and presented to the court.

Voluntary nonprofit nursing facility A nursing facility operated under voluntary or nonprofit auspices, including church-related facilities.

Waiver The intentional giving up of a right, such as allowing another person to testify to information that would ordinarily be protected as a privileged communication.

Will A legal declaration of the intentions a person wishes to have carried out after death concerning property, children, or estate. A will designates a person or persons to serve as the executor(s) responsible for carrying out the instructions of the will.

Witness A person who is called to give testimony in a court of law.

Writ A written order that is issued to a person or persons, requiring the performance of some specified act or giving authority to have it done.

Appendix B

Consent to Use of Restraints

Name of Resident:____

Notice of Some Consequences of Using/Not Using Restraints

The use of restraints can result in declines in functioning, including chronic constipation, incontinence, pressure sores, loss of muscle tone, loss of independent mobility, increased agitation, loss of balance, withdrawal or depression, reduced social contact, loss of bone mass and possibility of death by strangulation.

Some types of restraints, for some residents, can also promote mobility and a greater degree of socialization by allowing the resident a greater degree of independent functioning.

If a resident is likely to fall if not restrained, it is important to understand that falls are a leading cause of death in the elderly population. From 10 to 25 percent of falls by nursing home residents result in significant injury, such as hip, rib or other fractures. Injuries of this kind in an elderly person may result in complications that require even more extensive treatment or, in some instances, result in death.

If a resident is confused and likely to wander if not restrained, it is important to understand that although the facility takes reasonable precautions to have a safe environment and prevent confused residents from leaving the facility, it is not possible to individually monitor all residents at all times.

* * *

Source: Courtesy of Arden House Nursing Home, Hamden, CT.

The attending physician has recommended the use of the following restraints (specify):

The purpose of these restraints is to (specify for each recommended restraint):

I have read the Notice regarding the use/non-use of restraints and it was explained to me and discussed with me by________________________

________________________ on ________________________.
(name of staff) (date)

____ I understand the risks and benefits of using the restraints listed above and hereby give my consent to their use.

____ I understand the risks and benefits of using the restraints listed above and do not consent to their use.

Signed____
Resident

or

Signed____
Conservator, Power of Attorney for Health Care, or
Responsible Relative (please specify)

Witness____

Date____

Appendix C

Residents' Bill of Rights

EXERCISING YOUR RIGHTS

- You have the right to be fully informed, orally and in writing, in a language you understand, of your rights and the facility's rules governing resident conduct and responsibilities, and of changes in your rights and in the facility's rules.
- You have the right to exercise your rights as a resident and as a citizen. The facility must protect and promote your rights and encourage and assist you in exercising them.
- You have the right to be treated equally with other residents in receiving care and services, and regarding transfer and discharge, regardless of the source of payment for your care.
- You have the right to exercise your rights without fear of discrimination, restraint, interference, coercion or reprisal.

DIGNITY AND SELF-DETERMINATION

- You have the right to be treated with consideration, respect and full recognition of your dignity and individuality.
- You have the right to reasonable accommodation of your individual needs and preferences, except when your health or safety of others would be endangered.
- You have the right to choose activities, schedules and health care consistent with your interests and your assessment and plan of care.
- You have the right to make choices about aspects of your life that are significant to you.

- You have the right to keep and use your personal possessions, as space permits, unless doing so would infringe on the rights, health or safety of other residents.
- You have the right to notice before your roommate is changed.

PRIVACY

- You have the right to privacy in accommodations, in receiving personal and medical care and treatment, in written and telephone communications, in visits and in meetings with family and resident groups. However, the facility is not required to provide you with a private room.
- You have the right to associate and communicate privately with persons of your choice, including other residents.
- If you are married, you have the right to privacy for visits with your spouse.
- If you are married and your spouse is a resident of this facility, you have the right to share a room with your spouse, subject to his or her consent.

COMMUNICATING WITH OTHERS

- You have the right to privacy in written and spoken communications.
- You have the right to send and receive unopened mail promptly.
- You have the right to have stationery, stamps and writing implements made available by the facility for you to purchase.
- You have the right to a regularly available telephone that you can use in privacy.
- You have the right to interact with persons both inside and outside of the facility.
- You have the right to receive information from agencies that act as client advocates and to have the opportunity to contact such agencies.

Source: Reprinted by permission of Murtha, Cullina, Richter, and Pinney, Two Whitney Avenue, New Haven, CT 06510.

VISITS

- You have the right to be visited by your family.
- You have the right to be visited by your attending physician, by the nursing home Ombudsman, and representatives of federal and state agencies concerned with resident care.

- You have the right to be visited by any other person of your choice, including persons who provide services to nursing home residents, subject to reasonable restrictions.
- You have the right to refuse to receive any visitor you do not want to see.

GROUP ACTIVITIES

- You have the right to participate in social, religious and community activities that do not interfere with the rights of other residents.
- You have the right to organize and participate in resident groups in the facility.
- Your family has the right to meet with families of other residents in the facility.

GRIEVANCES

- You have the right to voice grievances and recommend changes in facility policies and services to staff or to outside representatives of your choice.
- You have the right to have prompt efforts made by the facility to resolve grievances you may have, including those about the behavior of other residents.
- You have the right to file a complaint with the Connecticut Department of Health Services or the Connecticut Department of Aging regarding abuse, neglect or misappropriation of residents' property.

CARE AND TREATMENT

- You have the right to choose your personal attending physician.
- You have the right to be fully informed, in a language you understand, about your total health status, including your medical conditions.
- You have the right to participate in planning your care and treatment and to be fully informed in advance about changes in your care and treatment that affect your well-being.
- You have the right to refuse treatment.
- You have the right to administer your own drugs, unless your care planning team has determined that it would not be safe for you to do so.
- You have the right to the opinions of two physicians concerning the need for surgery, prior to surgery, except in an emergency.
- You have the right to refuse to participate in experimental research.
- You have the right to be free from restraints and psychoactive drugs administered for discipline or convenience and not required to treat your medical symptoms. Physical and chemical restraints may be used only to ensure your physical safety or enable you to function better, and then only on the written order of a physician that states when and for how long they are to be used, except in an emergency.

- You have the right to have psychopharmacologic drugs administered only on orders of a physician, as part of a written care plan designed to eliminate or modify the symptoms the drug was prescribed to treat, and only if an independent external consultant reviews whether your drug plan is appropriate at least once a year.
- You have the right to be free from verbal, sexual, physical or mental abuse, corporal punishment and involuntary seclusion.
- You have the right not to perform work for the facility. If performing work for the facility is recommended as part of your care plan and suitable work is available, you have the right to choose to perform work for the facility and to choose whether you wish to work as a volunteer or for payment at prevailing rates, if your choice and the kind of work you will be doing are documented in your care plan.
- You have the right to see the results of current federal, state and local inspection reports and plans of correction.

PERSONAL AND CLINICAL RECORDS

- You have the right to privacy and confidentiality of your personal and clinical records.
- You have the right to approve or refuse the release of these records to anyone outside the facility, except when you are transferred to another health care institution or the release of your records is required by law or by third party payors such as Medicare, Medicaid or private insurers.

TRANSFER AND DISCHARGE

- You have the right to be allowed to stay in the facility and may not be discharged from the facility, except as provided by federal law and Connecticut General Statutes section 19a-535. Federal and State law permit an involuntary transfer or discharge only when the transfer or discharge is necessary for your welfare and your welfare cannot be met in the facility; or transfer or discharge is appropriate because your health has improved so that you no longer need the services provided by the facility; or the health or safety of individuals in the facility is endangered; or, if you are paying for your care, your account is more than fifteen days in arrears; or if the facility ceases to operate.
- You must be given thirty days notice of a transfer or discharge from the facility unless the transfer or discharge is made because the health or safety of individuals in the facility is endangered; your health has improved sufficiently to allow for a more immediate transfer or discharge; immediate transfer or discharge is necessary due to urgent medical need; or you have resided

in the facility for less than thirty days. In such cases, you must be given as much notice as practicable.

- You have the right to appeal an involuntary transfer or discharge from the facility to the Connecticut Department of Health Services.
- You may be involuntarily transferred from one room to another within the facility only for medical reasons or for your welfare or that of other residents, as documented in your medical record. You must be given thirty days written notice, except where the health, safety or welfare of other patients is endangered; where immediate transfer within the facility is required by your urgent medical needs; or you have resided in the facility for less than thirty days. In such cases, you must be given as much notice as practicable.
- You may not be involuntarily transferred or discharged from the facility or transferred within the facility if the transfer or discharge presents imminent danger of death.

PAYMENT FOR SERVICES

- You have the right to be fully informed of the services available in the facility, and, if you are paying for the cost of your care, of the per diem rate and charges for any services not covered by the per diem rate. If your care is paid for by Medicare or Medicaid, you have the right to be informed of the services that are not covered by Medicare or Medicaid and the charges for such services.
- You cannot be required to waive any rights you may have to receive Medicare or Medicaid, or to give assurances that you are not eligible or will not apply for Medicare or Medicaid, as a condition of admission to or continued residence in the facility.
- You cannot be required to have a third party guarantee payment for your care as a condition of admission to or continued residence in the facility.
- You cannot be required to pay or give the facility any gift, money, donation for their consideration as a condition of admission to or continued residence in the facility.
- You have the right to be informed of how to apply for and use Medicare and Medicaid and how to receive refunds for previous payments covered by these programs.

PERSONAL FUNDS

- You have the right to manage your personal financial affairs and cannot be required to deposit your personal funds with the facility.

- You have the right to have the facility manage your personal funds, if you authorize this in writing. You have the right to a quarterly accounting of your funds. A separate statement about how the facility manages residents's funds is provided.

RESIDENTS' RIGHTS REGARDING PERSONAL FUNDS

You have the right to manage your own personal financial affairs. You are not required to deposit your personal funds with the facility. However, you are entitled to have the facility manage your personal funds if you or your legally liable relative, guardian or Conservator give the facility your request or consent in writing. The facility must give you a quarterly accounting of financial transactions made on your behalf and follow other procedures prescribed by law in managing your funds. Pursuant to federal law and Connecticut General Statutes Section 19a-551, the facility must not commingle your personal funds with the facility's funds; must obtain a signed receipt for each expenditure from your personal funds and maintain an individualized itemized record of income and expenses and give you or your legally liable relative, guardian or Conservator access to this record; must give you a quarterly accounting; and, if you are receiving Medicaid assistance, must notify you or your legal representative in writing when the amount in the account reaches $1,400. If you are receiving Medicaid assistance, if the amount in your personal funds account plus the value of any other non-exempt assets reaches $1,600, you may lose your eligibility for assistance.

The facility must pay you interest at the rate of at least five (5) percent per year on any security deposit or other advance payment required by the facility prior to your admission. If the facility does not refund the amount of any such advance deposit due upon your discharge or death within thirty days of your discharge or death, the facility must pay interest at the rate of ten (10) percent from the date of discharge or death.

Lists of charges that are not covered by the basic self-pay per diem rate or by Medicare or Medicaid are attached.

I hereby acknowledge that I have received a copy of this residents' bill of rights and that it has been explained to me by the facility's staff.

____________________ ________________________________

Date Signature of Resident

or

____

Signature of Conservator, Power of Attorney or Relative (please specify)

I have received a copy of residents' rights regarding personal funds.

____
Signature of Resident
or

____
Signature of Conservator, Power of Attorney or Relative (please specify)

____
Date

Appendix D

National Practitioner Data Bank Forms

Exhibit D-1 Adverse Action Report

National Practitioner Data Bank
P.O. Box 6048
Camarillo, CA 93011-6048

ADVERSE ACTION REPORT

OMB NO. 0915-0126
EXP. DATE 3/31/91

FOR DATA BANK USE ONLY

Document Number of Previous Report (To be entered by Reporting Entity only when submitting a "Correction or Addition," or "Void Previous Report.")

SECTION A — REPORTING ENTITY INFORMATION

1. Data Bank ID (15)
2. Type of Report ☐ Initial Report ☐ Correction or Addition ☐ Revision to Action ☐ Void Previous Report
3. Type of Adverse Action Taken ☐ Licensure ☐ Clinical Privileges ☐ Society Membership
4. Entity Name (40)
5. Street Address (40)
6. City (28)
7. State (2)
8. Zip Code (5 or 9)

SECTION B — PRACTITIONER INFORMATION

Add'l info. (see instructions)

9. Practitioner Name Last (25) | First (15) | Middle (15) | Suffix (3)
10. Other Name Used Last (25) | First (15) | Middle (15) | Suffix (3)
11. Organization Name (40)
12. Work Address (40)
12. City (28)
14. State (2)
15. Zip Code (5 or 9)
16. County (if not U.S.) (10)
17. Home Address (40)
18. City (28)
19. State (2)
20. Zip Code (5 or 9)
21. County (if not U.S.) (10)
22. a. License Number (16)
22. b. State of Licensure (2)
22. c. Field of Licensure (3)
23. Date of Birth (mm/dd/yy)
24. Social Security Number (U.S.) (9)
25. Federal DEA No. (12)
26. a. Professional School Attended (40)
26. b. Year of Graduation (4)

SECTION C — ADVERSE ACTION INFORMATION

27. Date of Action (mm/dd/yy)
28. Adverse Action Classification Code (5)
29. Length of Action (in months)
30. Effective Date of Action (mm/dd/yy)
30. Description of the acts or omissions or other reasons for the action taken, and if known and if applicable, the reasons for surrender of clinical privileges (600)

SECTION D — CERTIFICATION

I certify that the reporting entity or individual identified in Section A of this report is authorized, under the provisions of P.L. 99-660, as amended, and as specified in 45 CFR Part 60, to provide this information to the National Practitioner Data Bank. I further certify that the reporting entity or individual has authorized me to submit this report to the Data Bank and that the information provided is true and complete.

WARNING: Any person who knowingly makes a false statement or misrepresentation to the National Practitioner Data Bank is subject to a fine and imprisonment under Federal statute.

32. Printed Name of Authorized Representative (40)
33. Title of Authorized Representative (40)
34. Telephone Number (15) ( ) , ext.
35. Signature Date (mm/dd/yy)
36. Signature of Authorized Representative

HRSA-530 (3/90) WHITE-DATA BANK YELLOW-STATE MEDICAL OR DENTAL BOARD PINK-OTHER STATE LICENSING BOARD GOLD-REPORTING ENTITY

Exhibit D-2 Additional Information

EXP. DATE 3/31/91

ADDITIONAL INFORMATION

FOR DATA BANK USE ONLY

1. Data Bank ID (15) (Repeat from item 1 on the main form)	2. Page of	3. Date (mm/dd/yy)	4. Initials

5. Practitioner Name Last (25)	First Init.	Middle Init.	Suffix

ADDITIONAL LICENSE NUMBERS Add'l info (see instructions)

a. License Number (16)	b. State of Licensure (2)	c. Field of Licensure (3)
a. License Number (16)	b. State of Licensure (2)	c. Field of Licensure (3)
a. License Number (16)	b. State of Licensure (2)	c. Field of Licensure (3)

ADDITIONAL FEDERAL DEA NUMBERS Add'l info (see instructions)

Federal DEA Number (12)	Federal DEA Number (12)

ADDITIONAL PROFESSIONAL SCHOOLS ATTENDED Add'l info (see instructions)

a. Professional School Attended (40)	b. Year of Graduation
a. Professional School Attended (40)	b. Year of Graduation
a. Professional School Attended (40)	b. Year of Graduation

ADDITIONAL HOSPITAL AFFILIATIONS Add'l info (see instructions)

a. Hospital Affiliation (40)	b. City (28)	c. State (2)
a. Hospital Affiliation (40)	b. City (28)	c. State (2)
a. Hospital Affiliation (40)	b. City (28)	c. State (2)

NARRATIVE DESCRIPTIONS CONTINUED

38. Description of the acts or omissions and injuries or illnesses upon which the action or claim was based

39. Description and total amount of judgment or settlement and any conditions attached thereto, including terms of payment

INSTRUCTIONS

Use this form as an addendum to one of the following National Practitioner Data Bank main forms: *Medical Malpractice Payment Report; Adverse Action Report; Request for Information Disclosure;* or *Request for Information Disclosure–Supplement.* Use this form only when you are providing more than one License Number, Federal DEA Number, Professional School Attended, or Hospital Affiliation, or are continuing the narrative descriptions requested in Items 38 and 39 of the *Medical Malpractice Payment Report.* Please be sure that you have placed an "X" in the "Add'l. Info." box in the appropriate section heading on the main form.

1. Please provide your Entity's Data Bank ID–report from Item 1 on the main form.
2. Enter this *Additional Information* form's page number in the first blank, and the total number of pages (including the main form) in the second blank.
3. Enter the same date you entered for the signature date on the main form.
4. Each *Additional Information* form must bear the initials of the same person who signed the main form.
5. Please provide the Practitioner's last name as stated on the main form, as well as the initials for the first and middle names, and a suffix, if used.
6. In the appropriate section, fill in the additional information items following the instructions for the main form. If more space is needed, place an "X" in the "Add'l. Info." box, and continue to provide all known information on another form.
7. After all information has been completed, enclose (do not attach) form(s) with the main form.

HRSA-531 (3/90) SEE MAIN FORM FOR COPY DISTRIBUTION

Exhibit D-3 Request for Information Disclosure

National Practitioner Data Bank
P.O. Box 6050
Camarillo, CA 93011-6050

REQUEST FOR INFORMATION DISCLOSURE

OMB. NO. 0915-0126
EXP. DATE 3/31/91

FOR DATA BANK USE ONLY

SECTION A–REQUESTING ENTITY INFORMATION

1. Data Bank ID (15)	2. Total Number of Practitioners	3. Page 1 of

4. Type of Query: ☐ Privileging or Employment ☐ Professional Review Activity ☐ Mandatory Two-Year ☐ State Licensing Board ☐ Self Query ☐ Other

5. Entity Name (40)

6. Street Address (40)

7. City (28)	8. State (2)	9. Zip Code (5 or 9)

SECTION B–PRACTITIONER INFORMATION

Add'l info (see instructions)

10. Practitioner Name Last (25)	First (15)	Middle(15)	Suffix (3)
11. Other Name Used Last (25)	First (15)	Middle(15)	Suffix (3)

12. Organization Name (40)

13. Work Address (40)

14. City (28)	15. State (2)	16. Zip Code (5 or 9)	17. County (if not U.S.) (10)

18. Home Address (40)

19. City (28)	20. State (2)	21. Zip Code (5 or 9)	22. County (if not U.S.) (10)

23. a. License Number (16)	23. b. State of Licensure (2)	23. c. Field of Licensure (3)

24. Date of Birth (mm/dd/yy)	25. Social Security Number (U.S.) (9)	26. Federal DEA No. (12)

27. a. Professional School Attended (40)	27. b. Year of Graduation (4)

SECTION C–CERTIFICATION

I certify that the requesting entity identified in Section A of this form is authorized, under the provisions of P.L. 99-660, as amended, and as specified in 45 CFR Part 60, to request and receive information from the National Practitioner Data Bank. I further certify that the information provided on this form is true and complete, and that the requesting entity identified in Section A of this form has authorized me to request this information.

If this is a self query, I certify that I am authorized to request this information, and I am the practitioner described in Section B of this form. I further certify that the information provided on this form is true and complete.

WARNING: Any person who knowingly makes a false statement or misrepresentation to the National Practitioner Data Bank is subject to a fine and imprisonment under Federal statute.

28. Printed Name of Authorized Representative/Agent/Self Querier (40)

29. Title of Authorized Representative or Agent (40)

30. Telephone Number (15) ( ) , ext.	31. Signature Date (mm/dd/yy)	32. Signature of Authorized Representative/Agent/Self Querier

SECTION D–AUTHORIZED AGENT INFORMATION

33. Agent Data Bank ID (15)	34. Agent Street Address (40)

35. City (28)	8. State (2)	9. Zip Code (5 or 9)

SECTION E–SELF QUERY NOTIFICATION

The individual named in Section A and further indentified in Section B of this form has appeared before me in person on the ______________ day of ______, 19___ and is known to me to be that individual. My notary seal appears in the lower right corner of this form.

38. Printed Name of Notary	39. Date Commission Expires (mm/dd/yy)
40. Signature of Notary	41. Notary Number

WHITE-DATA BANK YELLOW-REQUESTING ENTITY

HRSA-532 (3/90)

Exhibit D-4 Request for Information Disclosure–Supplement

National Practitioner Data Bank
P.O. Box 6050
Camarillo, CA 93011-6050

REQUEST FOR INFORMATION DISCLOSURE–SUPPLEMENT

OMB NO. 0915-0126
EXP. DATE 3/31/91

FOR DATA BANK USE ONLY

1. Data Bank ID (15)	2. Page of	3. Date (mm/dd/yy)	4. Intials

SECTION B — PRACTITIONER INFORMATION

10. Practitioner Name Last (25)	First (15)	Middle (15)	Suffix (3)
11. Other Name Used Last (25)	First (15)	Middle (15)	Suffix (3)
12. Organization Name (40)			
13. Work Address (40)			
14. City (28)	15. State (2)	16. Zip Code (5 or 9)	17. County (if not U.S.) (10)
18. Home Address (40)			
19. City (28)	20. State (2)	21. Zip Code (5 or 9)	22. County (if not U.S.) (10)
23. a. License Number (16)		23. b. State of Licensure (2)	23. c. Field of Licensure (3)
24. Date of Birth (mm/dd/yy)	25. Social Security Number (U.S.) (9)	26. Federal DEA No. (12)	
27. a. Professional School Attended (40)			27. b. Year of Graduation (4)

SECTION B — PRACTITIONER INFORMATION Add'l info. (see instructions)

10. Practitioner Name Last (25)	First (15)	Middle (15)	Suffix (3)
11. Other Name Used Last (25)	First (15)	Middle (15)	Suffix (3)
12. Organization Name (40)			
13. Work Address (40)			
14. City (28)	15. State (2)	16. Zip Code (5 or 9)	17. County (if not U.S.) (10)
18. Home Address (40)			
19. City (28)	20. State (2)	21. Zip Code (5 or 9)	22. County (if not U.S.) (10)
23. a. License Number (16)		23. b. State of Licensure (2)	23. c. Field of Licensure (3)
24. Date of Birth (mm/dd/yy)	25. Social Security Number (U.S.) (9)	26. Federal DEA No. (12)	
27. a. Professional School Attended (40)			27. b. Year of Graduation (4)

SECTION B — PRACTITIONER INFORMATION Add'l info. (see instructions)

10. Practitioner Name Last (25)	First (15)	Middle (15)	Suffix (3)
11. Other Name Used Last (25)	First (15)	Middle (15)	Suffix (3)
12. Organization Name (40)			
13. Work Address (40)			
14. City (28)	15. State (2)	16. Zip Code (5 or 9)	17. County (if not U.S.) (10)
18. Home Address (40)			
19. City (28)	20. State (2)	21. Zip Code (5 or 9)	22. County (if not U.S.) (10)
23. a. License Number (16)		23. b. State of Licensure (2)	23. c. Field of Licensure (3)
24. Date of Birth (mm/dd/yy)	25. Social Security Number (U.S.) (9)	26. Federal DEA No. (12)	
27. a. Professional School Attended (40)			27. b. Year of Graduation (4)

WHITE-DATA BANK YELLOW-REQUESTING ENTITY

HRSA-532-1 (3/90)

Appendix E

Living Will Forms

Exhibit E-1 Living Will Declaration

Right To Die 250 West 57th Street/New York, NY 10107	**Living Will Declaration**
INSTRUCTIONS *Consult this column for guidance.*	To My Family, Doctors, and All Those Concerned with My Care
This declaration sets forth your directions regarding medical treatment.	I, ______________________, being of sound mind, make this statement as a directive to be followed if I become unable to participate in decisions regarding my medical care. If I should be in an incurable or irreversible mental or physical condition with no reasonable expectation of recovery, I direct my attending physician to withhold treatment that merely prolongs my dying. I further direct that treatment be limited to measures to keep me comfortable and to relieve pain.
You have the right to refuse treatment you do not want, and you may request the care you do want.	These directions express my legal right to refuse treatment. Therefore I expect my family, doctors, and everyone concerned with my care to regard themselves as legally and morally bound to act in accord with my wishes, and in so doing to be free of any legal liability for having followed my directions.
You may list specific treatment you do not want. For example: *Cardiac resuscitation* *Mechanical respiration* *Artificial feeding/fluids by tube* *Otherwise, your general statement, top right, will stand for your wishes.*	I especially do not want: ______________________ ______________________ ______________________ ______________________
You may want to add instructions or care you do want—for example, pain medication; or that you prefer to die at home if possible.	Other instructions/comments: ______________________ ______________________ ______________________
If you want, you can name someone to see that your wishes are carried out, but you do not have to do this.	**Proxy Designation Clause:** Should I become unable to communicate my instructions as stated above, I designate the following person to act on my behalf: Name ______________________ Address ______________________ If the person named above is unable to act on my behalf, I authorize the following person to do so: Name ______________________ Address ______________________ This Living Will Declaration expresses my personal treatment preferences. The fact that I may have also executed a document in the form recommended by state law should not be construed to limit or contradict this Living Will Declaration, which is an expression of my common-law and constitutional rights.
Sign and date here in the presence of two adult witnesses, who should also sign.	Signed: ______________________ Date: __________ Witness: ______________ Witness: ______________ Address: ______________ Address: ______________ Keep the signed original with your personal papers at home. Give signed copies to doctors, family, and proxy. Review your Declaration from time to time: intial and date it to show it still expresses your intent.

Tear off and mail to: Society for the Right to Die, 250 W. 57th Street, New York, NY 10107.

The Annual Report of the Society for the Right to Die is available from NY State Dept. of State, Office of Charitable Contributions, 162 Washington Ave., Albany, NY 12230

Please send me __________ additional copies of the Living Will Declaration.

☐ I am enclosing my dues/contribution in support of the Society's program.

(Please make checks payable to Society for the Right to Die. *Minimum annual membership dues: $15.*)

☐ $15 ☐ $35 ☐ $100 ☐ Other $ ________

Name ______________________

Address ______________________

City ______________ State __________ Zip __________

☐ I am enclosing names and addresses of others to receive information from the Society.

Note: Forms may be purchased from Julius Blumberg, Inc., NYC 10013, or any of its dealers. Reproduction prohibited.

Source: Reprinted by permission of Society for the Right to Die, 250 West 57th Street, New York, NY 10107.

Exhibit E-1 continued

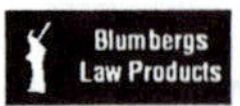

P 3202—LIVING WILL, 5-85

WARNING: This document may be legally binding. Consult an attorney as to its legal effect.

Living Will

To: My Family, my Physician, my Lawyer, my Clergyman, any Medical Facility in whose care I happen to be and any individual who may become responsible for my Health, Welfare or Affairs:

If the time comes when I can no longer take part in decisions concerning my life, I wish and direct the following:

If a situation should arise in which there is no reasonable expectation for my recovery from extreme physical or mental disability, I direct that I be allowed to die, and not be kept alive by medications, artificial means, life support equipment or "heroic measures". I do, however, ask that medication be mercifully administered to me to alleviate suffering even though this may shorten my remaining life.

This statement is made after careful consideration and is in accordance with my convictions and beliefs. I urge those concerned to take whatever action necessary, including legal action, to fulfill my wishes and directions. To the extent that the provisions of this document are not legally enforceable, I hope that those to whom it is addressed will regard themselves as morally bound by it.

Elective Provisions
Check the box and write initials next to each election you desire.

☐............ 1. I wish to live out my last days at home rather than in a hospital if it does not jeopardize the chance of my recovery to a meaningful and conscious life and does not impose an undue burden on my family.

☐............ 2. If any of my tissues or organs are sound and would be of value as transplants to other people, I freely give my permission for such donations.

In Witness Whereof, I state that I have read this, my living will, know and understand its contents and sign my name below.

Dated.. 19............ ....
Signature

Witness*.. Print or type full name, address & tel. no. of person signing.

....

....

....

Witness*..

....

....

....

....

*After each witness signature print or type full name, address and tel. no.

Copies of this document have been given to the following:

Name ____________________ Name ____________________
Address ____________________ Address ____________________
____________________ ____________________
Telephone ____________________ Telephone ____________________

Your state may have specific rules regarding this living will such as how long it will be effective, requirements for witnesses, etc. Consult your attorney before signing.

Optional Acknowledgement

STATE OF
COUNTY OF ss.:
On 19 before me personally came
to me known, and known to me to be the individual described in, and who executed the foregoing instrument, and he acknowledged to me that he executed the same. ____________________

Exhibit E-2 Missouri

MISSOURI

DECLARATION

I have the primary right to make my own decisions concerning treatment that might unduly prolong the dying process. By this declaration I express to my physician, family and friends my intent. If I should have a terminal condition it is my desire that my dying not be prolonged by administration of death-prolonging procedures. If my condition is terminal and I am unable to participate in decisions regarding my medical treatment, I direct my attending physician to withhold or withdraw medical procedures that merely prolong the dying process and are not necessary to my comfort or to alleviate pain. It is not my intent to authorize affirmative or deliberate acts or omissions to shorten my life rather only to permit the natural process of dying.

Other instructions:

Signed this ________ day of ____________________, __________.

Signature ____

City, County and State of Residence ______________________________

The declarant is known to me, is eighteen years of age or older, of sound mind and voluntarily signed this document in my presence.

Witness ____

Address ____

Witness ____

Address ____

REVOCATION PROVISION

I hereby revoke the above declaration.

Signed ________________________________
(Signature of Declarant)

Date ____________________.

Source: Reprinted by permission of Society for the Right to Die, 250 West 57th Street, New York, NY 10107.

Appendix F

Durable Power of Attorney Forms

Exhibit F-1 Durable Power of Attorney for Health Care

BE IT KNOWN, that ,
of , the
undersigned Grantor, does hereby grant a durable power of attorney for health care to
, of
, as my attorney-in-fact and Agent.

I hereby grant to my Agent full power and authority to make health care decisions for me to the same extent that I could make such decisions for myself if I had the capacity to do so. In exercising this authority, my Agent shall make health care decisions that are consistent with my desires as stated in this document or otherwisae made known to my Agent, including, but not limited to, my desires concerning obtaining or refusing or withdrawing life prolonging care, treatment, services, and procedures.

I hereby authorize all physicians and psychiatrists who have treated me, and all other providers of health care, including hospitals, to release to my Agent all information contained in my medical records which my Agent may request. I hereby waive all privileges attached to physician-patient relationship and to any communication, verbal or written, pertaining to my physical or mental health, including medical and hospital records, and to execute any releases, waivers or other documents that may be required in order to obtain such information, and to disclose such information to such persons, organizations and health care providers as my Agent shall deem appropriate. My Agent is authorized to employ and discharge health care providers including physicians, psychiatrists, dentists, nurses, and therapists as my Agent shall deem appropriate for my physical, mental and emotional well-being. My Agent is also authorized to pay reasonable fees and expenses for such services contracted.

My Agent is authorized to apply for my admission to a medical, nursing, residential or other similar facility, execute any consent or admission forms required by such facility and enter into agreements for my care at such facility or elsewhere during my lifetime. My Agent is authorized to arrange for and consent to medical, therapeutical and surgical procedures for me including the administration of drugs. The power to make health care decisions for me shall include the power to give consent, refuse consent, or withdraw consent to any care, treatment, service, or procedure to maintain, or treat a physical or mental condition.

Exhibit F-1 continued

I reserve unto myself the right to revoke the authority granted to my Agent hereunder to make health care decisions for me by notifying the treating physician, hospital, or other health care provider orally or in writing. Notwithstanding any provision herein to the contrary, I retain the right to make medical and other health care decisions for myself so long as I am able to give informed consent with respect to a particular decision. In addition, no treatment may be given to me over my objection, and health care necessary to keep me alive may not be stopped if I object.

This power of attorney shall not be affected by subsequent disability or incapacity of the principal. Notwithstanding any provision herein to the contrary, my Agent shall take no action under this instrument unless I am deemed to be disabled or incapacitated as defined herein. My incapacity shall be deemed to exist when so certified in writing by two licensed physicians not related by blood or marriage to either me or to my Agent. The said certificate shall state that I am incapable of caring for myself and that I am physically and mentally incapable of managing my financial affairs. The certificate of the physicians described above shall be attached to the original of this instrument and if this instrument is filed or recorded among public records, then such certificate shall also be similarly filed or recorded if permitted by applicable law. To the extent permitted by law, I herewith nominate, constitute and appoint my Agent to serve as my guardian, conservator and/or in any similar representative capacity, and, if I am not permitted by law to so nominate, constitute and appoint, then I request any court of competent jurisdiction which may be petitioned by any person to appoint a guardian, conservator or similar representative for me to give due consideration to my request.

Signed this ________ day of ________________________, 19___.

Signed in the presence of:

State of , 19____
County of SS.

Then personally appeared the foregoing , as Grantor, who known to me acknowledged the foregoing to be his or her free act and deed, before me.

____
Notary Public
My Commission Expires:

c. E-Z Legal Forms

Source: Courtesy of E-Z Legal Forms. Forms may be purchased from E-Z Legal Forms, 5401 NW 102nd Avenue, Suite 139, Sunrise, FL 33351.

Exhibit F-2 Texas Durable Power of Attorney for Health Care

INFORMATION CONCERNING THE DURABLE POWER OF ATTORNEY FOR HEALTH CARE. THIS IS AN IMPORTANT LEGAL DOCUMENT. BEFORE SIGNING THIS DOCUMENT, YOU SHOULD KNOW THESE IMPORTANT FACTS:

Except to the extent you state otherwise, this document gives the person you name as your agent the authority to make any and all health care decisions for you in accordance with your wishes, including your religious and moral beliefs, when you are no longer capable of making them yourself. Because "health care" means any treatment, service, or procedure to maintain,

Exhibit F-2 continued

diagnose, or treat your physical or mental condition, your agent has the power to make a broad range of health care decisions for you. Your agent may consent, refuse to consent, or withdraw consent to medical treatment and may make decisions about withdrawing or withholding life-sustaining treatment. Your agent may not consent to voluntary inpatient mental health services, convulsive treatment, psychosurgery, or abortion. A physician must comply with your agent's instructions or allow you to be transferred to another physician.

Your agent's authority begins when your doctor certifies that you lack the capacity to make health care decisions.

Your agent is obligated to follow your instructions when making decisions on your behalf. Unless you state otherwise, your agent has the same authority to make decisions about your health care as you would have had.

It is important that you discuss this document with your physician or other health care provider before you sign it to make sure that you understand the nature and range of decisions that may be made on your behalf. If you do not have a physician, you should talk with someone else who is knowledgeable about these issues and can asnwer your questions. You do not need a lawyer's assistance to complete this document, but if there is anything in this document that you do not understand, you should ask a lawyer to explain it to you.

The person you appoint as agent should be someone you know and trust. The person must be 18 years of age or older or a person under 18 years of age who has had the disabilities of minority removed. If you appoint your health or residential care provider (e.g., your physician or an employee of a home health agency, hospital, nursing home, or residential care home, other than a relative), that person has to choose between acting as your agent or as your health or residential care provider; the law does not permit a person to do both at the same time.

You should inform the person you appoint that you want the person to be your health care agent. You should discuss this document with your agent and your physician and give each a signed copy. You should indicate on the document itself the people and institutions who have signed copies. Your agent is not liable for health care decisions made in good faith on your behalf.

Even after you have signed this document, you have the right to make health care decisions for yourself as long as you are able to do so and treatment cannot be given to you or stopped over your objection. You have the right to revoke the authority granted to your agent by informing your agent or your health or residential care provider orally or in writing, or by your execution of a subsequent durable power of attorney for health care. Unless you state otherwise, your appointment of a spouse dissolves on divorce.

This document may not be changed or modified. If you want to make changes in the document, you must make an entirely new one.

You may wish to designate an alternate agent in the event that your agent is unwilling, unable, or ineligible to act as your agent. Any alternate agent you designate has the same authority to make health care decisions for you.

THIS POWER OF ATTORNEY IS NOT VALID UNLESS IT IS SIGNED IN THE PRESENCE OF TWO OR MORE QUALIFIED WITNESSES. THE FOLLOWING PERSONS MAY NOT ACT AS WITNESSES:

(1) the person you have designated as your agent;
(2) your health or residential care provider or an employee of your health or residential care provider;
(3) your spouse;
(4) your lawful heirs or beneficiaries named in your will or a deed; or
(5) creditors or persons who have a claim against you.

Exhibit F-2 continued

I have read and understood the contents of this disclosure statement.

______________________________ ________________
(Signature) (Date)

Source: Reprinted by permission for the Right to Die, 250 West 57th Street, New York, NY 10107.

DURABLE POWER OF ATTORNEY FOR HEALTH CARE

DESIGNATION OF HEALTH CARE AGENT.

I,______________________________(insert your name) appoint:

Name:______________________________
Address:______________________________
______________________________Phone:________________

as my agent to make any and all health care decisions for me, except to the extent I state otherwise in this document. This durable power of attorney for health care takes effect if I become unable to make my own health care decisions and this fact is certified in writing by my physician.

LIMITATIONS ON THE DECISION MAKING AUTHORITY OF MY AGENT ARE AS FOLLOWS:

____
____
____

DESIGNATION OF ALTERNATE AGENT.

(You are not required to designate an alternate agent but you may do so. An alternate agent may make the same health care decisions as the designated agent if the designated agent is unable or unwilling to act as your agent. If the agent designated is your spouse, the designation is automatically revoked by law if your marriage is dissolved.)

If the person designated as my agent is unable or unwilling to make health care decisions for me, I designate the following persons to serve as my agent to make health care decisions for me as authorized by this document, who serve in the following order:

A. First Alternate Agent
Name:______________________________
Address:______________________________
______________________________Phone:________________

B. Second Alternate Agent
Name:______________________________
Address:______________________________
______________________________Phone:________________

The original of this document is kept at:______________________________
The following individuals or institutions have signed copies:
Name:______________________________
Address:______________________________

Name:______________________________
Address:______________________________

Exhibit F-2 continued

DURATION.

I understand that this power of attorney exists indefinitely from the date I execute this document unless I establish a shorter time or revoke the power of attorney. If I am unable to make health care decisions for myself when this power of attorney expires, the authority I have granted my agent continues to exist until the time I become able to make health care decisions for myself.

(IF APPLICABLE) This power of attorney ends on the following date:____________

PRIOR DESIGNATIONS REVOKED.

I revoke any prior power of attorney for health care.

ACKNOWLEDGMENT OF DISCLOSURE STATEMENT.

I have been provided with a disclosure statement explaining the effect of this document. I have read and understood that information contained in the disclosure statement.

(YOU MUST DATE AND SIGN THIS POWER OF ATTORNEY)

I sign my name to this durable power of attorney for health care on______________day of

_________________________19____________at_____________________________

____

(City and State)

____

(Signature)

____

(Print Name)

STATEMENT OF WITNESSES.

I declare under penalty of perjury that the principal has identified himself or herself to me, that the principal signed or acknowledged this durable power of attorney in my presence, that I believe the principal to be of sound mind, that the principal has affirmed that the principal is aware of the nature of the document and is signing it voluntarily and free from duress, that the principal requested that I serve as witness to the principal's execution of this document, that I am not the person appointed as agent by this document, and that I am not provider of health or residential care, an employee of a provider of health or residential care, the operator of a community care facility, or an employee of an operator of a health care facility.

I declare that I am not related to the principal by blood, marriage, or adoption and that to the best of my knowledge I am not entitled to any part of the estate of the principal on the death of the principal under a will or by operation of law.

Witness signature:____

Print Name:____Date:__________

Address:____

Witness signature:____

Print Name:____Date:__________

Address:____

Exhibit F-3 Texas Directive to Physicians

Directive made this____________day of______________________________(month, year).

I____, being of sound mind, willfully and voluntarily make known my desire that my life shall not be artifiically prolonged under the circumstances set forth below, and do hereby declare:

1. If at any time I should have an incurable or irreversible condition caused by injury, disease, or illness certified to be a terminal condition by two physicians, and where the application of life-sustaining procedures would serve only to artificially prolong the moment of my death and where my attending physician determines that my death is imminent or will result within a relatively short time without application of life-sustaining procedures, I direct that such procedures be withheld or withdrawn, and that I be permitted to die naturally.

2. In the absence of my ability to give directions regarding the use of life-sustaining procedures, it is my intention that this directive shall be honored by my family and physicians as the final expression of my legal right to refuse medical or surgical treatment and accept the consequences from such refusal.

Other directions:

3. If I have been diagnosed as pregnant and that diagnosis is known to my physician, this directive shall have no force or effect during the course of my pregnancy.

4. This directive shall be in effect until it is revoked.

5. I understand the full import of this directive and I am emotionally and mentally competent to make this directive.

6. I understand that I may revoke this directive at any time.

Signed____________________________

City, County, and State of Residence____

I am not related to the declarant by blood or marriage; nor would I be to any portion of the declarant's estate on his/her decease; nor am I the attending physician of the declarant or an employee of the attending physician; nor am I a patient in the health care facility in which the declarant is a patient, or any person who has a claim against the portion of the estate of the declarant upon his/her decease. Furthermore, if I am an employee of a health facility in which the declarant is a patient, I am not involved in providing direct patient care to the declarant nor am I directly involved in the financial affairs of the health facility.

Witness__________________________

Witness__________________________

This Directive complies with the Natural Death Act, Tex. Stat. Ann art 4590h (1977, amended 1979, 1983, 1985, 1989).

Courtesy of the Society for the Right to Die, 250 W. 57th Street, New York, NY 10107

Exhibit F-3 continued

- -

Tear off and mail to: Society for the Right to Die, 250 W. 57th Street, New York, NY 10107

Please send me_________additional copies of the Texas Directive to Physicians.

M I am enclosing my tax-deductible dues/contribution in support of the Society's program.

(Please make checks payable to Society for the Right to Die.
Minimum annual memebership dues: $15.)

M $15 M $35 M $100 M Other $______

Name____

Street Address____

City___________________________________State___________Zip____________

M I am enclosing the names and addresses of others to receive information from the Society.

The Annual Report of the Society for the Right to Die is available from NY State Dept. of State, Office of Charitable Contributions, 162 Washington Ave., Albany, NY 12230

Appendix G

Health Care Proxy

(1) I,____

hereby appoint____________________________________

(name, home address and telephone number)

____

as my health care agent to make any and all health care decisions for me, except to the extent that I state otherwise. This proxy shall take effect when and if I become unable to make my own health care decisions.

(2) Optional instructions: I direct my proxy to make health care decisions in accord with my wishes and limitations as stated below, or as he or she otherwise knows. (Attach additional pages if necessary.)

____

____

____

(Unless your agent knows your wishes about artifical nutrition and hydration [feeding tubes], your agent will not be allowed to make decisions about artificial nutrition and hydration. See the preceding instructions for samples of language you could use.)

(3) Name of substitute or fill-in proxy if the person I appoint above is unable, unwilling or unavailable to act as my health care agent.

____

(name, home address and telephone number)

____

(4) Unless I revoke it, this proxy shall remain in effect indefinitely, or until the date or condition stated below. This proxy shall expire (specific date or conditions, if desired):

____

(5) Signature____________________________________

Address______________________________________

Date____

Source: New York State Department of Health, distributed by Society for the Right to Die, 250 West 57th Street, New York, NY 10107.

Statement by Witnesses (must be 18 or older)
I declare that the person who signed this document is personally known to me and appears to be of sound mind and acting of his or her own free will. He or she signed (or asked another to sign for him or her) this document in my presence.

Witness 1 ____________________

Address ____________________

Witness 2 ____________________

Address ____________________

New York State Department of Health

Distributed by **Society for the Right to Die**
250 West 57th Street, New York, NY 10107 (212) 246-6973

ABOUT THE HEALTH CARE PROXY

This is an important legal form. Before signing this form, you should understand the following facts:

1. This form gives the person you choose as your agent the authority to make all health care decisions for you, except to the extent you say otherwise in this form. "Health care" means any treatment, service or procedure to diagnose or treat your physical or mental condition.
2. Unless you say otherwise, your agent will be allowed to make all health care decisions for you, including decisions to remove or withhold life-sustaining treatment.
3. Unless your agent knows your wishes about artifical nutrition and hydration (nourishment and water provided by a feeding tube), he or she will not be allowed to refuse those measures for you.
4. Your agent will start making decisions for you when doctors decide that you are not able to make health care decisions for yourself.

You may write on this form any information about treatment that you do not desire and/or those treatments that you want to make sure you receive. Your agent must follow your instructions (oral or written) when making decisions for you.

If you want to give your agent written instructions, do so right on the form. For example, you could say:

> If I become terminally ill, I do/dont't want to receive the following treatments: . . .
>
> If I am in a coma or unconscious, with no hope of recovery, then I do/don't want . . .

If I have brain damage or a brain disease that makes me unable to recognize people or speak and there is no hope that my condition will improve, I do/don't want . . .

Examples of medical treatments about which you may wish to give your agent special instructions are listed below. This is not a complete list of the treatments about which you may leave instructions.

- artificial respiration
- artificial nutrition and hydration (nourishment and water provided by feeding tube)
- cardiopulmonary resuscitation (CPR)
- antipsychotic medication
- electric shock therapy
- antibiotics
- psychosurgery
- dialysis
- transplantation
- blood transfusions
- abortion
- sterilization

Talk about choosing an agent with your family and/or close friends. You should discuss this form with a doctor or another health care professional, such as a nurse or social worker, before you sign it to make sure that you understand the types of decisions that may be made for you. You may also wish to give your doctor a signed copy. You do not need a lawyer to fill out this form.

You can choose any adult (over 18), including a family member, or close friend, to be your agent. If you select a doctor as your agent, he or she may have to choose between acting as your agent or as your attending doctor; a physician cannot do both at the same time. Also, if you are a patient or resident of a hospital, nursing home or mental hygiene facility, there are special restrictions about naming someone who works for that facility as your agent. You should ask staff at the facility to explain those restrictions.

You should tell the person you choose that he or she will be your health care agent. You should discuss your health care wishes and this form with your agent. Be sure to give him or her a signed copy. Your agent cannot be sued for health care decisions made in good faith.

Even after you have signed this form, you have the right to make health care decisions for yourself as long as you are able to do so, and treatment cannot be given to you or stopped if you object. You can cancel the control given to your agent by telling him or her or your health care provider orally or in writing.

FILLING OUT THE PROXY FORM

Item (1) Write your name and the name, home address and telephone number of the person you are selecting as your agent.

Item (2) If you have special instructions for your agent, you should write them here. Also, if you wish to limit your agent's authority in any way, you should say so here. If you do not state any limitations, your agent will be allowed to make all health care decisions that you could have made, including the decision to consent or refuse life-sustaining treatment.

Item (3) You may write the name, home address and telephone number of an alternate agent.

Item (4) This form will remain valid indefinitely unless you set an expiration date or condition for its expiration. This section is optional and should be filled in only if you want the health care proxy to expire.

Item (5) You must sign and date the proxy. If you are unable to sign yourself, you may direct someone else to sign in your presence. Be sure to include your address.

Two witnesses at least 18 years of age must sign your proxy. The person who is appointed agent or alternate agent cannot sign as a witness.

Index of Cases

A

Abercrombie v. Roof, 208
Albertville Nursing Home v. Upton, 157
Amalgamated Association of Street, Electric Railway & Motor Coach Employees v. Lockridge, 365
American Hospital Association v. National Labor Relations Board, 363
American Medical Nursing Centers-Greenbrook v. Heckler, 324, 347
American Nurses Association v. Passaic General Hospital, 344
Anco, Inc. v. Human Services Finance Commission, 329
Arena v. Lincoln Lutheran of Racine, 370
Aurora v. Secretary of Health and Human Services, 324

B

Baker v. Vanderbilt University, 406
Banks v. Board of Pharmacy, 227
Barber v. Superior Court, 284
Battaglia v. Sisters of Charity Hospital, 394
Beach v. Western Medical Enterprises, Inc., 153
Beasley v. State Personnel Board, 77
Behnke v. Department of Health and Social Services, 330
Berger v. United States, 62
Berlin v. Nathan, 409
Bernardi v. Community Hospital Association, 209
Bielecki v. Perales, 70
Big Town Nursing Home, Inc. v. Newman, 50
Billups v. Methodist Hospital of Chicago, 384
Bird v. Pritchard, 102
Blackmon v. Langley, 184
Blanton v. United States, 240
Bleeker v. Dukakis, 164
Booty v. Kentwood Manor Nursing Home, Inc., 39
Bouvia v. Superior Court, 301
Boyd v. Bulala, 410
Boyer v. Grandview Manor Care Center, 179
Brinson v. Axelrod, 76
Brown v. Physicians Mutual Insurance Co., 382

Brown v. Shannon West Texas Memorial Hospital, 210
Bruner v. Oregon Baptist Retirement Home, 335
Buckley Nursing Home, Inc. v. Massachusettes Commission Against Discrimination, 361

C

Cardwell v. Rockford Memorial Hospital Association, 413
Carroll v. Gaddy, 161
Carry v. Laugh, 54
Caruso v. Pine Manor Nursing Center, 44
Celestine v. United States, 51
Chapman v. United States, Department of Health and Human Services, 68
Charlesgate Nursing Center v. State of Rhode Island, 369
Chester Extended Care Center v. DPW, 327
Choe v. Axelrod, 276
Churchill v. Waters, 380
City of Newport v. Fact Concerts, Inc., 324
Clark v. Wagoner, 42
Cleary v. American Airlines, Inc., 389
Cliff House Nursing Home, Inc. v. Department of Public Health, 164
Cohen v. Daughters of Sarah Nursing Home Company, Inc., 173
Cohran v. Harper, 106
Colorado Dept. of Social Services v. DHHS, 13
Commonwealth v. Hillhaven Corp., 78
Conrad v. Hackett, 336
Corning Glass Works v. Brennan, 361
Costal Health Services, Inc. v. Rozier, 100
Cruzan v. Director, Missouri Department of Health, 292
Cruzan v. Harmon, 291

D

Daniels v. Hillcrest Homes, Inc., 397
Darling v. Charleston Community Memorial Hospital, 45, 178
Deerings West Nursing Center v. Scott, 33
Dempsey v. Senior Services Division, 253
Department of Human Services v. Berry, 11
Department of Social Services v. Our Lady of Mercy, 326
Duldulao v. St. Mary of Nazareth Hospital Center, 380
Dunahoo v. Brooks, 38

E

Eales v. Tanana, 395
Eli v. Griggs County Hospital and Nursing Home, 387
Elwood v. SAIF, 367
Erie Care Center, Inc. v. Ackerman, 156
Estes Health Care Centers, Inc. v. Bannerman, 39, 108
Euclid Manor Nursing Home v. Board of Review, 390
Eufemio v. University of the State of New York, 78

F

Facey v. Merkle, 41
Fair Rest Home v. Commonwealth of Pa. Dept. of Health, 11
Ferguson v. Dr. McCarthy's Rest Home, 42
Feuereisen v. Axelrod, 164
Fleming v. Baptist General Convention of Oklahoma, 210
Flint City Nursing Home, Inc. v. Depreast, 159
Foley v. Interactive Data Corp., 399
Fondulac Nursing Home v. Industrial Commission, 367
Forbis v. Wesleyan Nursing Home, Inc., 391
Franklin v. Collins Chapel Correctional Hospital, 94

G

Garner v. Crawford, 101
Goff v. Doctors General Hospital, 214
Greer v. Medders, 58
Griggs v. Duke Power Co., 361, 384
Gunduy v. Commissioner of Education, 414
Gunn v. HI-C-Home, Inc., 43
Gust v. Pomeroy, 320

H

Hargrave v. Landon, 69
Harris v. Manor Healthcare Corp., 111
Harvet v. Unity Medical Center, Inc., 394
Hauptman v. Grand Manor Health Related Facility, Inc., 160
Hayes v. Shelby Memorial Hospital, 384
Haynes v. Hoffman, 42
Heller v. Ambach, 227
Heller v. Medine, 103
Henricks v. Sanford, 98
Henry v. Deen, 110
Henson v. Department of Consumer and Regulatory Affairs, 258
Heritage of Yankton, Inc. v. South Dakota Department of Health, 432
Hernandez v. Lutheran Medical Center, 91
Hinson v. Cameron, 398
Hobson v. McClean Hospital Corp., 389
Homes v. Department of Professional Regulation Board of Nursing, 212
Hoodkroft Convalescent Centers v. State of New Hampshire, Division of Human Services, 328

I

In re Beth Israel Medical Center, 299
In re Dinnerstein, 288
In re Eichner, 297
In re Estate of Brooks, 284
In re Estate of Dorone, 241
In re Estate of Longeway, 301
In re Estate of Smith v. O'Halloran, 71
In re Fosmire v. Nicoleau, 241
In re Hallock, 288
In re Hier, 299
In re Jobes, 300
In re Lydia Hall Hospital, 286
In re Melideo, 240
In re Quinlan, 284, 286, 287, 288, 290
In re Spring, 288
In re Storar, 286, 290
In re Welfare of Colyer, 289
In the Matter of Alaimo v. Ambach, 69
In the Matter of Axelrod, 77
In the Matter of Clair C. Conroy, 298, 300
In the Matter of Jascalevich, 274
In the Matter of Westchester County Medical Center ex. rel. O'Connor, 290

J

Jagust v. Brookhaven Memorial Association, Inc., 397
Jenkins v. Bogalusa Community Medical Center, 102
John F. Kennedy Memorial Hospital, Inc. v. Bludworth, 289
Johnson v. Terry, 110
Joiner v. Benton Community Bank, 381
Jones v. Hinds General Hospital, 384
Jones v. State Board of Medicine, 410
Judge v. Rockford Memorial Hospital, 55

K

Kallengerg v. Beth Israel Hospital, 210
Keller v. Miami Herald Publishing Co., 53
Kern v. Gulf Coast Nursing Home of Moss Point, Inc., 204
Keyes v. Humana Hospital Alaska, Inc., 405
Khanna v. Microdata Corp., 388
Kizer v. County of San Mateo, 12
Knutson v. Life Care Communities, Inc., 158
Koelbl v. Whalen, 155, 268
Krestview Nursing Home, Inc. v Synowiec, 158

L

Ladenheim v. Union County Hospital District, 178
Lagrone v. Helman, 32
Lambert v. Beverly Enterprises, Inc., 220
Lane v. Candura, 285
Langford v. Lane, 396
Larrimore v. Homeopathic Hospital Association, 210
Leach v. Akron General Medical Center, 289
Leal v. Simon, 188
Lipp v. United States, 9
Loren v. Board of Examiners of Nursing Home Administrators, 164
Love v. Heritage House Convalescent Center, 392
Lucas v. HCMF Corporation, 40
Lynch v. Redfield Foundation, 351

M

McGarrah v. SAIF, 367
McGillivray v. Rapides Iberia Management Enterprises, 33
Macleod v. Miller, 258
McQuary v. Air Convalescent Home, Inc., 385
Magnolias Nursing and Convalescent Center v. Department of Health and Rehabilitation Services, 149
Mankato Lutheran Home v. Miller, 391
Marbury v. Madison, 1, 17, 20
Masterson v. Pennsylvania Railroad, 270
May v. Marcus, 111
May v. Triple C Convalescent Centers, 49
Meech v. Hillhaven West, Inc., 399
Miller Home, Inc. v. Commonwealth, Department of Public Welfare, 76, 188
Monk v. Doctors Hospital, 215
Monroe County Nursing Home District v. Missouri Department of Social Services, 328, 338
Montclair Nursing Home v. Wills, 392
Montgomery Health Care Facility v. Ballard, 154, *155*, 212
Montgomery v. American Nursing Centers, Inc., 92
Moon Lake Convalescent Center v. Margolis, 147, 200, 204
Mort v. Unicare Health Facilities, Inc., 111
Mueller v. Mueller, 99
Mullen v. Axelrod, 78
Mulligan v. Lederle, 99
Murphy v. Senior Services Division, 253

N

National Health Corporation v. South Carolina Department of Health and Environmental Control, 431
National Labor Relations Board v. American Medical Services, Inc., 371
National Labor Relations Board v. Reed & Prince Manufacturing Co., 358
National Labor Relations Board v. Remington Rand, 276
National Labor Relations Board v. Res-Care Inc., 370
National Labor Relations Board v. Woodview-Calabasas Hospital, 358
Nepa v. Commonwealth Department of Public Welfare, 74
New York State Health Facilities Association, Inc. v. Axelrod, 331
Newman Brothers, Inc. v. McDowell, 157
Newman v. Emerson Radio Corp., 399
Nichols v. Green Acres Rest Home, 93, 156
Northeast Georgia Radiological Associates v. Tidwell, 179
Norton v. Argonaut Insurance Co., 209
Nursing Home of Dothan, Inc. v Alabama State Health Planning and Developement Agency, 431

O

O'Brien v. Cundard Steam Ship Co., 243
O'Connor v. Eastman Kodak Co., 379

Odomes v. Nucare Inc., 360
Our Lady of the Woods v. Commonwealth of Kentucky Health Facilities, 207

P

Palmateer v. International Harvester Co., 381
Palmer v. Intermed, Inc., 41
Pardazi v. Cullman Medical Center, 386
Paros v. Hoemako Hospital, 396
Parrish v. Clark, 211
Patrick v. Burget, 411
Payne v. Marion General Hospital, 302
Payton Health Care Facilities, Inc. v. Estate of Campbell, 111
Peete v. Blackwell, 48
Pena v. Brattleboro Retreat, 383
People ex rel. Vega v. Smith, 276
People v. Casa Blance Convalescent Homes, Inc., 148
People v. Coe, 75
People v. Eulo, 290
People v. Kendzia, 227
People v. Lancaster, 159
People v. Nygren, 211
People v. Smithtown General Hospital, 274
Pick v. Santa Ana-Tustin Community Hospital, 178
Pierce v. Ortho Pharmaceutical Corp., 379, 381
Pollack v. Methodist Hospital, 352
Poor Sisters of St. Francis v. Catron, 232
Powell v. Parkview Estate Nursing Home, Inc., 41, 101
Pugh v. See's Candies, Inc., 389

R

Reid v. Axelrod, 76
Renny v. Port Huron Hospital, 389
Roberson v. Provident House, 39
Rock v. Sear-Brown Associates, 379
Roe v. Wade, 286

S

St. Paul Insurance Companies v. Talladega Nursing Home, 347
Satz v. Perlmutter, 290
Sayes v. Pilgrim Manor Nursing Home, Inc., 48
Schloendorff v. Society of New York Hospital, 236, 286
Schmitt v. Pierce, 290
Scott v. Bradford, 237
Selan v. Commonwealth Unemployment Compensation Board of Review, 395
Sermchief v. Gonzales, 194
Severns v. Wilmington Medical Center, 289
Shores v. Senior Manor Nursing Center, 388
Sides v. Duke Hospital, 378
Silver Lake Nursing Home v. Axelrod, 329
Simonson v. Meader Distribution Company, 394
Slocum v. Berman, 156
Smith v. Gravois Rest Haven, Inc., 158
Smith v. Van Gorkum, 165
Speet v. Bacaj, 406
Starks v. Director of the Division of Employment Sec., 398
State Department of Human Services v. Northern, 286
State of Connecticut, Department of Income Maintenance v. Heckler, 330
State of North Carolina v. Beatty, 227
State v. Beatty, 67
State v. Brenner, 63
State v. Cargille, 68
State v. Heath, 67
State v. Pleasant Hill Health Facility, Inc., 79
State v. Serebin, 164
State v. Stuckey Health Care, Inc., 330
Stenger v. Brown, 323
Stevens v. Morris Communication Corp., 54
Stiegelmeier v. West Side Deutscher Frauen Verein, 334
Stiffelman v. Abrams, 76
Stocking v. Hall, 335

Stogsdill v. Manor Convalescent Home, Inc., 186
Stogsdill v. Manor Convalescent Home, Inc. and Hiatt, M.D., 36
Stoker v. Tarentino, 215
Summit Health Ltd. v. Pinhas, 420
Superintendent of Belchertown State School v. Saikewicz, 284, 287-288, 290

T

Tasker v. United States, 9
Theodore v. Department of Health & Human Services, 383
Truan v. Smith, 184
Tuma v. Board of Nursing, 195

U

United States v. Bay State Ambulance & Hospital Rental Services, Inc., 69
United States v. Hutcheson, 358
Utter v. United Hospital Center, Inc., 214

V

Valentine v. Kaiser Foundation Hospitals, 186
Valley View Convalescent Home v. Department of Social Services, 10–11
Voa Autumnwood Care Center v. Shiff 330–331
Volk v. Dept. of Human Resources, 326

W

Warra v. Masabi Regional Medical Center, 398
Washington State Nurses Association v. Board of Medical Examiners, 229
Watson v. Idaho Falls Consolidated Hospitals, Inc., 380, 387
Weiner v. McGraw-Hill, 380
Westhampton Nursing Home v. Whalen, 328
Wilde v. Houlton Regional Hospital, 396
Wilkinson v. Madera Community Hospital, 352
Wills v. Dekalb Area Retirement Center, 261
Wisconsin Association of Nursing Homes, 53
Wooten v. United States, 106

X

XYZ Nursing Home, Inc. v. Kurlansky, 272

Y

Yankee v. State Department of Health, 275
Yerry v. Ulster County, 398
Younger v. Southwestern Savings and Loan Assn., 383

Z

Zella Wahnon & Assoc. v. Bassman, 221
Zucker v. Axelrod, 228

Index

A

Abandonment
elements leading to recovery of damages, 183
physician liability, 182–183
Absolute privilege, 55
Abuse of residents
abusive search, 75
allegations not supported by evidence, 78
areas for investigation, 73–74
and discharged employees, 385–386
facts about, 71–72
forcible administration of medication, 77
forms of, 70
improper care, 78
intimidation of abusive resident, 77–78
Office of Inspector General study, 65–66
physical abuse, 76–77
and resident rights, 71
and revocation of license, 74–75
solutions to, 72–73
Acquired immunodeficiency syndrome (AIDS)
confidentiality, 427–428
discrimination, 428–429
education about, 430
employment issues, 429
and health care workers, 426–427
mandatory testing, 427
Occupational Safety and Health Act, 430
reporting requirements, 429–430
Ryan White Comprehensive AIDS Resources Emergency Act, 427
transmission of, 424–425
Adjudication, judicial branch, 16
Administration on Aging, 24
Administrative agencies
Department of Health and Human Services, 20–25
Department of Justice, 26
Department of Labor, 26
functions of, 8
National Institute on Aging, 25–26
National Labor Relations Board, 27
Administrative law, 8–13
conflicts among state laws, 12–13
nature of, 8–9
review of regulations by court, 9–12
Administrative Procedures Act, 8, 12
Administrators
cases related to, 164

CEO, role and responsibility of, 161–163
contract liability, 163
liability for acts of others, 163
tort liability, 163
Admissions, and resident rights, 251–253
Adult day care centers
financial difficulties of, 117
nature of, 117
Affirmative action, 371–372
Age discrimination, 362, 383
Age Discrimination in Employment Act of 1967, 362
Aging, of population, 114–116
AIDS. *See* Acquired immunodeficiency syndrome (AIDS)
Ambulance service kickback, 69
American Nurses Association, 197–198
purpose of, 197
standards of practice, 198
Answer, pleadings, 83–84
Appeals, 112
grounds for, 112
Appellate court, 17
appeals process, 112
Arbitration, malpractice, 405
Arraignment, 61
procedure in, 61
Arrest, 61
procedure in, 61
and type of complaint, 61
Assault, 47
definition of, 47
Assisted living facilities, nature of, 117–118
Assumption of risk defense, 102–103
Autopsy, 305–314
authorization by decedent, 312–313
authorization by person other than decedent, 313–314
consent statutes, 312
consent with limitations, 314
fraudulently obtained consent, 314

B

Baby boomers, 116
Bargaining units, per institution, 363–364
Battery, 47–49
definition of, 47
in health care setting, 48–49
Beds, falls, 158
Bench warrant, 91
Bidding, corporate duty related to, 156
Bill of particulars, 84–85
Billing fraud, 67–68
billing for services not furnished, 68
Breach of duty
criteria for, 38
in negligence, 38–39, 44
Burden of proof, 91–95
beyond a reasonable doubt, 92, 93
credible evidence, 92
in criminal case, 93
in negligence, 92
res ipsa loquitur, 93–95
violation of internal policy/procedures, 93
violation of statute, 93
Burns, duty related to nursing staff, 215

C

Case law, 5–6
Certificate of need, 430–433
disapproval of application, 431–432
Certification, of health care professionals, 232
Change in condition, duty related to nursing staff, 214
Child labor acts, 366
Civil rights, resident rights, 252
Claims, malpractice, settlement of, 352–353
Clinical nurse specialist, 202
Closing statements, trial, 107–108
Code of Napoleon, 5
Collateral source rule, malpractice, 406–407
Collective bargaining agreement, 372–373

Committees
  ethics, 303–305
  quality assurance, 419–420
  risk management, 422–423
Common law, 2–7
  history of
    England, 2–5
    United States, 5–7
Communicable disease, reporting of, 280
Comparative negligence, 103–104
  50 percent system, 103–104
  pure system, 103
Compensatory damages, 109–110
Complaint, 83
  elements of, 83
Computerized medical records, 273
Conference, criminal law, 61
Confidentiality
  AIDS and health care workers, 427–428
  medical records, 270
  as resident right, 261
Conflict of interest, corporate duty related to, 151–152
Consent
  for autopsy, 312–314
  and competent residents, 240–241
  definitions of, 235
  express consent, 235
  general consent, 238
  and guardian, 241
  implied consent, 235, 242–243
  and incompetent residents, 242
  and mentally ill, 242
  and minors, 241
  oral consent, 237
  parties for consent, 240
  proof of consent, 237–240
  refusal of treatment, 244
  restraints, use of, 448–449
  special consent, 238–240
    for experimental procedures/drugs, 239–240
    for nonroutine inoculations, 239
  written consent, 237, 238
  See also Informed consent
Conservatorship, 297
Constitution, 7
Consultation, physician liability, failure to seek consultation, 185–187
Contingency fee limitations, malpractice, 407
Continuing care retirement communities, nature of, 118
Contractual relationships in employment
  express agreements, 379
  implied contracts, 379–381
Contributory negligence, 101–102
Controlled Substances Act, 223
Corporate authority
  express authority, 144
  implied authority, 145
  ultra vires acts, 145
Corporate negligence, 45–47
Corporations, long-term care services as, 143
Counterclaims, pleadings, 84
Courts of appeals, 17–18
Credentialing, medical staff, 177
Crime, classification of, 60
Criminal law, 1, 60
  arraignment, 61
  arrest, 61
  conference, 61
  criminal negligence, 63–64
  criminal trial, 62
  defense attorney, 62
  drug abuse, 63
  falsification of records, 64
  fraud, 64–69
  murder, 69–70
  operating without operating certificate, 70
  petty theft, 78–79
  prosecutor, 62
  resident abuse, 70–78
  sexual improprieties, 79
Criminal negligence, 63–64
  definition of, 63
Criminal trial, 62

D

Damages, 109–112
  compensatory damages, 109–110
  joint and several liability, 111–112
  nominal damages, 109–110
  schedule of damages, 110–111
Day care centers
  Medicaid, 325–326
  private insurance, 332
Death
  autopsy, 305–314
  definition of, 289–291
  organ donation, 314–316
  reporting of, 280–281
  right to die, 258–259
  suspicious deaths, 281
  unclaimed dead bodies, 316–317
  wrongful handling of dead body, 305
  See also Euthanasia; Right to die
Decubitus ulcers, duty related to nursing staff, 212–213
Defamation actions, 387
Defamation of character, 53–56
  absolute and qualified privilege, 55
  defenses to defamation action, 55–56
  definition of, 53
  libel, 53–54
  slander, 54–55
Defense attorney, 62
  role of, 62
Defenses against recovery, 100–107
  assumption of risk, 102–103
  comparative negligence, 103–104
  contributory negligence, 101–102
  Good Samaritan laws, 104–105
  ignorance of law, 105–106
  intervening cause, 106
  statute of limitations, 105
Defensive medicine, 403–404
Delay in treatment, physician liability, 184
Demonstrative evidence, 97–98
Demurrer, 83
Dental services, nursing facilities, 219
Department of Health and Human Services, 20–25
  Administration on Aging, 24
  Family Support Administration, 23
  Federal Council on Aging, 24–25
  Health Care Financing Administration, 23
  Office of Human Development Services, 23–24
  organization of, 21
  Public Health Service, 22–23
  Social Security Administration, 23
Department of Justice, 26
  fraud section, 67
Department of Labor, 26
Diagnosis related groups, 337–338
  and medical records, 337–338
  nature of, 337
Diagnostic tests, physician liability, failure to order diagnostic tests, 185
Dietary services
  nursing facilities, 219–220
  OBRA requirements, 219–220
Direct evidence, 95–97
  examination of witnesses, 95–96
  expert witness, 96–97
Director of nursing services, requirements for, 199–200
Disabled
  employment discrimination, 363, 384–385
  Pepper Commission recommendations, 129–130
Discharge, and residents rights, 254–258
Disclaimers, and termination of employees, 393–395
Disclosure, failure to disclose, physician liability, 184
Discovery, 85–86
  examination before trial, 86–87
  malpractice, 408
Discrimination
  AIDS patients, 428–429
  in employment, 361–363, 383–385
  toward residents, 252
Dismissal, as motion, 87–88
District courts, 17

Do not resuscitate orders, 302
Documentary evidence, 98–99
Documentation, physician liability, lack of documentation, 187
Drug abuse, 63
Drug substitution, 226
Durable power of attorney, 295–296, 466–472
Duty to use due care
  in negligence, 32–38, 44
  and standard of care, 35–38

E

Employee rights, 368
Employment
  and AIDS infected, 429
  contractual relationships, 379–381
  employment practices, 400–401
  employment-at-will, 378–379
  public policy issues, 381–386
    age discrimination, 383
    defamation actions, 387
    fairness and discharge, 389–390
    handicapped discrimination, 384–385
    pregnancy discrimination, 384
    racial discrimination, 383–384
    reporting patient abuse, 385–386
    retaliatory discharge, 387–389
    sex discrimination, 384
    whistleblowing, 382
  termination of employees, 392–399
Equal employment opportunity, 371
Equal Employment Opportunity Act of 1972, 361–362
Equal Pay Act of 1963, 360–361
Equipment, corporate duty related to, 152–153
Ethics
  corporate duty related to, 160
  ethics committees, 303–305
    composition of, 304
    functions of, 304–305
  Hippocratic oath, 302–303
Euthanasia
  active euthanasia, 284
  definition of, 282–283
  history of, 282–283
  involuntary euthanasia, 286
  legal aspects, 286–289
  passive euthanasia, 284
  voluntary euthanasia, 285–286
  See also Right to die
Evidence, 95–100
  demonstrative evidence, 97–98
  direct evidence, 95–97
    examination of witnesses, 95–96
    expert witness, 96–97
  documentary evidence, 98–99
  hearsay evidence, 99–100
  judicial notice rule, 99
  and medical books, 100
Executive branch, 15–16
  operation of, 15–16
Expert witness, 96–97
  malpractice, 408
  situations for use of, 96–97
Express agreements, 379
Express consent, 235
Express corporate authority, 144

F

Facilities, corporate duty related to, 152–153
Failure to follow up, physician liability, 184
Fair Labor Standards Act, 360
Fairness, and employee discharge, 389–392
Falls
  from beds, 158
  corporate duty for protection against, 158–159
  duty related to nursing staff, 215–216
  and floors, 159
  from windows, 159
False imprisonment, 49–52
  conditions for, 49–50
  definition of, 49
  use of restraints, 51–52

Falsification of records, 64
  by nursing home stockholder, 68
Family Support Administration, 23
Federal Council on Aging, 24–25
Federal Mediation and Conciliation Service, 359
Federal Tort Claims Act, 106
Feeding tubes, and right to die, 291–292, 298–301
Felony
  and arrest, 61
  definition of, 60
Fenwick, Mrs. Bedford, 192
Financial rights, of residents, 259
Financing long–term care
  average cost of nursing facility, 313
  and diagnosis related groups, 337–338
  language of financial agreements, pitfalls, 337
  life care contracts, 333–336
  Medicaid, 324–331
  Medicare, 322–324
  private insurance, 320–321, 331–333
  resource utilization groups, 339–340
  spouse's financial obligation, 336–337
Floors, falls, 159
Food, Drug, and Cosmetic Act, 223–224
Formulary system, drug substitutions, 226
Forseeability
  and negligence, 42–43
  test for, 42
Fraud, 56, 64–69
  ambulance service kickback, 69
  billing for services not furnished, 68
  billing fraud, 67–68
  Department of Justice fraud section, 67
  falsification of records by nursing home stockholder, 68
  and joint ventures, 66–67
  kickback arrangements, 68–69
  and life care contracts, 333
  and Office of Inspector General, 65–66
Frivolous claims, malpractice, 408–409

G

Good Samaritan laws, 104–105
Government
  executive branch, 15–16
  judicial branch, 16–19
  legislative branch, 13, 15
  separation of powers, 19–20
Government facilities
  placement of residents, 253–254
  and resident rights, 253–254
Governmental controls, pharmaceutical services, 222
Governor, responsibilities of, 16
Grand jury, 61
Grievances, and residents, 262
Guardian
  and consent, 241
  and right to die, 297

H

Harvard Medical Practice study, 6, 29, 403
Health care expenditures, current/future expenditures, 318
Health Care Financing Administration, 23, 322
Health Care Policy Research study, 120
Health care proxy
  form for, 473–476
  and right to die, 296–297
Hearsay evidence, 99–100
Hippocratic oath, 302–303
Home health care, nature of, 116–117
House Select Committee on Aging, 128–130

I

Ignorance of law defense, 105–106
  independent contractor, 107
  sovereign immunity, 106–107
Implied consent, 235, 242–243
Implied contracts, 379–381
Implied corporate authority, 145
Improper care, as abuse, 78

Incident reports
legal obligations, 276
as subject to subpoena, 423
Incompetent residents, and consent, 242
Independent contractor, and liability, 107, 146
Infection control
corporate duty related to, 157–158
duty of nursing staff, 212
Informed consent, 260
failure to disclose, physician liability, 184
nature of, 236–237
proof in informed consent suits, 237
Injunctions, labor/management relations, 372
Injury
in negligence, 39–40, 45
scope of, 39
Institute of Medicine report, recommendations, 137–138
Insurance
categories of risk in, 343–344
corporate duty related to, 153
elements of policy, 343
liability insurance, 345–349
malpractice insurance, 350, 352
medical liability insurance, 349–350
and risk management, 353
self-insurance, 350–351
settlement of claims, 353
trustee coverage, 351–352
types of coverage for facilities, 351
Insurance for long-term care, 320–321, 331–333
day care centers, 332
Medigap policies, 332–333
Intentional torts, 47–58
assault, 47
battery, 47–49
defamation of character, 53–56
false imprisonment, 49–52
fraud, 56
intentional infliction of mental distress, 57–58
invasion of privacy, 56–57
Intermediate care facility, 119
Invasion of privacy, 56–57
definition of right to privacy, 57
rights to privacy, 56

J

Joint and several liability, 111–112
definition of, 409
malpractice, 409
Joint ventures
and fraud, 66–67
nature of, 66
Judge
charge to the jury, 108–109
role of, 89
Judicial branch, 16–19
appellate court, 17
courts of appeals, 17–18
district courts, 17
operation of, 16–19
Supreme Court, 18–19
Judicial notice rule, 99
Jury
judge's charge to, 108–109
role of, 90
voir dire, 90

K

Kickbacks, 68–69
definition of, 68
and Office of Inspector General, 65
types of arrangements, 69
See also Fraud

L

Labor laws
federal
Age Discrimination in Employment Act of 1967, 362
bargaining units per institution, 363–364

Equal Pay Act of 1963, 360–361
Fair Labor Standards Act, 360
federal, Equal Employment Opportunity Act of 1972, 361–362
Labor-Management Reporting and Disclosure Act of 1959, 359–360
National Labor Relations Act, 356–358
Norris-LaGuardia Act, 358–359
Occupational Safety and Health Act of 1970, 373–375
Rehabilitation Act of 1973, 363
state
child labor acts, 366
labor relations statutes, 365
right-to-work laws, 366
union security contract, 365–366
wage and hour laws, 366
worker's compensation, 366–367
Labor/management relations
affirmative action, 371–372
collective bargaining agreement, 372–373
employee rights, 368
equal employment opportunity, 371
injunctions, 372
management rights, 368–371
resident rights and labor disputes, 372
Laboratory services, nursing facilities, 221
Labor-Management Reporting and Disclosure Act of 1959, 359–360
Law
administrative law, 8–13
common law, 2–7
definition of, 1
sources of, 2
statutory law, 7–8
Legislative branch, 13, 15
operation of, 15
Liability
of administrators, 163
and health care professionals, 344–345
joint and several liability, 111–112
and nurse practitioner, 201–202
and respondeat superior, 146
and special duty nurse, 203
See also Physician liability
Liability insurance, 345–349
medical liability insurance, 349–350
common risks, 349
liability classes, 349
parts of
amount of coverage, 346–347
conditions of policy, 347–349
defense and settlement, 346
insurance agreement, 345
policy period, 346
and risk management, 353
trustee coverage, 351–352
Libel, 53–54
definition of, 53
Licensure
definition of, 232
of health care professionals, 232–233
nurses, 195–197
practicing without a license, 197
requirements for license, 196–197
suspension/revocation, 197
nursing facilities, 126
objectives of, 232–233
revocation after abuse of residents, 74–75
Life care communities, nature of, 118
Life care contracts, 333–336
death of resident in probationary period, 334
and extraordinary medical costs, 335–336
and fraud, 333
inability to perform contract, 335
and mutual obligation, 333
and property transfers, 334
termination of, 334
Living will, 295
execution of, 295
forms for, 462–465
Longevity, 137–139
Institute of Medicine report recommendations, 137–138
Long-term care corporations
authority of governing body, 144–145

express corporate authority, 144
implied corporate authority, 145
ultra vires acts, 145
business form, 143
CEO, role and responsibility of, 161–163
duties of administration
duties specified by corporate law, 148
duty to appoint administrator, 148–150
duty to avoid self-dealing/conflict of interest situations, 151–152
duty to be ethically/financially scrupulous, 160
duty to comply with statutes/rules/regulations, 147–148
duty to establish infection control program, 157–158
duty to propitious treatment, 151
duty to protect against falls, 158–159
duty to provide adequate facilities/equipment, 152–153
duty to provide adequate insurance, 153
duty to provide adequate staff, 155
duty to provide safe environment for residents and employees, 156–157
duty to provide satisfactory resident care, 153–154
duty to require competitive bidding, 156
duty to safeguard resident valuables, 159–160
duty to supervise and manage, 150
medical staff, bylaws, 160–161
respondeat superior, 145–146
Long-term care services
adult day care centers, 117
assisted living facilities, 117–118
continuing care retirement communities/life care communities, 118
home health care, 116–117
not-for-profit facilities, 143
nursing facilities, 18–126
skilled nursing services in hospitals/transitional care units, 118

M

Malfeasance, 38
Malpractice
arbitration, 405
caps on awards, 410
collateral source rule, 406–407
contingency fee limitations, 407
and defensive medicine, 403–404
discovery, 408
expert witness, 408
findings of study of, 402
first case, 6
frivolous claims, 408–409
joint and several liability, 409
mediation, 404
no-fault system, 411
peer review organizations, 411–413
precalendar conference, 408
pretrial screening panel, 405–406
professional misconduct, 413–414
statutes of limitations, 408
structured awards, 414
and tort system, 403, 404
Malpractice insurance, 350, 352
malpractice insurance associations, 350
mandated medical staff coverage, 352
Management, rights of, 368–371
Mandatory testing, AIDS, 427
Master-servant relationship, respondeat superior, 145–146
Mediation, malpractice, 404
Medicaid, 324–331
cases related to, 326–331
day care centers, 325–326
and Office of Inspector General, 65
patient quotas, 331
utilization review, 424
Medical books, as evidence, 100
Medical director, 173–176
position responsibilities for, 174–176
qualifications for, 173–174

responsibilities of, 173
Medical records
access to residents, 271
charge for reproduction of, 272
charting, guidelines for, 274–275
computerized, 273
confidentiality, 270
contents of, 267–268
and diagnosis related groups, 337–338
falsification of, 274
improper use of, 273
and legal proceedings, 269–270
legal reporting obligations, 275–281
communicable diseases, 280
death, 280–281
incident reporting, 276
National Practitioner Data Bank, 277–280
legal requirements, 268–269
Privacy Act of 1974, 272–273
purposes of, 266–267
request by third parties, 271
retention of, 275
Medical staff
bylaws, 160–161
credentialing, 177
disruptive physicians, 178
interference of facility with patient–physician relationship, 179–180
medical director, 173–176
physician liability, 182–198
physician monitoring, 178
physician services, 166–172
privileges, 176–177
survey process
interviewing of, 181
record review, 181
residents, interviewing of, 180
survey evaluation factors, 182
termination of privileges, 178–179
Medicare, 322–324
assignment of Part B claims, 322–323
cases related to, 323–324
Medigap policies, 332–333
and Office of Inspector General, 65
processing Part B claims, 323
utilization review, 423–424
Medication, 208–211
by nursing, 208–211
administration without prescription, 211
failure to administer medication, 210–211
failure to discontinue medication, 211
failure to note order change, 210
negligent injection, 209
unsterile needle, 210
wrong dosage, 209
wrong medication, 208
wrong route of administration, 210
errors, physician liability, 188
forcible administration of, 77
Medigap policies, 332–333
Memorandum of law, 89
Mental distress, intentional infliction of, 57–58
Mentally ill, and consent, 242
Minors, and consent, 241
Misdemeanors
and arrest, 61
definition of, 60
Misdiagnosis, physician liability, 187
Misfeasance, 38
Monitoring, of physicians, 178
Motions, 87–88
dismissal, 87–88
summary judgment, 88
Murder, 69–70
examples in health care settings, 69–70

N

National Health Planning and Resource Development Act of 1974, 430
National Institute on Aging, 25–26
National Labor Relations Act, 356–358
elections, 357–358
jurisdiction, 356–357
unfair labor practices, 358

National Labor Relations Board, 27
  on bargaining units, 363–364
National League for Nursing, 199
National Planning and Resource
  Development Act of 1974, 126
  parts of, 128
National Practitioner Data Bank
  forms for, 458–461
  limitations on disclosure, 280
  purpose of, 277
  queries to, 277–279
Negligence, 30–47
  breach of duty, 38–39, 44
  burden of proof, 31
  burden of proof in, 92
  comparative negligence, 103–104
  conditions for, 30–31
  contributory negligence, 101–102
  corporate negligence, 45–47
  criminal negligence, 63–64
  degrees of, 31
  duty to use due care, 32–38, 44
  elements of, 31
  injury/actual damages, 39–40, 45
  intentional vs negligent wrongs, 30
  ordinary and gross negligence, 31
  proximate cause/causation, 40–43, 45
  res ipsa loquitur, 93–94
Nightingale, Florence, 191
No-fault system, malpractice, 411
Nominal damages, 109–110
Nonfeasance, 38
Norris-LaGuardia Act, 358–359
Not-for-profit facilities, long-term care
  services, 143
Notice of trial, 89
Nurse practitioner, 200–202
  and liability, 201–202
  role of, 201
  training of, 201
Nursing
  American Nurses Association,
    197–198
  clinical nurse specialist, 202
  definitions of practice of, 192–195
  director of nursing services,
    requirements for, 199–200
  duties of nursing staff, 211–216
    duties to report changes in
      resident's condition, 214
    duty to follow established nursing
      procedures, 211–213
    duty to follow physicians orders, 214
    duty to take correct telephone orders,
      215
    duty to take safety precautions,
      215–216
  historical view, 191–192
  legislation related to, 193–194
  licensure, 195–197
  medication, 208–211
  National League for Nursing, 199
  nurse practitioner, 200–202
  nursing assistants, 203–205
  shortage of nurses, 194–195
  special duty nurse, 202–203
  student nurses, 205
  survey of nursing services, 205–207
Nursing assistants, 203–205
  and failure to follow procedures, 204
  functions of, 203
  and resident falls, 204–205
  training of, 203
Nursing facilities, 18–126
  certification of health care
    professionals, 232
  dental services, 219
  dietary services, 219–220
  intermediate care facility, 119
  laboratory services, 221
  licensing of health care professionals,
    126, 232–233
  need for, 120
  occupational therapy, 221
  Omnibus Budget Reconciliation Act of
    1987, major changes related to,
      131–132
  pharmaceutical services, 221–227
  physical therapy, 227–228
  physician's assistants, 228–229

population characteristics, 119–120
quality of life, improvement of, 138–139
radiology services, 229
reasons for admission to, 121
recreation services, 229
regulation of, 126
rehabilitation services, 229–230
respiratory therapy, 230–232
services of, 124
skilled nursing facility, 118
staffing characteristics, 124, 125
use of term, 119

O

Occupational Safety and Health Act of 1970, 373–375
and AIDS, 430
legal liability, 375
OSHA survey, 375
standards of, 373–374
state regulation, 375
Occupational therapy, nursing facilities, 221
Office of Human Development Services, 23–24
Office of Inspector General, 65–66
and Medicare/Medicaid kickbacks, 65
study of resident abuse, 65–66
Ombudsman, for residents, 263–264
Omnibus Budget Reconciliation Act of 1987, 119, 130–137, 166, 322
economic effects of, 132–133
major changes related to nursing facilities, 131–132
survey process, 133–137
Opening statements, trial, 91
Operating certificate, operating without, 70
Organ donations, 314–316
by person other than decedent, 316
revoking donation, 316
Uniform Anatomical Gift Act, 315–316

P

Patient Self-Determination Act of 1990, 297–298
Peer review
and malpractice, 411–413
misuse of process, 420
Pepper Commission, 128–130, 402
on disabled persons, 129–130
recommendations of, 128–129
Performance standards, quality assurance, 421
Petty theft, 78–79
Pharmaceutical services
case reviews, 226–227
Controlled Substances Act, 223
distribution/dispensing/administration of drugs, 225
drug substitution, 226
Food, Drug, and Cosmetic Act, 223–224
formulary system, 226
nursing facilities, 221–227
OBRA regulations, 222–223
state regulations, 224–225
storage of drugs, 226
Pharmacist, billing fraud, 67–68
Photographs, as evidence, 97
Physical abuse, 76–77
Physical therapy, nursing facilities, 227–228
Physician liability, 182–198
abandonment, 182–183
alternative procedures, 184
delay in treatment, 184
failure to disclose, 184
failure to follow up, 184
failure to order diagnostic tests, 185
failure to seek consultation, 185–187
lack of documentation, 187
medication, 188
misdiagnosis, 187
psychiatry, 187–188
treatment outside field of competence, 188–189
wrongful death, 183–184
Physician services, 166–172
guidelines for, 168–172
OBRA regulations, 166–168
Physician's assistants, nursing facilities, 228–229

Physicians orders, duty related to nursing staff, 214
Plea bargaining, 61
Pleadings, 81–85
  answer, 83–84
  bill of particulars, 84–85
  complaint, 83
  counterclaims, 84
  demurrer, 83
  summons, 81, 83
Pocket veto, 19
Population, aging population, 114–116
Power of attorney, 295–296
  durable, 296, 466–472
Precalendar conference, malpractice, 408
Pregnancy discrimination, 384
Pretrial screening panel, malpractice, 405–406
Privacy Act of 1974, 272–273
Privacy rights
  of residents, 260–261
  See also Invasion of privacy
Private law, 2
Privileges, medical staff, 176–177
Products liability, 58
  nature of, 58
  proof of, 58
Professional misconduct, 413–414
  acts of, 413
  penalties for, 413
Property transfers, and life care contracts, 334
Prosecutor, 62
  role of, 62
Prospective payment system, diagnosis related groups, 337–338
Proximate cause/causation
  and forseeability, 42–43
  in negligence, 40–43, 45
Psychiatry, physician liability, 187–188
Public Health Service, 22–23
Public law, 1–2
Pure system, 103

Q

Qualified privilege, 55
Quality assurance
  committees, 419–420
  and disclosure of information, 420
  and Medicaid/Medicare, 420
  OBRA regulations, 417–418
  performance standards, 421
  risk management, 421–423
  steps in monitoring quality of care, 418–419
  utilization review, 423–424
Quality of life, improving in nursing facilities, 138–139

R

Racial discrimination, in employment, 361–362, 383–384
Radiology services, nursing facilities, 229
Rehabilitation Act of 1973, 363
Recreation services, nursing facilities, 229
Refusal of treatment
  documentation of, 244
  as resident responsibility, 263
Rehabilitation services
  nursing facilities, 229–230
  OBRA requirements, 229–230
Reporting requirements
  AIDS, 429–430
  death, 280–281
Res ipsa loquitur, 93–95
  nature of, 93–94
  negligence, 93–94
  shifting burden if proof under, 94
Resident abuse, 70–78
Resident responsibilities
  compliance instructions, 262–263
  facility rules and regulations, 263
  financial obligations to facility, 263
  provision of information, 262
  refusal of treatment, 263
  respect for other's rights, 263
Resident rights
  and admissions, 251–253
  civil rights, 252
  classification of, 246

confidentiality of information, 261
and discharge/transfer, 254–258
financial rights, 259
and government facilities, 253–254
grievances, 262
informed consent, 260
and labor disputes, 372
listing of rights, 246–250
notice of rights, 261
privacy rights, 260–261
Resident's Bill of Rights, 450–456
right to die, 258–259
survey process, 246
violation of, 261
Resource utilization groups, 339–340
categories of, 339
purpose of, 339
Respiratory therapy
nursing facilities, 230–232
survey process, 230–232
Respondeat superior, 145–146
and liability, 146
nature of, 145–146
Restraints
consent for use of, 448–449
and false imprisonment, 51–52
principles related to use of, 52
Retaliatory discharge, of employees, 387–389
Right to die, 258–259
do not resuscitate orders, 302
and Dr. Kervorkian, 301
and durable power of attorney, 295–296
and feeding tubes, 291–292, 298–301
and guardian, 297
and health care proxy, 296–297
living will, 295
Patient Self-Determination Act of 1990, 297–298
right-to-die tag, 297
Right-to-work laws, 366
Risk management, 421–423
and administration, 422
and board of directors, 422
committees, 422–423
elements of program, 423
and insurers, 353–354
and medical staff, 422
purpose of, 421
Ryan White Comprehensive AIDS Resources Emergency Act, 427

S

Safety, corporate duty related to, 156–157
Search, abusive search, 75
"Second Fifty Years: Promoting Health and Preventing Disability," 137
Self-insurance, 350–351
Senate Subcommittee on Long-Term Care, 71–72
Separation of powers, 19–20
and lawmaking, 19–20
Sex discrimination, in employment, 384
Sexual improprieties, 79
Skilled nursing facility, 118
Skilled nursing services, in hospitals, 118
Slander, 54–55
definition of, 53
proof of damages, 55
Social Security Administration, 23
Social Security Amendments of 1965, 322, 324
Sovereign immunity, 106–107
Special duty nurse, 202–203
and liability, 203
role of, 202
Spouse, financial obligations for medical care, 336–337
Staff
corporate duty related to, 155
interviewing for survey, 181
Standard of care, 35–38
failure to follow, criteria for, 38
history of, 37
nature of, 35–36
Stare decisis, meaning of, 7
State laws. *See* Labor laws
State regulations, pharmaceutical services, 224–225

Statute of limitations, 105
  computation of period for, 105
  malpractice, 408
Statutory law, 7–8
  history of, 7
  interpretation by court, 8
Structured awards, malpractice, 414
Student nurses, 205
  functions of, 205
Subpoenas, 90–91
  parts of, 90
  subpoena ad testificandum, 91
  subpoena duces tecum, 91
Summary judgment, as motion, 88
Summons, 81, 83
Supreme Court, 18–19, 20
Survey process
  and experimental research, 239–240
  for medical staff, 180–182
  for nursing services, 205–207
  Omnibus Budget Reconciliation Act of 1987, 133–137
  resident rights, 246
  respiratory therapy, 230–232
Suspension
  license of nurse, 197
  of physicians, 178–179

T

Telephone orders, duty related to nursing staff, 215
Termination of employees, 392–399
  alternatives to, 392
  based on hostile attitude, 396
  based on improper billing practices, 397
  based on misconduct, 397
  based on poor work performance, 398–399
  based on theft, 398
  and damages sought by discharged employee, 399
  and disclaimers, 393–395
  and fairness, 389–390
  and financial necessity, 396
  retaliatory discharge, 387–389
  review guidelines, 393
  termination for cause clause, 395
  and unemployment compensation, 390–392
  and violation of published policies, 395–396
Termination of privileges, medical staff, 178–179
Theft, by employees, 78–79, 398
Tort reform, and malpractice, 403, 404
Torts, 2
  categories of torts, 30
  definition of, 29
  intentional torts, 47–58
  negligence, 30–47
  products liability, 58
Transfer
  elements of transfer agreement, 257–258
  and residents rights, 254–258
Transitional care units, nature of, 118
Trial
  appeals, 112
  burden of proof, 91–95
  closing statements, 107–108
  damages, 109–112
  defenses against recovery, 100–107
  discovery, 85–86
  evidence, 95–100
  execution of judgments, 112–113
  judge
    charge to the jury, 108–109
    role of, 89
  jury, role of, 90
  memorandum of law, 89
  motions, 87–88
  notice of trial, 89
  opening statements, 91
  overview of procedures, 82
  pleadings, 81–85
  preparation of witnesses, 86–87
  subpoenas, 90–91
  trial brief, 89
Trustees, liability insurance, 351–352

U

Ultra vires acts, 145
Unemployment compensation, and
  termination of employees,
    390–392
Uniform Anatomical Gift Act,
  315–316
Uniform Controlled Substances Act,
  222
Union security contract,
  365–366
Utilization review, 423–424
  Medicaid, 424
  Medicare, 423–424

V

Valuables of residents, corporate duty
  related to, 159–160
Voir dire, jury, 90

W

Wage and hour laws, 366
Whistleblowing, 382
  definition of, 382
Windows, falls, 159
Witnesses
  examination before trial, 86–87
  examination of, 95–96
  preparation for trial, 86–87
Worker's compensation, 366–367
  job stress, 367
  physical injury, 367
Written consent, 237, 238
Wrongful death, physician liability, 183–184

X

X-rays
  as evidence, 97–98
  and judicial notice, 185